W9-BWN-915

TOURO COLLEGE LIBRARY
Kings Highway

WITHDRAWN

Aging: Demographics, Health, and Health Services

Elizabeth Vierck and Kris Hodges

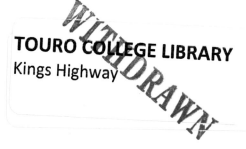

TOURO COLLEGE LIBRARY
Kings Highway

WITHDRAWN

An Oryx Book
Greenwood Press
Westport, Connecticut • London

BP45

Library of Congress Cataloging-in-Publication Data

Vierck, Elizabeth, 1945–
    Aging : demographics, health, and health services / Elizabeth Vierck and Kris Hodges.
      p. cm.
    Includes bibliographic references and index.
    ISBN 1–57356–547–4 (alk. paper)
    1. Aged—Health and hygiene. 2. Aging—Social aspects. 3. Aged—Services for. 4.
Aged—Medical care. 5. Longevity. I. Hodges, Kris. II. Title.
    RA564.8.V54 2003
    362.1'9897'00973—dc21   2002075342

British Library Cataloguing in Publication Data is available.

Copyright © 2003 by Elizabeth Vierck and Kris Hodges

All rights reserved. No portion of this book may be reproduced,
by any process or technique, without the express written
consent of the publisher.

Library of Congress Catalog Card Number: 2002075342
ISBN: 1–57356–547–4

First published in 2003

Greenwood Press, 88 Post Road West, Westport, CT 06881
An imprint of Greenwood Publishing Group, Inc.
www.greenwood.com

Printed in the United States of America

The paper used in this book complies with the
Permanent Paper Standard issued by the National
Information Standards Organization (Z39.48-1984).

10 9 8 7 6 5 4 3 2 1

7/20/04

To Craig
To Erik, Jeff, and Ken

Contents

List of Charts and Tables

CHAPTER 7 Nutrition

CHAPTER 8 Chronic Conditions and Common Health Problems

CHAPTER 9 Mental Health and Illness

CHAPTER 10 Prescription and Over-the-Counter Drugs

CHAPTER 11 Long-Term Care: An Overview

CHAPTER 12 Long-Term Care: Home Health Care

CHAPTER 13 Long-Term Care: Nursing Home Care

Acknowledgments

Many people helped in bringing this book to fruition. We would like to thank Martha Little Munson at the National Center for Health Statistics for her patience and assistance with the long-term care data; Tom Gabe for getting us to the right source in the federal government; Sherry Murphy at the Mortality Statistics branch for getting us more detailed death statistics; and Mary Darling at the University of Minnesota and Barbara Petroulis of Optima Research for their indispensable feedback on the nutrition chapter.

A very big thank you goes out to RoperASW and Mediamark Research for the use of their data, without which this book would be that much less comprehensive. Specific thank yous are in order for Diane Crispell and her crucial role in obtaining access to RoperASW's vast databank, and to Lancey Heyman for her similar role at Mediamark Research. Additionally, we thank Lacey for her patience while we bombarded her with requests for "just one more" tidbit of information.

Most importantly we acknowledge our family and friends who endured our endless hours dedicated to this book. We apologize for our seemingly antisocial behavior while we had our noses stuck in some lengthy report or were lost in thought about some aspect of the book. Thank you for your patience, understanding, and support.

Acronyms and Abbreviations

AARP	American Association of Retired Persons
ADE	Adverse Drug Events
ADEA	Age Discrimination in Employment Act
ADL	Activities of Daily Living
BMI	Body Mass Index
CBO	Congressional Budget Office
CMS	Centers for Medicare & Medicaid Services
DHKS	Diet and Health Knowledge Survey
EEOC	Equal Employment Opportunity Commission
ENP	Elderly Nutrition Program
ERISA	Employee Retirement Income Security Act
GAO	General Accounting Office
HI	Hospital Insurance
HIV	Human Immunodeficiency Virus
HMO	Health Maintenance Organization
IADL	Instrumental Activities of Daily Living
LTC	Long-term Care
M+C	Medicare+Choice
MRC	Medicare Rights Center
MSA	Metropolitan Statistical Area
NSAID	Nonsteroidal Anti-inflammatory Drugs
PACE	Programs of All-Inclusive Care for the Elderly
PFFS	Private Fee-for-Service
PPO	Preferred Provider Organization
QMB	Qualified Medicare Beneficiary
RDA	Recommended Daily Allowance
SIPP	Survey of Income and Program Participation
SLMB	Specified Low Income Medicare Beneficiary
SMI	Supplemental Medicare Insurance
SNF	Skilled Nursing Facility
USDA	U.S. Department of Agriculture

Introduction

Issues relating to age and aging are now dominant players in social policy in the United States and, indeed, the world. This book provides quick access to a wide range of facts about this phenomenon. It is designed to stand alone or to be used as a whole. This volume is intended for use by gerontologists, geriatricians, health policy analysts, researchers, information specialists, marketing professionals, journalists, students, and others doing research on aging, health, and health services.

Aging: Demographics, Health, and Health Services covers almost all topics relating to aging and health. This is not just a dry book of statistics. We have worked diligently to present the content in an easy-to-read and interesting format. We describe trends and offer insights to provide a cohesive framework for the vast amount of statistics now available on aging.

The book is designed for browsing and serendipitous discovery as well as to locate a specific piece of information. The text is exhaustive in its coverage of issues, highlighted by easy-to-follow subtitles, charts, and tables. Important definitions and key facts stand out from the text for easy access. Sources include government reports, private studies, and never-before-published statistics from RoperASW, Mediamark Research, the National Nursing Home Survey, and the National Home and Hospice Care Survey. Sources for all statistics are cited throughout the publication.

Aging: Demographics, Health, and Health Services is divided into topical areas covering the meaning of aging, demographics, life expectancy, health status, nutrition, health care services, long-term care, and health care coverage and financing. Chapter 1 is an essay titled "Aging in the Twentieth Century," which provides an overview of what we learned about aging in the United States in the last century and the incredible increases in the amount of attention paid to age and aging.

This volume represents many thousands of hours of work over a 2-year period, during which we reviewed more than 1,500 documents. The results of these efforts is a book that provides one definitive, comprehensive source of information about people aged 65 years and older.

TERMINOLOGY USED IN THIS BOOK

Unless otherwise stated, the data used in this book describe the elderly (senior population), defined as the group aged 65 years and older. Within the elderly population are three widely recognized age brackets:

- young-old (65 to 74 years)
- middle-old (75 to 84 years)
- oldest-old (85 years and older)

Unfortunately, not all data sources match this standard. Throughout the book, we identify the age categories used by data sources that differ from these. However, sometimes a source may refer to older people and not clearly define which age category that includes. The term "older" generally refers to the 55+ population. This book primarily describes the elderly or senior (65+) population. Note that the "+" symbol as used in this book refers to all ages above a particular age. Thus, 65+ means 65 years of age and older.

VALUE PROVIDED BY THE AUTHORS

As writers and analysts, we have designed this book for optimum use by the reader. Throughout the volume we go beyond just reporting data to provide analytical support and insight. We have computed and present percent changes and ratios, and we provide data from other age groups to aid in making comparisons. At times, the data have been calculated to provide more user-friendly statistics.

We also have included many data sources and insights that have never before been published. For example, comprehensive analyses were conducted on newly available nursing home, home health care, and hospice care data. An extensive interpretation of nutrition data by Kris Hodges provides new perspectives on the nutritional status of the elderly. Additionally, we have included proprietary attitudinal and behavioral data from RoperASW and Mediamark Research to provide other perspectives on today's elderly.

We have attempted to provide the most up-to-date statistics available. Data are current as of March 2002. Although some data sources are updated frequently and may have missed our deadline, much of the information provided here does not change substantially from year to year.

One of the benefits of today's "information highway" is the wide accessibility to data. Some government data sources are available on CD-ROM or as downloadable files from the Internet. When relevant, we have obtained such data and analyzed it (as with nursing home, home health, and hospice care data). In other cases, we culled information from the most recently available printed tables and reports.

We have taken the utmost care in reviewing and checking data numerous times. Occasionally, we have found erroneous material from data sources and have corrected these errors. We have also checked and rechecked our data and have tested for internal consistency and simple face validity (i.e., whether the data make sense). However, some inadvertent errors are possible. We urge all readers to be as vigilant as we have been, for we are not infallible. References are provided to allow users to delve into further detail.

We have also paid careful attention to interpret data properly. For clarity's sake, we use "increases with age" or "declines with age" to explain trends in which rates go up or down across age groups. For example, in Chapter 5, we describe the percentage of people who report that their health is very good or excellent and we say it "progressively declines with age." This is because the measurement is, indeed, lower for each succeeding age group; that is, at age 65 to 74, it is 48 percent; at age 75 to 84, it is 39 percent; and at age 85+, it is 33 percent.

By using the term "with age," we are not implying that as individuals age or in future generations the same effect will hold. The progression reflects one static point in time. Only longitudinal analysis, which follows the same group of people through a given time period, can determine a true age effect.

It is our hope that *Aging: Demographics, Health, and Health Services* will enable the reader to locate relevant data quickly and easily.

CHAPTER 1

Aging in the Twentieth Century

One of the twentieth century's most significant demographic events was the graying of America. This phenomenon sits alongside the discovery of "the wireless," air travel, radio, television, penicillin, birth control pills, silicon chips, two world wars, the depression, and the birth of the baby boom, as one of the key influences on American society throughout the twentieth century. This chapter covers some of the highlights and impacts of aging in the last century in the United States. Our access to statistics available from the early 1900s is limited; such data, unfortunately, are sorely lacking. However, with the facts that are available, we provide some key comparisons that are representative of the "age wave" that swept through the twentieth century.

AGING IN 1900

When the twentieth century began, no one saved for old age because old age was a rarity. No one worried about arthritis because few lived long enough to develop the "disease of old age." Retirement as we know it today did not exist. There was no Social Security to provide a safety net of income for former workers; no Medicare to cover hospitalization and other health needs; no system of community services such as Meals-on-Wheels or home health care. All these programs were more than half a century away.

In 1900, most elderly Americans did not have a high school education. There were no retirement communities or assisted-living centers. Most adults owned their own homes and lived with a spouse or other family member. One-third were poor, and many more had marginal incomes, often relying on family members for resources. For those who lived to older ages, ageism—the prejudice against elderly people—had reared its ugly head and was becoming entrenched in American attitudes and industry. An example comes from an article published by *Cosmopolitan* magazine in June 1903, in which the author, Edward Everett Hale, said: "There is no place in our working order for older men."[1]

TABLE 1.1
Aging America: Then and Now

1900	2000
Seniors as proportion of the population: 4%	Seniors as proportion of the population: 13%
Fastest growing age group: teens	Fastest growing age group: 85+
High mortality/high fertility	Low mortality/low fertility
Median age for males: 23 years	Median age for males: 34 years
Median age for females: 22 years	Median age for females: 37 years
Life expectancy at birth: 47 years	Life expectancy at birth: 77 years
Life expectancy at age 85: 4 years	Life expectancy at age 85: 6 years
Death rate: 17.2 per 1,000	Death rate: 8.6 per 1,000 (in 1998)
Population aged 85+: 122,000	Population aged 85+: more than 4 million
Centenarians were not counted	65,000 people aged 100+
Acute conditions dominated	Chronic conditions dominated
Influenza and pneumonia killed 202 out of 100,000	Influenza and pneumonia killed 34 out of 100,000 (in 1998)
Flu epidemic took 20 million lives worldwide (in 1917–1919)	AIDs projected to kill 2 million lives worldwide by 2010
Tuberculosis killed 194 out of 100,000	Tuberculosis killed 0.4 out of 100,000
Heart disease was number 4 killer in U.S.; influenza and pneumonia were top killers	Heart disease was top killer in United States
No pension system	56% covered by pensions
35% of all homes had telephones (in 1920)	97.5% of elderly households had phones
30% of elderly were poor (in 1930)	10.5% of elderly were poor
19% of women in workforce	60% of women in workforce
Median education level for baby born in 1900–1905: 8.8 years	Median education level for baby born 1931–1935: 12.3 years.
Social Security did not exist	27.5 million retired workers received Social Security
Medicare did not exist	19 million elderly were Medicare beneficiaries
AARP did not exist	AARP had 33 million members
Top-selling U.S. magazines (in 1910): *Saturday Evening Post* and *Life*.	Top-selling U.S. magazine for all audiences: *AARP Bulletin; Modern Maturity* is second.

Sources: U.S. Bureau of the Census; National Center for Health Statistics; David Hackett Fischer, *Growing Old in America* (New York: Oxford University Press, 1978), 157.

SIZE AND GROWTH OF THE OLDER POPULATION

The population at the start of the twentieth century was younger than at the start of the twenty-first century, as shown in Table 1.1. The early 1900s were characterized by high mortality and high fertility, and this kept the nation young. In 1900, 1 in 25 Americans was aged 65+. As the twenty-first century dawns, 1 in 8 Americans is in this age group, and every fifth American is 55+, compared with 1 in 10 in 1900. The following facts highlight how America has "grayed" from 1900 to 2000:

The age wave.   From 1900 to the end of the twentieth century, the size of the entire U.S. population increased three times, while the population aged 65+ increased eleven times.

Increase in the very old.   The oldest-old population grew rapidly during the twentieth century. In 1900, only 122,000 people were aged 85 and older compared with 4 million in 2000, a more than 30-fold increase.[2]

Changed age composition of the population.   Today's combination of low fertility and low mortality has greatly changed the age composition of the U.S. population. In 1900, there were 73 children and 7 elderly people per 100 workers; in 2000, this changed to 42 children and 21 elderly for every 100 workers.

Median age.   In 1900, the median age of the population was 23 years versus 35.8 in 2000.[3]

THIRTY YEARS ADDED TO LIFE EXPECTANCY

One of the major accomplishments in the twentieth century in the United States is that three decades have been added to life expectancy. In fact, it is only in the twentieth century that older age became an expected part of the life cycle.

In 1900, life expectancy at birth was 47 years. A married couple could expect that one or the other would die before all of their children left home. Now a husband and wife who are 60 can expect to reach age 65 together. A baby born in 2000 could expect to live 77 years, surpassing the previous record high of 76.5 years recorded in 1997.

The twentieth century's advances in life expectancy occurred in two stages. The first stage occurred in the first half of the century, caused by decreases in the death rate of children largely due to improvements in the prevention and treatment of infectious diseases. This resulted in the century's greatest gains in longevity; the expected lifetime of a newborn advanced 21 years.

The second stage was the result of decreases in the death rates of adults. In fact, declines in deaths among the middle-aged and elderly populations have been responsible for most advances in longevity since 1970. Between 1950 and 1998, 8.5 years were added to life expectancy at birth.

The net result of the gains in life expectancy since 1900 is that today, 75 percent of the deaths occur to the elderly, compared with 19 percent at the beginning of the twentieth century.

Gains in longevity at the oldest end of the life cycle have been modest compared with those at birth.[4] In 1900, for those lucky enough to survive to age 65, on average life expectancy was 12 more years. Americans who reached their sixty-fifth birthdays in 1998 could expect, on average, to live another 17.7 years. A similar trend occurs for those aged 85+. In 1900, life expectancy at age 85 was 4 years; in 2000 it was 6 years.

HEALTH AND MEDICINE

Seniors of the twentieth century were healthier than the elderly in any previous generation. Medical advances resulted in increasingly more people living into their eighties and nineties. In the past century, many debilitating conditions and diseases were eliminated. The introduction of antibiotics and the virtual eradication of smallpox and polio, along with improved sanitation, nutrition, and health care, greatly reduced deaths from numerous diseases. Table 1.2 summarizes the number of deaths and death rates from various conditions for 1900, and Table 1.3 does the same for 2000.

Many conditions that were not curable decades ago can now be treated before they do permanent damage or take a life. Today's treatments include medications to lower blood pressure and cholesterol; vaccines to help control rubella, tetanus, diphtheria, influenza, pneumonia, and other infectious diseases; and advances in the prevention and early detection of heart disease and certain forms of cancer.

The past century also saw improved surgical techniques, such as open-heart procedures, which have saved numerous lives. Practices and policies designed to pre-

TABLE 1.2
Deaths and Death Rates (per 100,000) for Leading Causes for All Ages: 1900

Cause of Death	Number of Deaths	Death Rate
All causes	343,217	1,719.1
Pneumonia and influenza	40,362	202.2
Tuberculosis	38,820	194.4
Diarrhea, enteritis, and ulceration of the intestines	28,491	142.7
Diseases of the heart	27,427	137.4
Intracranial lesions of vascular origin	21,353	106.9
Nephritis	17,699	88.6
All accidents	14,429	72.3
Cancer and other malignant tumors	12,769	64
Senility	10,015	50.2
Diphtheria	8,056	40.3

Source: National Office of Vital Statistics, 1947.

TABLE 1.3
Deaths and Death Rates (per 100,000) for Leading Causes for All Ages: 2000

Cause of Death	Number of Deaths	Death Rate
All causes	2,404,624	873.6
Diseases of heart	709,894	257.9
Malignant neoplasms	551,833	200.5
Cerebrovascular diseases	166,028	60.3
Chronic lower respiratory diseases	123,550	44.9
Accidents	93,592	34.0
Diabetes mellitus	68,662	24.9
Pneumonia and influenza	67,024	24.3
Alzheimer's disease	49,044	17.8
Nephritis, nephrotic syndrome, and nephrosis	37,672	13.7
Septicemia	31,613	11.5

Note: Not age adjusted.

Source: National Center for Health Statistics, National Vital Statistics System. Arialdi M. Minino and Betty L. Smith, "Deaths: Preliminary Data for 2000," *National Vital Statistics Reports* 49, no. 12 (October 19, 2001): Table 7.

vent deaths in the workplace and in transportation were introduced. They have helped to reduce the death rate from accidents and, for example, to reduce the occurrence of black lung and silicosis, which were common ailments among miners in the early 1900s. In addition, the understanding that tobacco causes lung cancer and other diseases has led to requirements that all public and many private buildings be smoke free.

FROM ACUTE TO CHRONIC ILLNESS

For older Americans, the twentieth century's advances in controlling acute conditions have resulted in dramatic changes in illness and disability patterns. Acute conditions dominated at the turn of the twentieth century, while chronic conditions are now the most common health problem for the elderly.

The pattern of health in an individual's lifetime has also changed. As people grow older, acute conditions become less frequent and chronic conditions become more prevalent.

Today, 79 percent of seniors aged 70+ suffer from at least one of seven chronic conditions, with arthritis and hypertension being the most common.[5] In addition, at least one-third report some activity limitation caused by a chronic condition.

EDUCATION

Educational levels of the elderly population improved throughout the past century. Individuals born during the period 1901 to 1905 have a median educational level of 8.8 years, whereas those born between 1931 and 1935 have a median educational level of 12.3 years.[6] In 1950, 17 percent of people aged 65+ were high school graduates and 3 percent had 4 or more years of college education.[7] Today, 67 percent are high school graduates and 15 percent have bachelor's degrees or higher.[8]

EMPLOYMENT AND RETIREMENT

Retirement, as an expected part of the life cycle, came into being in the twentieth century. In 1900, 63 to 68 percent of elderly men were in the labor force.[9] By 1998, only 16.9 percent were in the labor force (see Table 1.4). These century-wide figures cloud a recent increase in the working patterns of older men. Since 1985, labor force participation rates for men 65 and older have increased. For example, the rates for men aged 65 to 74 increased by 1.3 percentage points from 1988 to 1998.[10]

In 1935, when Social Security was established for people aged 65 and older, a small number of workers were expected to draw from the system. At that time, life expectancy at birth was lower than age 62. Today, Social Security provides benefits to 27.5 million retired workers.

TABLE 1.4
Percent Labor Force Participation Rates,
Males 65 and Over

Year	Percentage
1900	63.1%
1920	55.6
1930	54
1940	44.2
1950	45.8
1960	33.1
1970	26.8
1978	20.4
1988	16.5
1998	16.9

Source: Howard N. Fullerton Jr., "Labor Force
Projections to 2008: Steady Growth and
Changing Composition," *Monthly Labor Review*
(November 1999): 22.

WOMEN'S ROLES

As Americans approached the twentieth century, there was no such concept as the "empty nest." In 1850, the average mother was aged 59 when her last child was married, 2 years younger than the mean age of death for that year.[11] This contrasts with today's women, who can look forward to living more than 20 years after their children leave home.

Throughout the twentieth century, women increasingly participated in the labor force. In 1999, 34 percent of women aged 62 to 64 worked outside the home, compared with 29 percent in 1963. However, increased labor force participation has not resulted in incomes equivalent to those of men. In 1997, the median money income of men aged 65+ was $17,768, compared with $10,062 for women in this age group.[12]

DEFINITION: Money income includes income from Social Security and other sources. It does not include noncash benefits, such as food stamps, health benefits, rent-free housing, and goods produced and consumed on a farm. It also does not include benefits such as use of business transportation and facilities, full or partial payments by business or retirement programs, medical and education expenses, and so on. Data users should consider these elements when comparing income levels.

POVERTY, INCOME, AND THE MATURE MARKET

In the last 40 years, the percentage of the elderly living in poverty dropped from 35 percent to 10.5 percent. However, this statistic masks the fact that at the end of the twentieth century many elderly subgroups faced enormous economic hurdles. For example, in 1998, 26 percent of non-Hispanic blacks aged 65+ were poor. Moreover, divorced black women aged 65 to 74 had a poverty rate of 47 percent.

Although such statistics show that many elderly are poor, American businesses have discovered that enough of the elderly are well off to represent an important consumer market. By the end of the twentieth century, it had become clear that Americans aged 50 and over were worth a total of $7 trillion, making up 70 percent of the U.S. total wealth.[13]

FAMILY STRUCTURES

Increased life expectancy has changed the structure of families. In 1900, less than 20 percent of families could expect to have three living generations. By 1976, 55 percent of teenagers had three or four living grandparents, and 47 percent of middle-aged couples had at least two parents still alive.

LIVING ARRANGEMENTS AND FAMILY CONTACTS

During the twentieth century, an increasing number of elderly people formed one-person households. In 1880, only 1 in 8 people aged 64+ lived alone, compared with almost one-half of today's seniors aged 65+.[14] Additionally, less than 7 percent of elderly people in 1999 lived in a relative's household, nearly one-half the 1970 level.[15] This is in part due to the opportunities presented by the burgeoning of retirement housing, assisted living, and other age-segregated communities.

HOME OWNERSHIP

Owning one's home is an integral part of the American dream, as Michael R. Haines and Allen C. Goodman stated in their article, "A Home of One's Own."[16] Using data from New York, the authors pointed out that, among urban working-class families in the late nineteenth century, home ownership peaked at age 40 to 50. Into the twentieth century, however, this pattern changed. Profiles from the 1890, 1900, and 1930 censuses show that home ownership continued well into 70 and 80 years of age. As Table 1.5 shows, in 1900, more than one-third of people aged 70+ owned their own homes. According to Haines and Goodman, "Age was proving to be no barrier to the achievement of this part of the American dream. Increasingly, wealth in the form of homes was characteristic of the later years of the life course." At the beginning of

TABLE 1.5
Home Ownership by Age: 1900

Age Group	Home Owners
60–64 years	61%
65–69	67
70+	36

Source: U.S. Census tabulations by R. Haines and Allen C. Goodman. Reported in "A Home of One's Own," in David I. Kertzer and Peter Laslett (editors), *Aging in the Past* (Berkeley: University of California Press, 1995), Table 7.2.

TABLE 1.6
Home Ownership by Age: 1999

Age Group	Home Owners
60–64 years	81%
65–69	83
70–74	83
75+	77
65+	80

Source: U.S. Census Bureau, "Housing Vacancies and Home Ownership Annual Statistics: 1999," Table 15. Available online at www.census.gov.

the twenty-first century, as shown in Table 1.6, 80 percent of the elderly own their own homes.[17]

WIDOWHOOD

The age at which widowhood occurs for women improved greatly in the past century. In 1910, about one-fifth of women aged 50 who had ever been married were widows, and more than half of those aged 65 to 69 were widowed.[18] In 1940, however, this age was around 70, and by 1970, it was well past 70. Today about 30 percent of women aged 65 to 74 are widowed.[19]

AGEISM

During the twentieth century, many programs and protections—such as Social Security, Medicare, and Older Americans Act programs—were implemented. Today, however, the situation of the elderly seems bittersweet. While aging and aging services have clearly dominated much of the politics of the last century, gerontologists point out that, paradoxically, the elderly are still objects of ageism as the new century unfolds.

What exactly is ageism? It is the systematic stereotyping of and discriminating against people because they are old. Ageism is manifested in our society's worship of youth and its anxiety over wrinkles, in the contradictions of our desire for longevity and reluctance to grow old. When Eddie Mannix, an old-time executive at Warner Brothers, saw a screen test of 34-year-old Fred Astaire, he reportedly said, "He's too old and too bald."

Many older people fall victim to ageism by becoming prejudiced against themselves. An episode of the long-running comedy, *The Mary Tyler Moore Show*, reminded us of this when a delightful white-haired older man explained to perky, youthful Mary that part of his daily routine was going to a park and sitting on a bench. He found it rather boring, he said, but ever since he was little he had found old men sitting on benches, and felt it was his obligation to the younger generation to do the same. A child learns to expect old men to take to benches, and faithfully, in older age, sits out his expectation.

Thomas R. Cole described the twentieth century's lack of progress against ageism in his 1992 history of aging, *The Journey of Life:* "In our century vastly improved medical and economic conditions for older people have been accompanied by cultural disenfranchisement—a loss of meaning and vital social roles."[20]

Evidence of ageism exists today in the media and the workplace. For example, many older people who desire to work hit a "gray ceiling." More than 15,000 complaints about age discrimination in employment are made per year with the Equal Employment Opportunity Commission (EEOC).[21] Statistics from 1997 show, however, that the commission files suit in fewer than 1 percent of such cases. The EEOC has been greatly criticized by advocates of the aging for this meager record.

Recent results of a groundbreaking study conducted at Yale University Medical School demonstrated the effect that the negative stereotypes of aging have on older people.[22] This study included 54 participants between the ages of 62 and 82, who performed tasks such as recalling the most stressful event in the last 5 years. Participants were divided into two groups, one of which was exposed to positive stereotypes of aging (words such as "wisdom" and "creative") and the other exposed to negative stereotypes of aging (words such as "senile" and "dying").

After such exposure, the positive-stereotype group showed a significant decrease in two cardiovascular measures: systolic and diastolic blood pressure. In contrast, participants in the negative-stereotype group showed a significant increase in these measures, even before they performed any stressful tasks. The study also found that the elderly participants who were exposed to positive aging stereotypes demonstrated significantly higher self-confidence and higher mathematical performance than those exposed to the negative aging self-stereotypes.

According to Becca Levy, one of the authors of the study,

> Negative stereotypes of aging are found in many aspects of our culture, from casual conversations to television advertisements that often present the elderly either as close to childhood or close to death. . . . The study suggested that negative stereotypes of aging may contribute to health problems in the elderly without their awareness. This, in turn, could lead to older individuals mistakenly attributing decline in their health to the inevitability of aging, which might then reinforce the negative stereotypes and prevent successful aging.

PROGRAMS TO PROTECT THE ELDERLY

In his book *Growing Old in America*, noted historian David Hackett Fischer summed up the dynamic role that the emerging poverty of the growing elderly population played in the politics and policies of the twentieth century: "Early in the twentieth century, Americans learned to think of old age in a new way. That stage of life began to be seen as a problem to be solved by the intervention of 'society.'"[23]

The past century's new concentration on the bleak economic situation of the elderly as a social and health policy "problem" resulted in a burgeoning of organizations whose sole purpose was to pull seniors out of poverty, to advocate for them, and to assist in passing a number of government programs to protect them. The turn of the century to 1965—the landmark year in which Medicare, Medicaid, and the Older Americans Act were passed—saw the following chronology of events:

- The first public commission on aging in the United States was established in Massachusetts in 1909.
- The first old age pension system was created by the state of Arizona in 1915.
- The science of geriatrics was born in 1909 and the first textbook in the field was published in 1914.
- Social Security was established in 1935. (In fact, the United States created its federal retirement system late in the game; most European countries had enacted old age insurance decades earlier.)
- The first senior center was established in 1943.
- The Gerontological Society was established in 1945.
- The Friendly Visitors Program was founded in 1946.
- The National Retired Teachers Association was founded in 1947.
- The National Council on the Aging was founded in 1950.
- The American Association of Retired Persons was founded in 1958.
- In 1961, the first White House Conference on Aging was convened, the U.S. Senate Special Committee on Aging was formed, and the National Council of Senior Citizens was founded.
- In 1965, Medicare, Medicaid, the Older Americans Act, the Foster Grandparent Program, the Service Corps of Retired Executives, and Green Thumb had their beginnings.

These events reflect a momentum in which programs, services, and advocacy for the elderly became dominant forces in American life. Other key legislation passed during the twentieth century is listed in Table 1.7. Now, in the new millennium, we are seeing the effects of these landmark advances, such as the following:

- The United States boasts a vast network of agencies on aging that advocate on behalf of, and coordinate programs for, the elderly. Funded through the Older Americans Act, the network includes 57 state agencies on aging, 660 area agencies on aging, and more than 27,000 service providers.[24]
- Since the first textbook on gerontology was released in 1914, a large volume of literature on aging has been published by all branches of science. Seminal works on aging include Robert Butler's Pulitzer Prize–winning *Why Survive? Be-*

TABLE 1.7

Landmark Legislation Related to Aging: Twentieth Century

Year	Act/Institution	Description
1935	Social Security Act	Provides income benefits for the disabled, the retired, and upon death.
1937	U.S. Housing Act	Through Section 202, creates housing for the elderly and disabled; through Section 8, provides payments to landlords of low-income persons.
1949	Housing Act of 1949	Under Section 504, provides loans and grants to low-income households to eliminate safety hazards.
1964	Civil Rights Act of 1964	Created the Equal Employment Opportunity Commission to eliminate discrimination based on race, color, religion, sex, national origin, disability, or age in hiring, promoting, firing, wages, testing, apprenticeship, and all other terms and conditions of employment.
1965	Medicare	Provides health insurance for persons 65 and over, people of any age with permanent kidney failure, and qualifying disabled persons. Medicare was established as Title XVIII of the Social Security Act.
1965	Medicaid	Provides health care for low-income persons of all ages. Medicaid was established as Title XIX of the Social Security Act.
1965	Older Americans Act	Established objectives and funding to improve the lives of the elderly through federal, state, and local agencies.
1967	Age Discrimination in Employment Act (ADEA)	Prohibits employers, employment agencies, and unions from discriminating against individuals between ages 40 and 65 on account of their age.
1970	Urban Mass Transit Act	Assures availability of mass transportation for elderly and disabled persons.
1974	Authorization of Supplemental Security Income	Provides a guaranteed minimum income for persons aged 65+. Authorized under Title XVI of the Social Security Act.

ing Old in America, published in 1975, and the best-selling *Age Wave* by Ken Dychtwald. In 2000, AgeLine, a bibliographic database in social gerontology, had 50,000 citations related to aging. Most of the data are North American in origin.

- Hundreds of national and local interest groups advocate for the elderly. By 1971, the White House Conference on Aging's invitation list included 400 interest groups on aging. In 2000, AARP alone had a membership of more than 33 million.[25]

- Medicare and Social Security touch the lives of nearly every American, and the politics behind the programs are on the forefront of every politician's mind. Today, Social Security, Medicare, and Medicaid account for 40 percent of the federal budget.

TABLE 1.7
Continued

Year	Act/Institution	Description
1974	National Institute on Aging	Established by Congress to conduct and support biomedical, social, and behavioral research and training related to the aging process and the diseases and other special problems and needs of the aged.
1974	Employee Retirement Income Security Act (ERISA)	Established regulations to protect pensions from mismanagement and created a federal agency, the Pension Benefit Guarantee Corporation, to insure them.
1975	Age Discrimination Act	Prohibits discrimination, except employment, based on the age of any recipient of federal financial assistance.
1976	Energy Conservation and Production Act	Authorized the Weatherization Assistance Program, which among other things, reduces the impact of high fuel costs on low-income households, particularly those of the elderly and the handicapped.
1978	Amendments to the Age Discrimination in Employment Act	Raises the upper age limit of the ADEA to 70 for certain employers.
1978	Housing and Community Development Act	Authorized the Congregate Housing Services Program to demonstrate cost-effective assisted independent living.
1984	Retirement Equity Act of 1984	Amended ERISA to reduce the age at which workers must be allowed to participate in a pension plan, and implemented other pension protections.
1986	Amendments to the Age Discrimination in Employment Act	Raised the upper age limit of the ADEA to 70 for all workers.
1987	Housing and Community Development Act	Authorized the Congregate Housing Services Program as a permanent program.
1987	Omnibus Budget Reconciliation Act	As part of this legislation, Congress enacted comprehensive nursing home quality care provisions.
1990	Americans with Disabilities Act of 1990 (ADA)	Provides protection to persons of all ages who have disabilities, whether physical or mental. Prohibits discrimination in employment, public services, public accommodations, transportation, and telecommunications.

- Today Medicare covers 98 percent of the elderly, or 39 million older Americans.[26] In 1998, Medicare, the largest public payer for health care, financed $216.6 billion of spending for the health care of 38.8 million elderly and disabled beneficiaries.[27]

- In 1998, 27.5 million retired workers were receiving monthly Social Security checks, and the program paid out $326.8 billion in old age and survivors' benefits.[28]

NOTES

1. David Hackett Fischer, *Growing Old in America* (New York: Oxford University Press, 1978), 158.
2. Bureau of the Census, "Projections of the Resident Population by Age, Sex, Race, and Hispanic Origin, 1999 to 2100" (Washington, DC: U.S. Government Printing Office, 2000).
3. *World Almanac and Book of Facts* (New York: Scripps Howard, 1988), 533. Bureau of the Census, "Resident Population Estimates of the United States by Age and Sex: April 1, 1990 to June 1, 1999" (Washington, DC: U.S. Government Printing Office, 1999), 1.
4. U.S. Senate Special Committee on Aging, *Aging America* (Washington, DC: U.S. Government Printing Office, 1991), 20. Bureau of the Census, *65+ in the United States* (Washington, DC: U.S. Government Printing Office, 1996), 3-3. Bureau of the Census, "Component Assumptions of the Resident Population by Age, Sex, Race, and Hispanic Origin: Lowest, Middle, and Highest Series, 1999 to 2100," Mortality (Life Tables), middle series projections. Available online at www.census.gov.
5. National Center for Health Statistics, *Health, United States, 1999 With Health and Aging Chartbook* (Hyattsville, MD: U.S. Government Printing Office, 1999).
6. Fischer, *Growing Old in America*, 157.
7. U.S. Senate Special Committee on Aging, *Aging America*, 189.
8. Bureau of the Census, "Educational Attainment in the United States: March 1998," *Current Population Reports*, P-20-513 (October 1998): 2.
9. Fischer, *Growing Old in America*, 142.
10. Howard N. Fullerton Jr., "Labor Force Projections to 2008: Steady Growth and Changing Composition, *Monthly Labor Review* (November 1999): 22.
11. Fischer, *Growing Old in America*, 145.
12. Bureau of the Census, *Statistical Abstract of the United States: 1999* (119th edition) (Washington, DC, 1999).
13. Ken Dychtwald, *Age Power* (New York: Tarcher, 1999).
14. Bureau of the Census, "National Households and Families Projections, 1995 to 2010 (Series 2 projections for 2000)." Available online at www.census.gov.
15. Martha Farnsworth Riche, "America's Diversity and Growth: Signposts for the 21st Century," *Population Bulletin* 55, no. 2 (Washington, DC: Population Reference Bureau, June 2000): 31.
16. Michael R. Haines and Allen C. Goodman, "A Home of One's Own," in David L. Kertzer and Peter Laslett (editors), *Aging in the Past* (Berkeley: University of California Press, 1995), 213.
17. Bureau of the Census, "Housing Vacancies and Home Ownership Annual Statistics: 1999," Table 15. Available online at www.census.gov.
18. Tamara K. Haraven and Peter Uhlenberg, "Transition to Widowhood and Family Support Systems in the Twentieth Century, Northeastern United States," in David I. Kertzer and Peter Laslett (editors), *Aging in the Past* (Berkeley: University of California Press, 1995).
19. Federal Interagency Forum on Aging-Related Statistics, *Older Americans 2000: Key Indicators of Well-Being*. Available online at www.agingstats.gov.
20. Thomas R. Cole, *The Journey of Life* (New York: Cambridge University Press, 1992), xix.
21. U.S. Senate Special Committee on Aging, *Developments in Aging: 1997 and 1998, Volume 1* (Washington, DC: U.S. Government Printing Office, 2000), 84.
22. Becca Levy, Jeanne Y. Wei, and Jeffrey M. Hausdorff, "Reducing Cardiovascular Stress with Positive Self-stereotypes of aging," *Journal of Gerontology: Psychological Sciences* 55 (2000): 205–213.
23. Fischer, *Growing Old in America*, 157.

24. U.S. Senate Special Committee on Aging, *Developments in Aging: 1997 and 1998*, 255.

25. Encyclopedia Britannica website, britannica.com.

26. MEDPAC, "Beneficiaries' Financial Liability and Medicare's Effectiveness in Reducing Personal Spending," *Report to the Congress: Selected Medicare Issues* (Washington, DC: U.S. Government Printing Office, 1999).

27. Katherine Levit et al., "Health Spending in 1998: Signals of Change," *Health Affairs* 19, no. 1 (March, April 2000): 131.

28. Social Security Administration, *Social Security Bulletin Annual Statistical Supplement* (Washington, DC: U.S. Government Printing Office, 1999). Available online at www.ssa.gov.

CHAPTER 2

The Meaning of Aging

To Oliver Wendell Holmes, growing older was the urge to call policemen "sonny." Henry Wadsworth Longfellow likened aging to opportunity. This chapter presents survey data from the RoperASW organization that shed light on how adults of all ages view growing older today. Highlights from these findings include the following facts:

- Almost two-thirds of older adults (those aged 60+) say that they are not concerned about growing older.
- Two-thirds of older adults feel that the "good old days" were better than the present.
- People aged 60+ think old age begins at age 77, a decade later than that designated by people 18 to 29 years of age.
- One-half of people aged 60+ associate getting older with poor health, whereas younger adults associate aging with wisdom and time to enjoy themselves.
- Young and old alike report that the age-related condition that bothers them the most is having trouble taking care of oneself.
- When asked what product or activity they have used or have considered using to look younger, the most frequent answer for both young and old is regular exercise.

■ Most older adults show little concern about growing older

Close to two-thirds of today's older adults express little concern with growing older. Fewer than 1 in 10 is very concerned about this. In contrast, younger adults report slightly higher levels of concern about aging (see Table 2.1).

■ Most older and younger people say the "good old days" were better

Adults aged 60+ are more likely than younger generations to feel that the "good old days" were better than the present. Specifically, 63 percent of older adults feel this way versus 45 percent of those aged 18 to 29, 56 percent of those aged 30 to 44, and 57 percent of those aged 45 to 59.

TABLE 2.1
Level of Concern about Growing Older, by Age: 1998

	18–59 Years	60+ Years	Ratio of Older to Younger	Ratio of Younger to Older
Very or somewhat concerned	46%	37%	0.80	1.24
Very concerned	11	8	0.73	1.38
Somewhat concerned	35	29	0.83	1.21
Not at all or not too concerned	54	63	1.17	0.86
Not too concerned	30	31	1.03	0.97
Not at all concerned	24	32	1.33	0.75

Source: RoperASW data, 1998.

Not surprisingly, adults most commonly find the decade of their youth to be the "good old days." For older adults, this most commonly translates to the 1940s or 1950s, compared to the 1980s for the young adults aged 18 to 29 (see Chart 2.1).

■ Old age begins at 67; No! Make that 77

When does older age begin? People aged 18 and older believe that old age begins at 72* (see Table 2.2). The perception of when people become "old," however, shifts

CHART 2.1   Time Period Perceived as the "Good Old Days," by Age: 1998

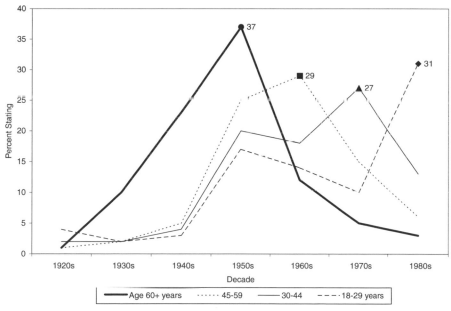

Source: RoperASW data, 1998.

----

*
  The specific question asked by RoperASW in their survey was: "We hear a lot about old age and old people. How old does a person have to be before you think of them as old?"

TABLE 2.2

The Age at Which Adults Think of Others as Being "Old," by Age: 1998

	Average Age at Which Others Are Thought of as Being "Old"
18+ years	72
18–29	67
30–44	72
45–59	74
60+	77

Source: RoperASW data, 1998.

by age group. For example, people aged 60+ think of others as old at age 77, while those aged 18 to 29 think old age starts 10 years earlier, at age 67. One in five people aged 60 and older (20 percent) says they can't pick an age at which they think of others as old because it varies too much. The perception of old age also differs by gender. Among people aged 18 and older, men think of age 71 as the beginning of old age, whereas women think it is age 74.

Older adults are more likely to be afraid of public speaking or walking outside alone at night than they are of their own death.

■ Aging is wisdom, poor health

RoperASW respondents were also asked to identify items on a list that they associated with the meaning of getting older (see Table 2.3). One-half of the respondents aged 60+ identify poor health with getting older. The next most common associations with older age happen to be positive, such as being a good role model, having more time, and wisdom. Younger adults actually have a more positive outlook, with wisdom and time to enjoy themselves outranking poor health.

About 3 in 10 older adults identify lack of mental acuity and being alone with getting older. Least associated with getting older are such negative attributes as being poor, unattractive, or useless.

Older people are more likely than younger people to associate poor health with getting older, and older people also have a greater tendency to identify being a role model for young people with aging. Younger people, in contrast, have a greater tendency than older people to associate wisdom, more free time, and greater dependency with aging.

Older men's impressions about aging are similar to those of older women with the exception that older women are more likely to mention "being a good role

TABLE 2.3

Aspects Most Commonly Associated with the Meaning of Getting Older, by Age: 1998

	18–59 Years	60+ Years	Ratio of Older to Younger	Ratio of Younger to Older
Poor health	39%	49%	1.26	0.80
Having more time to enjoy oneself	46	41	0.89	1.12
Wisdom	49	38	0.78	1.29
Being a good role model for young people	29	35	1.21	0.83
Having closer ties to family and friends	29	32	1.10	0.91
Having time to help others	28	32	1.14	0.88
Not being very sharp mentally	26	29	1.12	0.90
Being alone	27	27	1.00	1.00
Being dependent on other people	26	22	0.85	1.18
Being of no use to others	9	10	1.10	0.90
Being poor	9	9	1.00	1.00
Being unattractive	11	7	0.64	1.57

Source: RoperASW data, 1998.

model" (40 percent versus 26 percent) or "having time to help others" (38 percent versus 24 percent), and they have greater concerns about being dependent on others (25 percent versus 18 percent).

Older adults are more truthful about their age than younger adults—14 percent of older adults have ever lied about their age versus 22 percent of younger adults.[1]

◼ Ability to take care of oneself is the top concern about growing older

Young and old alike report that the age-related condition that bothers them the most is having trouble taking care of themselves (see Table 2.4). Body aches and pains, mental acuity, and increased risk of serious disease are also among the top aging-related concerns of adults.

Older adults are less bothered by various old-age ailments and conditions than are younger adults. The greatest differences are for such physically noticeable conditions as gray hair, wrinkles, and tooth loss. Although loss of sex drive is not high on the list of concerns, younger adults are substantially more bothered by it than older adults are, and older men are more bothered by it than older women are (15 percent versus 6 percent). Interestingly, both younger and older adults view losing muscle tone or teeth as more bothersome prospects than losing sexual drive.

TABLE 2.4
Selected Conditions Associated with Growing Older That Bother People the Most, by Age:
1998

	18–59 Years	60+ Years	Ratio of Younger to Older
Having trouble taking care of oneself	51%	45%	1.13
Having body aches or arthritis	44	43	1.02
Not being mentally alert	46	32	1.44
Being more at risk for serious disease	44	30	1.47
Losing muscle tone	30	24	1.25
Losing teeth	31	17	1.82
Having digestive problems or irregularity	21	12	1.75
Having gray hair	25	10	2.50
Getting wrinkles	21	10	2.10
Losing sexual drive or capability	19	10	1.90

Source: RoperASW data, 1998.

■ Regular exercise is the most frequently used measure for looking younger

When asked what product or activity they have used, or have considered using, to look younger, the most frequent answer for both young and old is regular exercise (see Table 2.5). However, younger adults are substantially more likely than older adults (47 percent versus 30 percent) to have used or considered regular exercise.[2] In fact, younger people are more likely than older people to have considered or used all of the methods mentioned in the survey (such as hair color, cosmetic surgery, and cosmetics), except wigs or toupees. Only 1 in 20 people (old and young alike) uses or has considered using wigs or toupees to look younger.

■ Women are much more likely than men to use or consider youth-enhancing methods

Women of all ages are more likely than men to use or consider using youth-enhancing methods. Among older adults, women are twice as likely as men to do so (see Table 2.6). Older men mostly use or consider a regular exercise routine as an option; hair color is a very distant second. Older women are eight times more likely than older men to use or consider hair coloring, and they are also substantially more likely than older men to have or consider having a regular exercise routine or various cosmetic options.

TABLE 2.5
Products or Methods Used or Considered to Look Younger, by Age: 1998

	18–59 Years	60+ Years	Ratio of Older to Younger	Ratio of Younger to Older
Net of all methods	65%	48%	0.74	1.35
Regular exercise	48	30	0.63	1.60
Hair color to hide the gray	33	24	0.73	1.38
Cosmetics	22	13	0.59	1.69
Skin products to reduce or prevent wrinkles	17	6	0.35	2.83
Cosmetic surgery	14	6	0.43	2.33
Wigs and toupees	5	5	1.00	1.00
Suntanning products to prevent wrinkles	17	4	0.24	4.25
Hair-replenishing lotions	7	1	0.14	7.00
Hair transplantation	4	<1	NA	NA

Source: RoperASW data, 1998.

■ Older women are less likely than younger women to use youth-enhancing methods

Older women are less likely than younger women to have used or considered using various youth-enhancing methods (see Table 2.7). Many factors can contribute to this fact, including older women's greater acceptance of their age-related physical

TABLE 2.6
Products or Methods Used or Considered for Use to Look Younger, by Age and Sex: 1998

	Men 60+ Years	Women 60+ Years	Ratio of Women to Men
Net of all methods	29%	62%	2.14
Hair color to hide the gray	5	39	7.80
Regular exercise	24	35	1.46
Cosmetics	1	21	21.00
Cosmetic surgery	<1	11	NA
Skin products to reduce or prevent wrinkles	1	9	9.00
Suntanning products to prevent wrinkles	<1	8	NA
Wigs and toupees	<1	8	NA
Hair-replenishing lotions	<1	2	NA

Note: NA = Not Available.
Source: RoperASW data, 1998.

TABLE 2.7

Products or Methods Used or Considered for Use to Look Younger among Women, by Age: 1998

	18–59 Years	18–29 Years	30–44 Years	45–59 Years	60+ Years	Ratio of Older to Younger Women	Ratio of Younger to Older Women
Net of all methods	69%	67%	71%	67%	62%	0.90	1.11
Hair color to hide the gray	49	47	50	49	39	0.80	1.26
Regular exercise	48	50	47	38	35	0.73	1.37
Cosmetics	34	33	35	35	21	0.62	1.62
Cosmetic surgery	17	24	17	18	11	0.65	1.55
Skin products to reduce or prevent wrinkles	28	32	27	24	9	0.32	3.11
Suntanning products to prevent wrinkles	25	27	25	22	8	0.32	3.13
Wigs and toupees	6	8	6	6	8	1.33	0.75
Hair-replenishing lotions	6	7	4	8	2	0.33	3.00

Source: RoperASW data, 1998.

changes, resignation that many aging-related aspects can no longer be affected, and the unavailability of products during their younger years when they could have been more effective. These dynamics are especially apparent in wrinkle reduction or prevention products that are three times more likely to be or have been in the antiaging arsenal of younger women.

NOTES

1. RoperASW data, 1997.
2. RoperASW data, 1998.

CHAPTER 3

Size and Growth of the Older Population

The growth and change of America's older population rank among the most important demographic developments of the twentieth century.[1]

> —*Judith Treas, "Older Americans in the 1990s and Beyond"*

Population aging represents, in one sense, a human success story—societies now have the luxury of aging.

> —*Bureau of the Census,* An Aging World, *2001*

One of the most dramatic changes occurring in our nation is the aging of our population. Increasing numbers of older people present enormous opportunities and challenges to all components of our society—individuals, families, business, government, and volunteer groups.

> —*Senator David Pryor,* Aging America, *1991 Edition*

Referred to as the graying of America, the emerging gerontocracy, and the age wave, this century's historical growth in the elderly population will dominate society, economics, and public policy well into the first century of the new millennium.

Highlights of this chapter include:

- Currently, 1 in 8 people in the United States is elderly.
- The number of people aged 65+ is projected to swell from about 40 million in 2010 to 54 million in 2020 to 82 million in 2050.
- In 2000, the elderly population was almost evenly split between seniors aged 65 to 74 and those aged 75+.
- Between 1990 and 2000, the number of people aged 85+ increased from 3 million to 4 million.
- Currently, about 65,000 centenarians live in the United States.

- Elderly women outnumber elderly men by a ratio of 3 to 2.
- Today, 38 percent of the overall veteran population is elderly.
- Worldwide in 2000, about 606 million people were aged 60+, the equivalent of the entire current populations of the United States, United Kingdom, and Netherlands combined.

EVERY EIGHTH AMERICAN

The aging of the population is a powerful demographic event with wide-reaching implications for society. At the beginning of the twentieth century, only 1 in 25 Americans was aged 65+. By the turn of the next century, 1 in 8 Americans was in this age group. When the 2000 census was conducted, 35 million people were aged 65 years and older, representing 12.4 percent of the population (see Table 3.1).[2]

Since 1960, the population aged 65+ has increased by more than 100 percent, in contrast to the 50 percent growth of the total population. This dramatic rate of increase is often attributed to the fact that Americans are living longer. In fact, longevity explains only part of the phenomenon. A primary cause is an increase in the annual number of births prior to 1920 and after World War II.[3] The aging of the pre-1920s population, along with a dramatic decline in the birth rate after the mid-1960s, contributed to the rise in the median age of the population from 28 in 1970 to 35.3 in 2000.[4]

TABLE 3.1
Population 65 Years and Older by Age: 1990 and 2000

Age	1990		2000		Percent of U.S. Total		Percent Change, 1990 to 2000
	Number	Percent	Number	Percent	1990	2000	
65+ years	31,241,831	100.0%	34,991,753	100.0%	12.6%	12.4%	12.0%
65–74	18,106,558	58.0	18,390,986	52.6	7.3	6.5	1.6
65–69	10,111,735	32.4	9,533,545	27.2	4.1	3.4	−5.7
70–74	7,994,823	25.6	8,857,441	25.3	3.2	3.1	10.8
75–84 years	10,055,108	32.2	12,361,180	35.3	4.0	4.4	22.9
75–79	6,121,369	19.6	7,415,813	21.2	2.5	2.6	21.1
80–84	6,121,369	19.6	7,415,813	21.2	2.5	2.6	21.1
85–94 years	2,829,728	9.1	3,902,349	11.2	1.1	1.4	37.9
85–89	2,060,247	6.6	2,789,818	8.0	0.8	1.0	35.4
90–94	769,481	2.5	1,112,531	3.2	0.3	0.4	44.6
95+ years	250,437	0.8	337,238	1.0	0.1	0.1	34.7

Source: U.S. Census Bureau, Census 2000 Summary File 1; 1990 Census of Population, General Population Characteristics, United States (1990 CP-1-1).

WANTED: CRYSTAL BALL

Population projections vary widely, depending on the assumptions that forecasters use about three factors: fertility, death rates, and immigration. Reflecting the tenuous nature of demographic predictions, the U.S. Census Bureau uses three different sets of assumptions to make three different projection series about the size of the U.S. population. These predictions may differ by 150 million people or more. Most analysts use the Census Bureau's "middle series" projections to plan for the future. We use this series throughout this book.

■ Growth is presently slow

Americans presently reaching age 65 were born during the 1930s when the song "Brother Can You Spare a Dime?" was a hit. They are children of the depression, a period of declining birth rate. As a result, the growth of the elderly population now is the slowest that it has been in U.S. history,[5] and it will remain slow until about 2005. This phenomenon is almost entirely due to a lack of growth in the group aged 65 to 74.

■ The grandparent boom will replace the baby boom

When the baby boomers begin to turn age 65+ in 2011, we will experience a grandparent boom—a rapid growth in the elderly population. The number of people aged 65+ is projected to swell from 39.7 million in 2010 to 53.7 million in 2020 to 81.9 million in 2050 (see Chart 3.1). About 1 in 6 Americans will be aged 65+ in 2020, compared with 1 in 8 now. This ratio will reach 1 in 5 in 2030 and remain at

CHART 3.1   Population 65+ by Age: 1900–2050

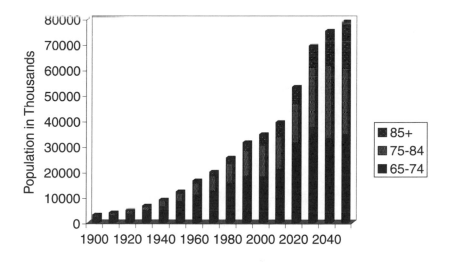

Source: Bureau of the Census.

that level through 2050. Incredibly, in 100 years, the number of persons aged 65+ will be 131.2 million—equivalent to the total U.S. population in 1940.

■ The elderly population is aging

Like the general population, the 65+ population is aging. In 1990, the young-old (aged 65 to 74) outnumbered the 75+ population by more than 4 to 3.[6] In 2000, 53 percent of all seniors were aged 65 to 74 (18.4 million people), and 47 percent were aged 75+ (16.2 million people) (see Table 3.1).[7] By 2050, the 75+ population will outnumber the group aged 65 to 74 by 10 million.

■ The group aged 85+ is small, but increasing rapidly

A major achievement of medical advances and health services in the twentieth century is the increase in the 85+ population. The oldest-old age group is small, but increasing rapidly. In the coming decades, the oldest-old will be the fastest-growing age group. Between 1990 and 2000, the number of people aged 85+ increased from 3 to 4.2 million. This number is expected to grow almost fivefold by 2050, when a projected 19.3 million people will be aged 85+.[8]

The proportion of oldest-old people in the population will also increase over the next 50 years. By 2050, the population aged 85+ is expected to reach 5 percent of the total population and 24 percent of the elderly population.[9]

■ One million centenarians are projected for 2050

The fact that an increasing number of people are living to be age 100+ has become a media sensation, in part due to the publication in 1999 of the results of a centenarian study conducted by two Harvard Medical School professors. Estimates on the number of centenarians in the United States vary. The Administration on Aging reported that 50,545 persons were aged 100+ in 2000.[10] The U.S. Census Bureau projects that 235,000 Americans will live to this age in 2020, and 1 million by 2050.[11]

■ Grandparent-maintained households increased 19 percent since 1990

As the elderly population has increased, more seniors have maintained households with two and three generations. In 1997, 3.9 million children were living in homes maintained by grandparents—5.5 percent of all children under age 18.[12] Among grandparent-maintained households, 15 percent of the grandmothers and 21 percent of the grandfathers are aged 65+.

■ The senior population will become more racially and ethnically mixed

The number and proportion of minority elderly is now relatively small. In 2000, 16.4 percent of persons aged 65+ were minorities:[13] 8 percent were African Americans, 2.4 percent were Asian and Pacific Islanders, and less than 1 percent were Native Americans. Minority populations are younger than nonminority populations. Only 6.6 percent of minority race and Hispanic populations were aged 65+ in 2000. Within the ethnic groups, 8.2 percent of African Americans, 7.8 percent of Asians and Pacific Islanders, 6.0 percent of American Indians and Native Alaskans, and 4.9 percent of Hispanics were aged 65+, compared with 15.0 percent of whites.

The disparity between white and minority seniors is expected to narrow beginning in the early part of the twenty-first century when the minority population aged 65+ will increase more rapidly than the corresponding white population. Minority populations are projected to represent 25.4 percent of the elderly population in 2030, up from 16.4 percent in 2000.[14] Between 1999 and 2030, the white population aged 65+ is projected to increase by 81 percent compared with 219 percent for older minorities, including Hispanics (328 percent), African Americans (131 percent), American Indians, Eskimos, and Aleuts (147 percent), and Asians and Pacific Islanders (285 percent). The growth of the minority elderly population will be the result of higher fertility for the nonwhite and Hispanic populations than for the white population. This growth will also reflect the changing composition of today's younger generations, which are more racially diverse.

■ More than 3 million elderly were born in foreign countries

In 2000, more than 3 million elderly Americans had been born in foreign countries (see Table 3.2), representing a slight increase from 2.8 million elderly immigrants in 1995. Almost two-thirds of all immigrants aged 65+, and three-fourths of those aged 85+, came to the United States prior to 1970.

■ Elderly women outnumber elderly men 3 to 2

Women greatly outnumber men in the group aged 65+, and this disparity increases with age. These statistics reflect the fact that women, on average, live longer than men. Women do not dominate all age groups, however. Males slightly outnumber females in the younger age groups. For example, for individuals aged 18 and younger in the United States in 2000, 35.2 million were female and 37.1 million were male.[15] Beginning in the early adult years, however, the ratio begins to shift, and by age 65+, women outnumber men 3 to 2 (see Table 3.3). After age 85, there are seven women for every three men.

TABLE 3.2
Foreign-Born Population Aged 65+ Years by Year of Entry and Age: March 2000 (numbers in thousands)

Year of Entry	65+ Years		65–74 Years		75–84 Years		85+ Years	
	Number	Percent	Number	Percent	Number	Percent	Number	Percent
1990–1999	363	11.6%	244	13.7%	94	9.7%	25	6.7%
1980–1989	446	14.3	282	15.9	129	13.4	35	9.4
1970–1979	380	12.2	239	13.4	109	11.3	32	8.8
Before 1970	1,925	61.8	1,013	57	632	65.6	280	75.3
Total	3,116	100	1,778	100	965	100	373	100

Source: Bureau of the Census, *Current Population Survey*, March 2000.

TABLE 3.3

**Number of Men per 100 Women by Age for the
Age 65+ Population: 1990 and 2000**

	1990	2000
65+ years	67	70
65–74	78	82
75–84	60	65
85+	39	41

Source: Bureau of the Census, "The 65 Years and Over
Population" (October 2001). Available online at
www.census.gov.

■ The ratio of oldest-old to people aged 50 to 64 triples in 50 years

People in their fifties and sixties are more and more likely to have living parents and other relatives who are aged 85+. Therefore, an increasing number of older people have the responsibility of caring for the oldest-old, who are likely to be frail and in need of extensive financial, medical, social, and emotional support.

In 1950, the ratio of the oldest-old people to persons aged 50 to 64 was 3 to 100. Today that ratio has more than tripled to 10 to 100.[16] The Census Bureau estimates that the ratio could reach 29 to 100 by 2050.[17]

■ The elderly are an increasing share of those not in the workforce

The support ratio is a statistical calculation to describe the economic responsibility that workers bear for people who are not in the workforce, taken to be children and the elderly. The instrument is crude because many younger and older people actually are in the labor force and, additionally, many people of working age are not employed. The support ratio for 1900 is estimated to have been 80 children and elderly for every 100 people of working age.[18] By 2000, the estimate for this ratio had decreased to 62 per 100. Forecasts of the support ratio are 68 per 100 in 2020, and a return to the 1900 level of 80 children and elderly per 100 workers in 2050.

The balance of children and elderly within the support ratio is expected to change dramatically as well. In 1900, the ratio was skewed toward children, with 73 children and 7 elderly people per 100 workers.* In 2000, children were less dominant, with 42 children and 21 elderly for every 100 workers. Projections for 2020 are 40 children and 28 elderly per 100 workers, and by 2050, 44 children and 36 elderly for every 100 workers.

■ U.S. veteran population shrinks and ages

The U.S. veteran population is growing smaller and older. In 2000, 9.5 million veterans were aged 65+, making up 37.4 percent of the overall veteran population of

---

* Numbers may not add up to the total support ratio figure due to rounding.

25.5 million.[19] The total veteran population is expected to decrease to 16.8 million in 2020. In addition, the median age of the veteran population will increase from 57 in 2000 to 62 in 2020. At that time, 45 percent of all veterans (7.6 million) will be aged 65+.

Today, a very small percentage of veterans are aged 85+. In 2000, 506,000 veterans were in this age group, representing 5 percent of the veteran population aged 65+. However, by 2020, the Veterans Administration estimates that 1 million veterans will be aged 85+, representing 13 percent of the 65+ veteran population.

■ The world is aging

Population aging is a global phenomenon. According to demographer David E. Redburn, "practically all of the countries of Southern, Western, and Northern Europe are 'older' than the United States if we look at the percentages of their populations over 60."[20]

According to the UN's Population Division, in 2000 about 606 million people globally were aged 60+, the equivalent of the entire current populations of the United States, United Kingdom, and Netherlands combined.[21] This number included 69 million people aged 80+. The number of people aged 60+ worldwide is expected to more than triple by 2050 to 2 billion, and the number of people aged 80+ is projected to increase more than fivefold to 379 million by that time.

In 2000, the population aged 60+ in the more-developed regions equaled about 20 percent of the population; by 2050, it is expected to account for 33 percent of the population.[22] In the less-developed regions, the proportion of the population aged 60+ is expected to rise from 8 percent in 2000 to close to 20 percent in 2050.

■ Older people outnumber children in the developed world

The older population of the more-developed regions has already surpassed the child population, defined as ages 0 to 14 years.[23] The UN Population Division predicts that by the year 2050 the ratio of older persons to children in the more-developed regions will be 2 to 1.

■ Ten years will be added to the world's median age by 2050

The population of the world will age faster in the next 50 years than it did in the past 50 years (Table 3.4).[24] Over the past half century, the median age for the world increased by 3 years, from 23.6 years in 1950 to 26.5 years in 2000. The UN Population Division predicts that in the next 50 years, the median age will rise by almost 10 years, reaching 36.2 years in 2050.

■ The proportion of children and older people in the world will be equal by 2050

The percentage of children aged 0 to 14 years in the world has declined from 34 percent in 1950 to 30 percent in 2000, just as the proportion of the 60+ population has increased globally from 8 percent to 10 percent.[25] In the next 50 years, the percentage of children is expected to drop by one-third, reaching 21 percent in 2050. At

TABLE 3.4
Median Age by Area: 1950, 2000, and 2050 (medium variant)

	Median Age in Years		
	1950	2000	2050
World total	23.6	26.5	36.2
Less-developed countries	24	27	36
More-developed countries	21	24	35
Least-developed countries	20	37	46
Africa	19	18	27
Asia	22	26	27
Europe	29	38	50
North America	30	36	41
Latin America and the Caribbean	20	24	38
Oceania	28	31	38

Source: UN Population Division, "World Population Prospects: The 2000 Revision."
Available online at www.un.org/esa/population/unpop.htm.

the same time, the proportion of older persons in the world is expected to more than double to 21 percent.

■ Europe is the leader in population aging

Population aging is most advanced in Europe. In 2000, children were 17 percent and people aged 60+ were 20 percent of the population. Japan is currently the country with the oldest population, with a median age of 41 years. Italy, Switzerland, Germany, and Sweden, each with median ages of 40 years, have the next oldest populations. In 2050, populations in which persons age 50+ dominate are projected to be Spain, with a median age of 55 years, and Italy, Slovenia, and Austria, with projected median ages of 54 years. Africa remains the major area with the youngest population. In 2000, 43 percent of the African population were children and only 5 percent were aged 60+.

NOTES

1. Judith Treas, "Older Americans in the 1990s and Beyond," *Population Bulletin* 50 (1995): 2.
2. Bureau of the Census, "The 65 Years and Over Population" (2001). Available online at http://factfinder.census.gov.
3. Jacob S. Siegel and Maria Davidson, "Demographic and Socioeconomic Aspects of Aging in the United States," in *Current Population Reports* P-23, No. 138 (Washington, DC: Bureau of the Census, 1984).
4. Bureau of the Census, "Age: 2000" (September 2001). Available online at http://factfinder.census.gov. U.S. Senate Special Committee on Aging, *Aging America: Trends and Projections, 1991 Edition* (Washington, DC: GPO, 1991), 4.

5. Bureau of the Census, "Projections of the Resident Population by Age, Sex, Race, and Hispanic Origin, 1999 to 2100" (2000). Available online at www.census.gov.
6. U.S. Senate Special Committee on Aging, *Aging America.*
7. Bureau of the Census, "Projections" (2000).
8. Ibid.
9. Ibid.
10. U.S. Administration on Aging, "Profile of Older Americans, 2001" (December 2001). Available online at www.aoa.dhhs.gov.
11. Bureau of the Census, *Aging America.*
12. Ken Bryson and Lynne M. Casper, *Coresident Grandparents and Grandchildren* (Washington, DC: Bureau of the Census, 1998), 23–198.
13. U.S. Administration on Aging, "Profile."
14. Administration on Aging, *A Profile of Older Americans: 2001.* Available online at www.aoa.gov/STATS/profile/default.htm.
15. Bureau of the Census, *Age: 2000.*
16. Ibid.
17. Bureau of the Census, *65+ in the United States* (Washington, DC, 1996), 2–19.
18. Jennifer Cheeseman Day, "Population Projections of the United States by Age, Sex, Race, and Hispanic Origin: 1995 to 2050" in *Current Population Reports* P-25-1130 (Washington, DC: Bureau of the Census, 1996), 9.
19. U.S. Department of Veterans Affairs, "National Veteran Population by Age (1990–2000)," Supplemental Tables 3 and 4. Available at www.va.gov.
20. David E. Redburn, "The 'Graying' of the World's Population," in *Social Gerontology* (Westport, CT: Auburn House, 1998), 1.
21. UN Population Division, "World Population Prospects: The 2000 Revision." Available at www.un.org/esa/population/unpop.htm.
22. Ibid.
23. Ibid.
24. Ibid.
25. Ibid.

CHAPTER 4

Life Expectancy: Three Decades in 100 Years

Never before in human history have so many lived for so long.

—Ken Dychtwald and Julie Penfold, the "New
Mature Market," in Social Gerontology

This chapter provides information about the dramatic increase in life expectancy that occurred during the twentieth century. It also covers many of the nuances of longevity in the United States, including the fact that the seemingly remarkable three-decade increase in life expectancy of the last century is not particularly impressive when stacked up against the rest of the world. In fact, the United States ranks eleventh in life expectancy among countries with populations of 10 million or more.

One of the most intriguing areas of research on aging is the examination of such factors as gender, race, income, education, and lifestyle, all of which influence how long we live. Many of the findings from this research are what one would expect. For example, exercising and refraining from smoking both prolong life. Likewise, affluent and highly educated people live longer than those who are poor and have less education. However, other findings are surprising; some delightfully so. Who would have suspected this welcome news: indulging your sweet tooth and having fun can prolong life?

Highlights from this chapter include:

- Thirty years were added to life expectancy during the twentieth century.
- The gap in life expectancy between men and women is decreasing.
- In the 1900s, life expectancy at age 65 increased by 5.8 years.
- Although Americans have enjoyed remarkable increases in life expectancy, the United States is outranked by 10 other developed countries with populations of 10 million or more.
- A white child born in 2000 could expect to live almost 6 years longer than a black child born that year.

LIFE EXPECTANCY IN THE TWENTIETH CENTURY

■ Thirty years were added to life expectancy in the twentieth century

One of the major accomplishments of the twentieth century in the United States is that 30 years have been added to life expectancy (Table 4.1).

A baby born in the United States in 1900 could expect to live an average of only 47 years.[1] A baby born in 2000 could expect to live 76.9 years, surpassing the previous record high of 76.7 recorded in 1999.[2] About 80 percent of babies born today can expect to survive to age 65, and roughly one-third to age 85.[3] As mentioned in Chapter 1, the greatest gains in longevity occurred in the first 50 years of the twentieth century, when the expected lifetime of a newborn advanced 21 years.

■ Life expectancy is forecast to increase 5 years by 2050

The Census Bureau's middle series projections are that life expectancy overall in the United States will increase to 82 years by 2050. According to the bureau's alter-

TABLE 4.1
Life Expectancy at Birth and Age 65: 1900–2000

At Birth	All Races Both Sexes	Men	Women	White Both Sexes	Men	Women	Black Both Sexes	Men	Women
1900	47.3	46.3	48.3	47.6	46.6	48.7	33.03	32.5	33.5
1950	68.2	65.6	71.1	69.1	66.5	72.2	60.7	58.9	62.7
1960	69.7	66.6	73.1	70.6	67.4	74.1	63.2	60.7	65.9
1970	70.9	67.1	74.8	71.7	68	75.6	64.1	60	68.3
1980	73.7	70	77.4	74.4	70.7	78.1	68.1	63.8	72.5
1990	75.4	71.8	78.8	76.1	72.7	79.4	69.1	64.5	73.6
2000***	76.9	74.1	79.5	77.4	74.8	79.9	71.8	68.3	75
At Age 65									
1900**	11.9	11.5	12.2	—	11.5	12.2	—	10.4*	11.43
1950	13.9	12.8	15	—	12.8	15.1	13.9	12.9	14.9
1960	14.3	12.8	15.8	14.4	12.9	15.9	13.9	12.7	15.1
1970	15.2	13.1	17	15.2	13.1	17.1	14.2	12.5	15.7
1980	16.4	14.1	18.3	16.5	14.2	18.4	15.1	13	16.8
1990	17.2	15.1	18.9	17.3	15.2	19.1	15.4	13.2	17.2
2000***	17.9	16.3	19.2	17.9	16.3	19.2	16.2	14.6	17.5

*Death registration area only. The death registration area increased from 10 states and the District of Columbia in 1900 to the coterminous United States in 1933.

**Includes deaths of nonresidents of the United States.

***Preliminary 2000 data.

Source: 1900 to 1990 data from *Health United States, 1999, Health and Aging Chartbook,* PHS 99-123.

native series, however, life expectancy could reach a high of 89.4 years or drop to a low of 74.8 years in 2050.[4]

■ The United States lags behind other developed countries

Although Americans have enjoyed remarkable increases in life expectancy at birth, the United States is outranked by 10 other countries. A baby born in any of the following countries in 2001 could expect to outlive a baby born the same year in the United States: Australia, Belgium, Canada, France, Germany, Italy, Japan, Netherlands, Spain, and the United Kingdom.[5] Japan had the highest life expectancy, at 80.8 years.

Countries with the lowest life expectancies are those in undeveloped regions. In 2000, the country of Malawi in southeast Africa had the world's lowest projected life expectancy at birth, only 36 years.[6]

According to a comprehensive study conducted by the World Health Organization, Harvard School of Public Health, and World Bank, in the next two decades, life expectancy at birth is expected to advance for women in all regions of the world. However, life expectancy for men will "grow much more slowly, mainly because of the impact of the tobacco epidemic."[7] The study predicted that by 2020, females born in established market economies will have a life expectancy of almost 88 years, whereas males will have a life expectancy of about 78 years.

■ A large gap exists in life expectancy across U.S. counties

A county-by-county study found as much as a 40-year discrepancy in the average longevity of U.S. residents.[8] The research, conducted by the Centers for Disease Control and Harvard University, projected that the differences in life expectancy in U.S. counties are parallel to those found between Japan and Sierra Leone. A review of county death certificates issued from 1959 to 1994 found that Asian American women in parts of New York, New Jersey, and Florida live, on average, into their late nineties, whereas Native American men in six South Dakota counties live only until their mid-fifties. Black men in Washington, DC, had a life expectancy of only 57.9 years.

■ The gap in life expectancy between men and women remains, but is decreasing

Through much of the twentieth century, improvements in life expectancy have benefited women more than men. This disparity appears to be a natural phenomenon. Females in the animal kingdom also tend to outlive males, whether they are mice or elephants.[9] From 1950 to 1980, life expectancy at birth for the total population rose by 5.5 years. It advanced by about 6.3 years for women, whereas the improvement was 4.4 years for men.

Since 1980, however, males have advanced in longevity faster than females. Between 1980 and 2000, 4.1 years were added to life expectancy for men, but only 2.1 years were added for women. In 2000, record high life expectancies of 74.1 years for men and 79.5 years for women were reached (see Table 4.1).

Differences in life expectancy at birth for males and females are expected to narrow in the next 50 years. According to Census Bureau middle series projections, a baby boy born in 2050 can expect to live 79.7 years, and a baby girl born in 2050 can expect to live 84.3 years. This represents a life-expectancy difference of 4.6 years, compared with 6.7 years in 2000.

◼ Life expectancy at age 65 continues to improve

Since the beginning of the twentieth century, 6 years have been added to life expectancy at age 65. Americans who reached their 65th birthdays in 2000 could expect, on average, to live another 17.9 years (see Table 4.1). Elderly males, whose life expectancy at age 65 was 16.3 years in 2000, have gained 4.8 years since the beginning of the twentieth century. Elderly females, who had a life expectancy of 19.2 years in 2000, have gained 7 years.

Differences in remaining years of life at age 65+ for both sexes are expected to narrow in the next 50 years. According to Census Bureau middle series projections, by 2050, males who reach their 65th birthdays can expect to live another 20.3 years, and females this age have a remaining life expectancy of 22.4 years. This represents a difference of 2.1 years between the sexes, compared with a 3.6-year difference in 2000.

◼ Life expectancy differs between blacks and whites

Life expectancy at birth differs by race. A white child born in 2000 could expect to live 5.6 years longer than a black child born in 2000 (life expectancy for whites was 77.4 years compared to 71.8 years for blacks; see Table 4.1). However, if blacks live to age 65, their life expectancy is much closer to that of whites than it was at birth. In 2000, life expectancy at age 65 was 17.9 years for whites and 16.2 years for blacks.

White females have a longevity advantage over black women as well as over men of both races. A white girl born in 2000 had a life expectancy of 79.9 years, while a black girl born in the same year could expect to live to age 75. Life expectancy at birth for white males was close to that of black females (74.8 years), and life expectancy for black males was 68.3 years.

The longevity hierarchy also holds true for the population aged 65+. In 2000, life expectancy at age 65 for white females was 19.2 years, followed by 17.5 years for black females, 16.3 years for white males, and 14.6 years for black males (see Table 4.1).

Despite the claims made for the exceptional longevity of Russian Georgians or Bolivian mountaineers, there is no reliable record of any human being surviving past 120 years of age. According to the National Institute on Aging, Shirechiyo Izumi of Japan reached the age of 120 years 237 days in 1986. His age of death has been verified by documents that most experts believe are authentic. He died after developing pneumonia.

CHARACTERISTICS, LIFESTYLE, AND LIFE EXPECTANCY

■ People who live longer and/or have a lower risk of death have certain characteristics

Death rates and longevity vary greatly for people with different characteristics and lifestyles. The good news is that some of these factors are within individual control. Recent findings on longevity show that people who have a lower risk of death and/or who live longer are those who:

Have fun.   They enjoy going to movies, eating out, playing cards, and taking part in other social activities. A study of 2,761 residents of New Haven, Connecticut, conducted by Thomas Glass of the Harvard School of Public Health, found that those who were most socially active lived an average of 2 years longer than those least engaged in such activities.[10]

Have high IQs as children.   A study of 2,792 Scottish children tested the association between and mortality over the normal human lifespan.[11] Researchers found that childhood mental ability is positively related to survival to at least age 76 years in both women and men. The authors concluded that childhood mental ability is a significant factor among the variables that predict age at death.

Indulge in sweets.   More than 7,800 men in a study of Harvard University alumni were asked about their candy consumption. After adjusting for age and other health habits, researchers found that men who indulged their sweet tooth lived almost a year longer than those who did not.[12]

Eat a healthy diet.   In the late 1980s, in the first study to look at the impact of overall dietary patterns, investigators at Queen's College (City University of New York) gave 42,254 women questionnaires regarding their food intake.[13] The respondents had a mean age of 61 years.* Those with the highest consumption of healthy foods cut their mortality risk by 31 percent.

In addition, a British study of 19,496 men and women aged 45 to 79 years showed that just a slight increase in vitamin C intake can reduce the risk of mortality.[14] According to the study's authors, even an increase of one serving daily of fruits and vegetables has encouraging prospects for longevity.

Refrain from smoking.   An analysis conducted by scientists at the National Institute on Aging (NIA) involving 8,604 nondisabled elderly persons found that male and female nonsmokers survived about 1.5 to 4 years longer than nonsmokers, depending on their level of activity. Moreover, most nonsmokers did not become disabled even when close to death.[15]

---

* The women were divided into quartiles based on how many times per week they consumed foods recommended by current dietary guidelines, which included fruits, whole grains, low-fat dairy, lean meats, and poultry. The data were adjusted for education, ethnicity, age, body mass index, smoking status, alcohol use, level of physical activity, menopausal hormone use, and history of disease.

In addition, Richard Rogers and colleagues, in a groundbreaking study on longevity patterns in the United States, found that 25 percent of the differential in male and female longevity is due to the high rates of males who smoke.[16]

Researchers from the University of Bristol estimated how much life is lost in smoking cigarettes.* They found that one cigarette reduces life by 11 minutes, a pack of 20 cigarettes reduces life by 3 hours 40 minutes, and a carton of cigarettes reduces life by 1.5 days.[17]

Research conducted at Duke University and funded by the National Institute on Aging found that stopping smoking at any age provides life extension. Life expectancy among smokers who quit at age 35 exceeded that of continuing smokers by 6.9 to 8.5 years for men and 6.1 to 7.7 years for women. Even those who quit much later in life gained some benefits. Among smokers who quit at age 65 years, men gained 1.4 to 2.0 years of life, and women gained 2.7 to 3.7 years.[18]

Have favorable levels of cholesterol and blood pressure and do not smoke.   A study of 366,559 subjects aged 18 to 59 found that those who did not smoke and had low blood pressure (less than or equal to 120/80 mm Hg) and low cholesterol (serum cholesterol level less than 200 mg/dL) could expect to live 5.8 years to 9.5 years longer than those who did not fit this profile.[19]

In addition, an analysis of three prospective studies, including the Multiple Risk Factor Intervention Trial (MRFIT), found that men with favorable baseline serum cholesterol levels had a life expectancy 3.8 to 8.7 years greater than men with unfavorable levels.[20]

Keep physically active.   The previously mentioned NIA analysis, which involved 8,604 nondisabled elderly persons, found that physical activity means longer lives for smokers and nonsmokers. Physical activity in elderly nonsmokers added 11 to 18 years of life, and 9 to 15 years for smokers. Higher physical activity also reduced the amount of disability before death.

In a Finnish study of 7,925 healthy men and 7,977 healthy women who are twins, leisure-time physical activity was associated with a reduced risk of premature death, even after genetic disorders were taken into account.[21] The researchers found that conditioning exercisers had a 43 percent lower risk of death when compared with those who were sedentary, and the occasional exercisers had a 29 percent reduced risk of death when compared with the sedentary.

DEFINITION: Conditioning exercisers are defined as those who reported exercising at least six times per month, with an intensity corresponding to at least vigorous walking for a mean duration of 30 minutes; occasional exercisers were those who were neither sedentary nor conditioning exercisers. Sedentary people were those who reported no leisure physical activity.

---

*
The life-lost calculation is for men only and based on the difference in life expectancy between male smokers and nonsmokers and an estimate of the total number of cigarettes a male smoker consumes in his lifetime.

Researchers at the University of Virginia School of Medicine examined the association between, and mortality in, a group of men 61 to 81 years of age who were nonsmokers and physically capable of participating in low-intensity activities on a daily basis. After adjustment for age, the mortality rate among the men who walked less than 1 mile per day was nearly twice that of those who walked more than 2 miles per day. Walking as little as 1 mile a day was found to lower the death rate by 19 percent. The results were adjusted for overall measures of activity and other risk factors.

In a study of Harvard graduates, researchers found that men who burned 2,000 or more calories a week by walking lived an average of 1 to 2 years longer than those who burned fewer than 500 calories a week by exercising.[22]

Are joggers.   A Dutch study found that joggers have a lower risk of death than nonjoggers do. The research is part of the Copenhagen City Heart Study, a prospective population study of cardiovascular disease. Researchers examined 4,658 Danish men over a period of 5 years. Persistent joggers had a lower incidence of death than nonjoggers and infrequent joggers. The results were independent of such factors as smoking, weight, blood pressure and cholesterol.[23] According to the authors, the study showed that a vigorous activity such as jogging is associated with a beneficial effect on mortality.

Are "healthy agers."   Data gathered from nearly 16,000 individuals demonstrate that "healthy agers"—those who do not have physical performance and/or related limitations—have longer life expectancies than those who are limited. For example, the gap in life expectancy for those who can and cannot walk a quarter of a mile is more than a decade.[24]

Have "healthy habits."   A study comparing members of the Seventh-Day Adventist Church to nonmembers suggested that "healthy habits" can lead to longer lives.[25] Researchers examined data from a 12-year study of health and lifestyle habits of more than 34,000 California Adventists. The subjects were aged 30 and older. Thirty percent of the Adventists were vegetarians, about 40 percent exercised vigorously for 15 minutes at least three times per week, and none smoked cigarettes. The researchers compared the Adventists data to those of white Californians who were not Adventists. They found that, compared to the non-Adventists, male Adventists' life expectancy was 7.2 years longer and female Adventists' life expectancy was 4.4 years longer.

Have a high income level.   Numerous studies have shown that higher incomes mean longer lives.[26] One recent longitudinal study found that at age 65, white men in the highest income families could expect to live 3.1 years longer than white men in the lowest income families; the difference between income groups was 2.5 years for black men, and 1.3 years for black women.[27] In addition, Richard E. Rogers and colleagues found that men living in affluent families have a mortality rate that is only marginally higher than that for women with similar incomes.[28]

Have a high educational level.   Many studies have shown that higher educational levels mean higher life expectancies.[29] Data from the National Institutes of Health (NIH) showed that among adults aged 25 to 64, deaths due to chronic diseases, communicable diseases, and injuries were all higher for men and women with lower educational levels.[30] Specifically, deaths due to chronic diseases for men with less than 12 years of education were 2.5 times those for men with more than 12 years of education. Among women, the comparable multiple was 2.1.

Have a high socioeconomic status.   In a classic mid-1960s study that tracked 17,530 British male civil servants over 10 years, researchers found that variations in mortality rates mirrored socioeconomic status. Mortality rates for men in the lowest civil service classification were three times higher than for those with the highest grades. In a subsequent 25-year tracking of the subjects, these results held true well past retirement.[31]

Volunteer in moderate amounts.   A study at the University of Michigan's Institute for Social Research found that volunteering for one organization for up to 40 hours a year has a protective effect on the mortality of older adults. Volunteering does not have the same benefit, however, if the older adult takes on too much and the activity becomes more like employment.[32]

Are Asian American.   Asian Americans, particularly among the elderly, have the lowest odds of death of any racial or ethnic group, including Caucasians.[33] Controlling for age and sex, Asian Americans exhibit 31 percent lower mortality compared with Caucasians.[34]

Are foreign born.   In a recent analysis, foreign-born U.S. residents demonstrated 20 percent lower odds of mortality than native-born persons.[35]

Live in the Midwest.   U.S. counties with the highest life expectancies are in mostly rural Midwestern or Western counties in Minnesota, South Dakota, Iowa, Colorado, Montana, and Utah.[36] This finding is controversial, however, because it may be a result of younger people moving out of these areas

Are married and living with two children.   Family composition affects mortality. According to Rogers and his colleagues, those who are married and living with only a spouse are 21 percent more likely to die than those who are married and living with a spouse and two children.[37]

Have a sibling who is a centenarian.   In a resounding confirmation of the effect of "good genes," a study conducted by Thomas Perls and reported in *The Lancet* found that siblings of centenarians had a fourfold greater chance of surviving into their nineties than siblings of a similar birth cohort who died in their early seventies.[38] A subsequent study conducted by Perls and his colleagues found that brothers of centenarians are at least 17 times and sisters 8 times more likely to live to be 100 years old than the general population.[39]

Attend religious services.   According to a meta-analysis of 42 studies that examined 125,826 people, the odds of survival for people who scored higher on measures of public and private religious involvement were 29 percent higher than those for people who scored lower on such measures.[40]

A number of other studies have found similar results. Over a 5-year period, researchers studied more than 2,000 residents aged 55+ living in California's affluent Marin County. Almost one-quarter of the subjects died in that period. The one factor that predicted survival was attending religious services. The researchers also found that people who engaged in volunteer work, along with attending religious services, were even more likely to live longer. Visiting museums and art galleries were also marginally protective.[41]

Other evidence on the effects of religious attendance on mortality varies, but confirms these studies in spirit. By one estimate, people who never attend religious services have about 80 percent higher odds of death than those who attend one or more times a week.[42] In addition, researchers studying people over a period of 28 years found that those who attended religious services at least weekly were 25 percent less likely to die than infrequent attendees.[43]

Are women in the labor force.   Several studies have shown that, considering women only, housewives have a higher mortality rate than women who work.[44]

Are women who have had children later in life.   A study by researchers at Harvard Medical School in Boston found that women who survived to age 100 were four times as likely to have had children while in their forties than women who survived to only the age of 73.[45]

Are women who are wafer thin.   A study of 115,195 women enrolled in the Nurses' Health Study examined the association between body-mass index (BMI) (defined as weight in kilograms divided by the square of the height in meters) and mortality.[46] The lowest mortality rate was observed among women who weighed at least 15 percent less than the U.S. average for women of similar age and among those whose weight had been stable since early adulthood. (Note: This finding is controversial. See Chapter 6 for information on weight and longevity.)

■ People who do not live as long and/or have a higher risk of death have other certain characteristics

People who have a higher risk of death and/or who live shorter lives are those who:

Are African Americans.   African Americans of all ages have the highest odds of death, mostly due to their disadvantaged social and economic situations.[47] A white child born in 1998 could expect to live 5.8 years longer than a black child born then. The discrepancy is in large part due to high rates of heart disease, cancer, and homicide among blacks.[48]

Are overweight.   In an American Cancer Society study of more than 1 million adults in the United States, researchers examined the relation between body-mass index and mortality. Results showed that the risk of death from all causes and all age groups increases for men and women who are moderately to severely overweight. This risk is greater for whites than for blacks.[49]

DEFINITION: Body mass index (BMI) correlates to fatness, and applies to both men and women. To determine BMI, weight in kilograms is divided by height in meters, squared. A BMI of 25 to 29.9 is considered overweight and 30 or above is considered obese.

However, another large study found that greater BMI was associated with higher mortality only up to 75 years of age, and then the risk declined. The latter research was part of the American Cancer Society's Cancer Prevention Study and included both men and women.[50]

Using data from the Third National Health and Nutrition Examination Survey, the Framingham Heart Study, and other secondary sources, researchers found that the life expectancy of moderately obese men aged 45 to 54 is reduced by 1 year compared to their nonobese peers.[51]

The prospective Nurse's Health Study, which involved only women, confirmed the relationship between overweight and higher risk of mortality. The study's authors found that excess body weight increases the risk of death from any cause, and the risk is higher among younger subjects.[52]

Have a tendency to "catastrophize." A 1998 study found that people with pessimistic attitudes appear to not live as long as those with more positive attitudes.[53] For example, the study found that men who "catastrophize" appear 25 percent more likely to die before age 65 than those who do not.

Live in urban center areas including Baltimore; Bronx, New York City; Washington, DC; New Orleans; and St. Louis. The previously mentioned county-by-county study by the Centers for Disease Control and Harvard University found that these urban counties all have life expectancies that are low.[54]

Life expectancy trivia

During the twentieth century, 10,840 days were added to life expectancy at birth. Fifty-eight percent of women born in 1900 survived to age 65, and 25 percent survived to age 85. Now, 90 percent of women born in 1990 are expected to live to age 65, and more than half will live to age 85.[55]

NOTES

1. National Center for Health Statistics, *Health, United States, 1988*, PHS 89-1232 (Hyattsville, MD, March 1989).
2. National Center for Health Statistics, *National Vital Statistics Report* 49, no. 12 (Hyattsville, MD, October 9, 2001).

3. National Center for Health Statistics, *Health, United States, 1999* (Hyattsville, MD, 1999), 30.
4. Bureau of the Census, *Resident Population Estimates of the United States by Age and Sex: April 1, 1990 to June 1, 1999* (Washington, DC, July 30, 1999), 4.
5. Bureau of the Census, *Statistical Abstract of the United States: 2001*, 121 edition (Washington, DC, 2001).
6. Bureau of the Census, *Statistical Abstract of the United States: 1998*, 118 edition (Washington, DC, 1998).
7. Christopher J. L. Murray and Alan D. Lopez, *The Global Burden of Disease* (Cambridge, MA: Harvard School of Public Health, 1996), 32.
8. C. J. L. Murray et al., *U.S. Patterns of Mortality by County and Race: 1965–1949* (Cambridge, MA: Harvard Center for Population and Development Studies, 1998), 8–11.
9. Ruth Larsen, "Gender Gap Dooms Men to Shorter Life Spans," *Insight on the News* 15, no. 21 (June 7, 1999): 40.
10. "Having Fun Extends Life for the Elderly," *Jet* 96, no. 16 (September 20, 1999): 40.
11. "Longitudinal Cohort Study of and Survival up to Age 76," *British Medical Journal* 322 (April 7, 2001): 819–822.
12. "Sweets and Chocolates Help You Live Longer," *Chemist and Druggist* (January 23, 1999): viii.
13. Ashima K. Kant, "A Prospective Study of Diet Quality and Mortality in Women," *Journal of the American Medical Association* 283, no. 16 (2000): 2109–2115.
14. Kay-tee Khaw et al., "Relation between Plasma Ascorbic Acid and Mortality in Men and Women in EPIC–Norfolk Prospective Study: A Prospective Population Study," *The Lancet* (March 3, 2001).
15. Luigi Ferruucci et al., "Smoking, Physical Activity, and Active Life Expectancy," *American Journal of Epidemiology* 149, no. 7 (April 1, 1999): 645.
16. Richard G. Rogers, Robert A. Hummer, and Charles B. Nam, *Living and Dying in the USA* (San Diego, CA: Academic Press, 1995), 49.
17. Mary Shaw and Richard Mitchell, *Time for a Smoke? One Cigarette Reduces Your Life by 11 Minutes* (British Medical Association and the Gale Group, January 1, 2000).
18. Donald H. Taylor et al., "Benefits of Smoking Cessation for Longevity," *American Journal of Public Health* 92 (2002): 990–996.
19. Jeremiah Stamler et al., "Low Risk-Factor Profile and Long-Term Cardiovascular and Noncardiovascular Mortality and Life Expectancy," *Journal of the American Medical Association* 282, no. 21 (December 1, 1999): 2012–2018.
20. Jeremiah Stamler et al., "Relationship of Baseline Serum Cholesterol Levels in Three Large Cohorts of Younger Men to Long-Term Coronary, Cardiovascular, and All-Cause Mortality and to Longevity," *Journal of the American Medical Association* 284 (2000): 311–318.
21. Urho M. Kujala, "Exercise Reduces Risk of Premature Death Even after Genetics Taken into Account," *Journal of the American Medical Association* 279 (1998): 440–444.
22. "Walk Your Way to Fitness," *Mayo Clinic Health Letter* (1996).
23. Peter Schnohr et al., "Mortality in Population Based Study of 4658 Men," *British Medical Journal* 321 (September 9, 2000): 602–603.
24. Richard G. Rogers, "Sociodemographic Characteristics of Long-Lived and Healthy Individuals," *Population and Development Review* 21, no. 1 (March 1995): 33–58.
25. G. E. Fraser and D. J. Shavlik, "Ten Years of Life: Is It a Matter of Choice?" *Archives of Internal Medicine* 161, no. 13 (2001): 1645.
26. S. H. Preston et al., "African-American Mortality at Older Ages: Results of a Matching Study," *Demography* 33, no. 2 (1996): 193–209.
27. E. Pamuk et al., "Socioeconomic Status and Health Chartbook," *Health United States* (Hyattsville, MD: National Center for Health Statistics, 1998), 88.

28. Rogers et al., *Living and Dying*, 304.
29. I. T. Elo and S. H. Preston, "Educational Differentials in Mortality: United States, 1979–85," *Social Science and Medicine* 42, no. 1 (1996): 47–57.
30. E. Pamuk et al., "Socioeconomic Status," 6.
31. I. Whitehall, Department of Epidemiology and Public Health, Royal Free and University College Medical School, London. Available online at www.ucl.ac.uk/ epidemiology/.
32. Mark A. Musick et al., "Volunteering and Mortality among Older Adults: Findings from a National Sample," *Journal of Gerontology, Social Sciences* 54B, no. 3 (1999): S173–179.
33. Rogers et al., *Living and Dying*, 304.
34. Ibid., 61.
35. Ibid., 53.
36. Murray et al., *U.S. Patterns: 1965–1994*, 8–11.
37. Rogers et al., *Living and Dying*, 84.
38. Thomas T. Perls et al., "Siblings of Centenarians Live Longer," *The Lancet* 351, no. 9115 (May 23, 1998): 1560.
39. Thomas Perls et al., "Exceptional Familial Clustering for Extreme Longevity in Humans," *Journal of the American Geriatrics Society* 48 (2000): 1483–1485.
40. Michael E. McCullough et al., "Religious Involvement and Mortality: A Meta-Analytic Review," *Health Psychology* 19, no. 3 (2000).
41. Douglas Oman and Dwayne Reed, "Religion and Mortality among the Community-Dwelling Elderly," *American Journal of Public Health* 88, no. 10 (1999): 1469–1475.
42. Rogers et al., *Living and Dying*, 103.
43. W. J. Strawbridge et al., "Frequent Attendance at Religious Services and Mortality over 28 Years," *American Journal of Public Health* 87, no. 6 (1997): 957–961.
44. Rogers et al., *Living and Dying*, 121.
45. Thomas T. Perls, "Middle-Aged Mothers Live Longer," *Nature* 389, no. 133 (September 11, 1997).
46. JoAnn E. Manson et al., "Body Weight and Mortality among Women," *The New England Journal of Medicine* 333, no. 11 (September 14, 1995).
47. Rogers et al., *Living and Dying*, 304.
48. L. Potter et al., "Influence of Homicide on Racial Disparity in Life Expectancy: United States, 1998," *Morbidity and Mortality Weekly Report* 50 (2001): 780–783.
49. Eugenia E. Calle et al., "Body-Mass Index and Mortality in a Prospective Cohort of U.S. Adults," *Department of Epidemiology and Surveillance Research* (Atlanta: American Cancer Society).
50. June Stevens et al., "The Effect of Age on the Association between Body-Mass Index and Mortality," *The New England Journal of Medicine* 338, no. 1 (January 1, 1998): 1–7.
51. David Thompson, "Lifetime Health and Economic Consequences of Obesity," *Archives of Internal Medicine* 159 (1999): 2177–2183.
52. Manson et al., "Body Weight and Mortality," 677–685.
53. "Catastrophizing and Untimely Death," *Psychological Science* 9, no. 2: 127–130 (1998).
54. Murray et al., *U.S. Patterns: 1965–1994*, 8–11.
55. John W. Rowe and Robert L. Kahn, *Successful Aging* (New York: Random House, 1998), 5.

CHAPTER 5

Health Status, Use of Health Services, and Attitudes toward Health Care Providers

The first wealth is health.

—Ralph Waldo Emerson

Health—The first of all liberties.

—Henry F. Amiel

This chapter covers seniors' perception of their health, disability levels, and use of a wide range of health care services. Much of the information we report is good news. Contrary to popular opinion, the majority of the elderly view their health positively. Although many are limited in activity, their rates of disability have actually declined in recent years. However, many subgroups of the older population are less hearty and report more unhealthy days. In addition, blacks and Hispanics are more likely than other elderly to rate their health as fair or poor.

The elderly heavily use hospital, physician, and other health services. Tragically, other essential health care needs may go unattended. For example, most hearing-impaired elderly do not use hearing aids.

Highlights of this chapter include:

- Almost three-quarters of people aged 65+ rate their health as good, very good, or excellent.
- Throughout the 1980s and 1990s, disability rates among the elderly declined.
- Seniors are disproportionately heavy users of hospital inpatient services.
- More than 9 in 10 elderly report visiting a physician at least once during the previous year.
- Seniors are the most likely age group to visit eye doctors.
- Older adults consider doctors and pharmacists to be the most believable sources of information about health care problems and issues.
- Two-thirds of seniors had a flu shot within the past year.

SELF-ASSESSMENT OF HEALTH

■ **Three-fourths of the elderly rate their health as good, very good, or excellent**

Self-assessed health ratings provide an indication of the overall physical, emotional, and social aspects of health and well-being and have been found to correlate highly with mortality. Contrary to popular opinion, older people, on average, view their health positively. Three-quarters of elderly Medicare beneficiaries rate their health as excellent, very good, or good; only one-quarter (26 percent) rate it as fair or poor. (See Chart 5.1 and detailed data provided in Table 5.1.)[1] Elderly Medicare beneficiaries most commonly report their health as good—about one-third do so. These good ratings remain relatively stable in the older age groups. In contrast, the top two health ratings (excellent and very good) progressively decline with age, whereas the bottom two ratings (fair and poor) progressively increase from 21 percent among the youngest-old to 36 percent among the oldest-old.

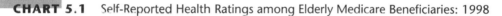

CHART 5.1   Self-Reported Health Ratings among Elderly Medicare Beneficiaries: 1998

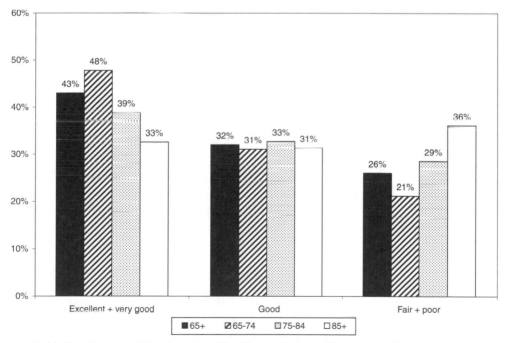

Source: Health Care Financing Administration, "The Characteristics and Perceptions of the Medicare Population (1998)," *Medicare Current Beneficiary Survey* (2001): Section 2. Available online at www.hcfa.gov/survey/mcbs/PubCNP98.htm.

TABLE 5.1

Detailed Data for Chart 5.1: Self-Reported Health Ratings among Elderly
Medicare Beneficiaries: 1998

Health Status	65+ Years	65–74 Years	75–84 Years	85+ Years
Excellent	15%	18%	13%	11%
Very good	27	30	25	21
Good	32	31	33	31
Fair	18	15	20	25
Poor	7.7	6.4	8.5	11
Excellent + very good	43	48	39	33
Fair + poor	26	21	29	36

Note: Numbers may not add up to 100 due to rounding.

Source: Health Care Financing Administration, "The Characteristics and Perceptions of the Medicare Population (1998)," *Medicare Current Beneficiary Survey,* (2001): Section 2. Available online at www.hcfa.gov/survey/mcbs/PubCNP98.htm. Additional calculations made by authors.

■ Seniors are more likely than younger people to rate their health as fair or poor

The elderly are more likely than younger people to rate their health as fair or poor. In 1999, only 19 percent of people aged 55 to 64 reported their health as fair or poor compared with 23 percent of those aged 65 to 74 and 30 percent of those aged 75+.[2]

■ Older blacks and Hispanics are more likely than whites to rate their health as fair or poor

According to the Medicare Current Beneficiary Survey and the Behavioral Risk Factor Surveillance Survey, elderly men and women assess their health similarly. However, blacks and Hispanics are more likely than whites to rate their health as fair or poor (see Table 5.2).[3] Poorer health ratings are also evident among those who have less education, have lower incomes, are not married, live in the South, have diabetes or high blood pressure, are underweight or obese, are smokers, or lack leisure-time physical activities (see Table 5.2).

■ Unhealthy days and health status are related

As might be expected, self-rated health status and average number of unhealthy days correlate highly among adults aged 65+. Those with excellent, very good, or good health report, on average, 1.4 to 4.3 unhealthy days in a 30-day period, whereas those with fair health report 9.1 unhealthy days and those with poor health report 23 such days in a 30-day period.[4]

TABLE 5.2
Percentage of Total Population Reporting Fair or Poor Health by Selected Characteristics:
1993–1997

	Men		Women	
	65–74 Years	75+ Years	65–74 Years	75+ Years
Total population	26%	33%	27%	34%
White	25	32	25	34
Black	40	43	43	47
Hispanic	33	40	39	46
Less than high school graduate	41	43	42	45
College graduate	13	23	13	22
Annual household income less than $15,000	43	43	38	42
Annual household income $50,000 or more	17	27	26	32
Widowed	35	34	30	35
Live in the South	29	37	32	39
Have diabetes	47	51	55	57
Told at least twice they have high blood pressure	34	41	38	44
Underweight	49	51	38	40
Obese (35–39.9 BMI)	40	55	48	50
Current smoker (less than one pack a day)	35	37	29	35
Current smoker (one or more packs a day)	33	39	29	36
Do not participate in leisure-time activity	38	43	39	43

Source: Centers for Disease Control and Prevention, "Surveillance for Sensory Impairment, Activity Limita-
tion, and Health-Related Quality of Life among Older Adults—United States, 1993–1997," *MMWR, CDC
Surveillance Summaries* 48, no. SS-8 (December 17, 1999): Table 5. Data from the Behavioral Risk Factor
Surveillance System.

DEFINITION: "Unhealthy days" are days when a respondent reports his or her
physical or mental health as "not good."

The average number of unhealthy days is highest among seniors aged 75+.
Younger seniors, aged 65 to 74, report about the same number of unhealthy days as
do the younger cohort aged 55 to 64 (see Chart 5.2).[5] Women report about one more
unhealthy day per month than men do. More unhealthy days are reported by seniors who are black or Hispanic; have less education or income; are divorced, widowed, or separated; have diabetes or breast cancer; are underweight or obese; are
current smokers; or do not participate in leisure-time physical activity.

Over a 12-month period, the elderly experience an average of 7.0 days where an
illness or injury keeps them in bed for more than half of the day.[6] This ranges from
6.5 days for those aged 65 to 74 and 8.0 days for those aged 75+ and is substantially
higher than the 3.7 days experienced by those aged 18 to 44 or the 5.7 days by those
aged 45 to 64. Elderly women experience more days (7.8 on average) in bed than do
elderly men (6.3 days on average).

CHART 5.2   Average Number of Unhealthy Days Reported during the Preceding 30 Days, by Age and Sex: 1993–1997

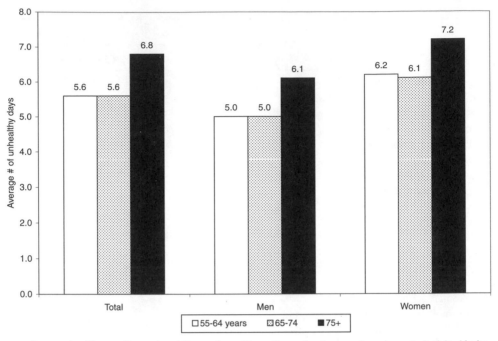

Sources: Centers for Disease Control and Prevention, "Surveillance for Sensory Impairment, Activity Limitation, and Health-Related Quality of Life among Older Adults—United States, 1993–1997," *MMWR, CDC Surveillance Summaries* 48, no. SS-8 (December 17, 1999): Table 7. 1993–1997 data from the Behavioral Risk Factor Surveillance System.

PHYSICAL ACTIVITY LIMITATION

■ Two-thirds of seniors have physical activity limitations

Sixty-five percent of noninstitutionalized elderly report at least some difficulty performing any one of nine tasks.[7] This ranges from 59 percent of people aged 65 to 74 and 74 percent of those aged 75+ (see Table 5.3). The elderly are substantially more likely to have activity limitations than are younger adults—23 percent of adults aged 18 to 44 and 42 percent of adults aged 45 to 64 are limited in some way.

The elderly are most limited in endurance activities such as lengthy standing or walking and least limited in small motor skill and less strenuous tasks (see Table 5.3). Physical activity limitations are most pronounced among the elderly aged 75+ as well as among elderly women.

To determine the level and type of activity limitation, important tasks of daily living are often classified into two categories, activities of daily living (ADLs) and instrumental activities of daily living (IADLs).

TABLE 5.3
Percentage of Elderly with Activity Limitations: 1997

	65–74 Years	75+ Years	Ratio of 75+ to 65–74 Years	Men, 65+ Years	Women, 65+ Years	Ratio of Women to Men
Any limitation in doing any one of the following nine tasks	59%	74%	1.25	60%	70%	1.17
Very difficult or impossible to:						
Stand or be on feet for 2 hours	18	32	1.73	20	27	1.34
Walk a quarter of a mile	16	31	1.90	19	25	1.35
Stoop, bend, or kneel	18	30	1.64	19	26	1.37
Push or pull large objects	16	28	1.71	14	27	1.90
Climb up 10 steps without resting	11	24	2.10	13	19	1.50
Lift or carry something as heavy as 10 pounds	11	20	1.85	8.9	19	2.17
Reach over one's head	5.2	9.9	1.90	5.8	8.3	1.43
Sit for 2 hours	4.7	6.4	1.36	4.1	6.4	1.56
Use fingers to grasp or handle small objects	3.9	5.8	1.49	3.9	5.3	1.36

Source: National Center for Health Statistics, "Summary Health Statistics for U.S. Adults: National Health Interview Survey, 1997," *Vital and Health Statistics,* series 10, no. 205 (Hyattsville, MD, May 2002): Table 19.

DEFINITION: *Activities of daily living (ADLs)* include bathing, dressing, eating, getting in or out of bed or chairs, walking, or using the toilet. *Instrumental activities of daily living (IADLs)* include making meals, shopping, managing money, doing light or heavy housework, or using the telephone.

The 1998 Medicare Current Beneficiary Survey indicated that 45 percent of elderly Medicare beneficiaries had some ADL/IADL limitation.[8] This ranged from 32 percent of those aged 65 to 74, to 79 percent of those aged 85+ (see Chart 5.3). The oldest beneficiaries were most often afflicted with three or more ADL limitations.

■ ADL limitations are most common in older age groups

ADL limitations are more pronounced in the oldest age groups, and women have more limitations than men do (see Table 5.4). Women aged 85+ display the greatest disability levels, with 70 percent exhibiting at least one ADL limitation.

■ Disability rates for the elderly are higher than for younger adults

According to the Census Bureau's 2000 Supplemental Survey, 41 percent of non-institutionalized elderly have a disability.[9] Disability rates increase with age: 14 percent of people aged 21 to 64 are disabled, compared with 34 percent of those aged 65 to 74 and 50 percent of those aged 75+. Disability rates are similar for men and

CHART 5.3   Percentage of Elderly Medicare Beneficiaries with Various Functional Limitations, by Age: 1998

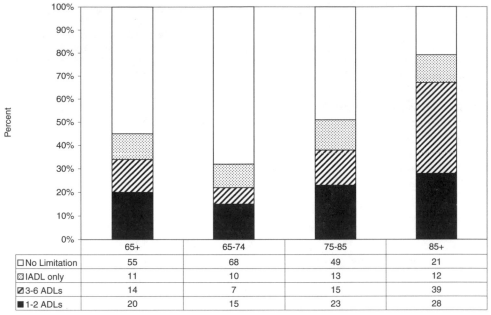

ADL/IADL Status	65+	65-74	75-85	85+
☐ No Limitation	55	68	49	21
☒ IADL only	11	10	13	12
◪ 3-6 ADLs	14	7	15	39
■ 1-2 ADLs	20	15	23	28

Source: Health Care Financing Administration, "The Characteristics and Perceptions of the Medicare Population (1998)," *Medicare Current Beneficiary Survey* (2001): Section 2. Available online at www.hcfa.gov/surveys/mcbs/PubCNP98.htm.

TABLE 5.4

Percentage of Elderly Medicare Beneficiaries with Various Functional Limitations, by Age and Sex: 1998

	IADL Limitation Only				ADL Limitation			
	Total	Men	Women	Ratio of Women to Men	Total	Men	Women	Ratio of Women to Men
65+ years	11%	9.1%	13%	1.41	34%	28%	38%	1.36
65–74	10	7.2	12	1.63	22	20	24	1.20
75–84	13	12	15	1.27	38	32	42	1.31
85+	12	12	12	0.98	67	60	70	1.17

Source: Health Care Financing Administration, "The Characteristics and Perceptions of the Medicare Population (1998)," *Medicare Current Beneficiary Survey* (2001): Section 2. Available online at www.hcfa.gov/surveys/mcbs/PubCNP98.htm.

What is "disability"?

In the 2000 Supplemental Survey, the Census Bureau defined disability based on the answers to these questions:

1. Does this person have any of the following long-lasting conditions: (a) blindness, deafness, or a severe vision or hearing impairment? or (b) a condition that substantially limits one or more basic physical activities such as walking, climbing stairs, reaching, lifting, or carrying?
2. Due to a physical, mental or emotional condition lasting six months or more, does this person have any difficulty in doing any of the following activities: (a) learning, remembering, or concentrating? (b) dressing, bathing, or getting around inside the home? (c) going outside the home alone to shop or visit a doctor's office? or (d) working at a job or business?

women, except at the oldest age group, in which women slightly edge out men (51 percent of women versus 47 percent of men aged 75+ are disabled).

Data from the Census Bureau's 1999 Survey of Income and Program Participation (SIPP) indicated somewhat higher disability rates than that found in their 2000 Supplemental Survey. According to the SIPP, 50 percent of noninstitutionalized elderly reported difficulty with one or more of six measures (see Table 5.5).[10]

TABLE 5.5
Percentage of Noninstitutionalized Elderly Reporting Disability: 1999

Any disability	50%	Difficulty with IADLs	20
Difficulty with specified functional activities	46	Getting around outside of the home	15
Walking three city blocks	31	Doing light housework	10
Climbing a flight of stairs	30	Preparing meals	7.7
Lifting or carrying 10 pounds	22	Taking care of money and bills	7.0
Hearing normal conversation	12	Using the telephone	4.9
Seeing words or letters in newsprint	11	Reporting selected impairments	8.2
Having speech understood	2.0	Alzheimer's disease, senility, or dementia	3.6
Difficulty with ADLs	13	Use of assistive aid	18
Getting in or out of the bed or chair	8.4	Cane, crutches, or walker	14
Bathing	8.1	Wheelchair	3.9
Getting around inside the home	6.1	Limitation in ability to work around the house	22
Dressing	5.4		
Toileting	3.5		
Eating	2.0		

Source: Centers for Disease Control, "Prevalence of Disabilities and Associated Health Conditions among Adults—United States, 1999," *MMWR Weekly,* 50, no. 7 (March 2, 2001): 121–125. Data from the Survey of Income and Program Participation.

■ The good news is that disability is declining

An analysis of the 1999 National Long-Term Care Survey by Duke University researchers indicated that 19.7 percent of the total elderly population was chronically disabled.[11] This represents a 25 percent reduction over 17 years (age-standardized rates were 26.2 percent in 1982). This translates into 7.0 million chronically disabled elderly in 1999—2.3 million fewer than if the 1982 rates had remained unchanged.

DEFINITION: A chronic disability is one that lasts for more than 90 days.

The Duke study also found that placement in nursing homes decreased from 6.2 percent to 3.4 percent of the elderly from 1982 to 1999. This decrease occurred despite a more than 30 percent increase in the elderly population over the same period. Researchers attribute the decline to lower rates of disability.

■ The bad news is that more than one-third of the elderly who need long-term care do not get help

Thirty-seven percent of elderly people living in the community who need long-term care (LTC) report that they do not receive it or receive less help than necessary.[12] Most of the unmet needs involve IADLs, such as meal preparation and outdoor mobility. Only 1.4 percent of the elderly report unmet ADL needs, and another 13.1 percent report undermet ADL needs.

DEFINITION: People living in the community are those who do not live in institutions such as nursing homes.

USE OF HEALTH CARE SERVICES

Inpatient Hospital Services

■ Seniors are disproportionate users of hospitals

Although seniors make up only 12 percent of the total U.S. population, they account for 39 percent of all hospital discharges and 48 percent of all days of care in nonfederal, short-stay hospitals.[13] In 2000, an estimated 12.4 million hospitalizations occurred among seniors—a 23 percent increase from 1970. In contrast, hospital stays shortened dramatically, with the average length of hospitalization among the elderly decreasing 31 percent, from 8.7 days in 1990 to 6.0 days in 2000.[14]

Hospital discharge rates increase dramatically with age, and gender differences narrow dramatically after age 44 (see Chart 5.4 and Table 5.6).[15] The youngest-old (aged 65 to 74) have a discharge rate nearly twice that of the next younger age bracket (aged 55 to 64). In turn, the oldest-old (85+) have a discharge rate that is more than twice that of the youngest-old.

CHART 5.4   Discharge Rates from Short-Stay, Nonfederal Hospitals: 1999

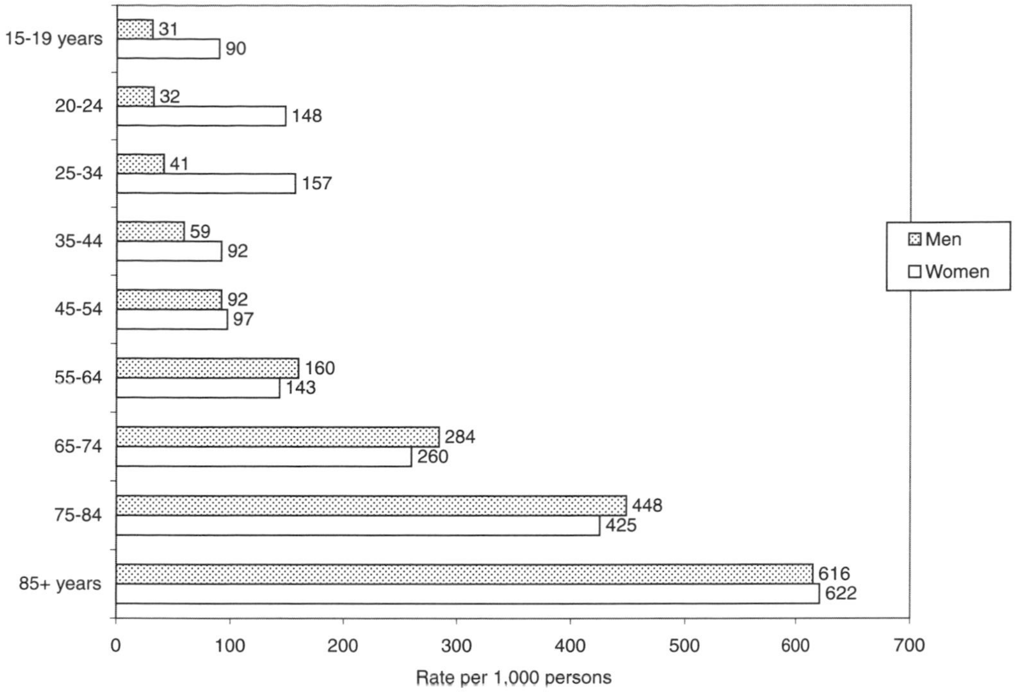

Source: Jennifer Popovic, "1999 National Hospital Discharge Survey: Annual Summary with Detailed Diagnosis and Procedure Data," *Vital and Health Statistics,* series 13, no. 151 (Hyattsville, MD: National Center for Health Statistics, 2001): Table 2.

TABLE 5.6
Detailed Data for Chart 5.4: Discharges Rates (per 1,000 Persons) from Short-Stay, Nonfederal Hospitals: 1999

	Total	Men	Women	Ratio of Women to Men
15–19 years	60	31	90	2.90
20–24	90	32	148	4.63
25–34	99	41	157	3.83
35–44	76	59	92	1.56
45–54	95	92	97	1.05
55–64	151	160	143	0.89
65+ years	370	368	372	1.01
65–74	271	284	260	0.92
75–84	434	448	425	0.95
85+	620	616	622	1.01

Source: Jennifer Popovic, "1999 National Hospital Discharge Survey: Annual Summary with Detailed Diagnosis and Procedure Data," *Vital and Health Statistics,* series 13, no. 151 (Hyattsville, MD: National Center for Health Statistics, 2001): Table 2.

TABLE 5.7

Number of Discharges and Average Length of Stay for Selected Major Causes of Hospitalization (First Listed Diagnosis) among Seniors: 2000

	Discharges		
	Number (000s)	Percent	Average Length of Stay (Days)
Total hospital discharges	12,396	100%	6.0
Heart disease	2,854	23	5.1
Pneumonia	763	6.2	6.5
Cancer	695	5.6	7.0
Cerebrovascular disease	711	5.7	5.4
Fractures	521	4.2	6.6
Osteoarthritis	303	2.4	4.7
Septicemia	216	1.7	7.8
Diabetes mellitus	192	1.5	5.9

Source: Margaret J. Hall and Maria F. Owings, "2000 National Hospital Discharge Survey," *Advance Data from Vital and Health Statistics*, no. 329 (Hyattsville, MD: National Center for Health Statistics, June 19, 2002): Tables 2 and 4.

■ Heart disease is the leading cause of hospitalization among the elderly

Heart disease accounts for 1 in 4 hospitalizations (as measured by hospital discharges) among the elderly (see Table 5.7).[16] Pneumonia, cancer, and strokes each account for about 6 percent of the hospitalizations. Seniors admitted with heart disease, cerebrovascular disease, or osteoarthritis have a lower than average length of hospitalization.

Among the elderly, the oldest-old are substantially more likely than their younger counterparts to be hospitalized due to heart disease, cerebrovascular disease, pneumonia, or fractures (see Chart 5.5).[17] Hospitalizations due to cancer or diabetes remain relatively stable across the age groups, whereas those for osteoarthritis actually are lowest among people aged 85+. Elderly men are more likely than women to be hospitalized due to heart disease, cancer, or pneumonia (see Table 5.8).[18] In contrast, senior women of all ages are more likely to be hospitalized due to fractures or osteoarthritis.

■ The elderly are five times more likely than younger people to die in the hospital

Among the elderly, 5.2 percent of discharges are due to death, compared with the 1 percent rate for those under age 65.[19] Elderly hospitalizations due to acute myocardial infarctions; lung, tracheal, or bronchus cancer; and septicemia are substantially

CHART 5.5   Discharge Rates for Selected Major Causes of Hospitalization, by Age: 1996

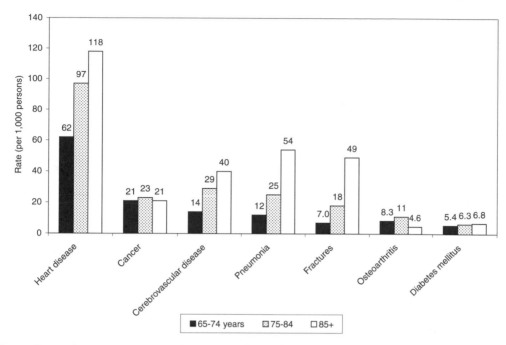

Source: Centers for Disease Control and Prevention, "Surveillance for Morbidity and Mortality among Older Adults—United States, 1995–1996." *MMWR, CDC Surveillance Summaries* 48, no. SS-8 (December 17, 1999): Table 2. Data from the National Hospital Discharge Survey.

TABLE 5.8
Elderly Discharge Rates (per 1,000 Persons) for Selected Major Causes of Hospitalization, by Sex: 1996

Cause of Hospitalization	Men	Women	Ratio of Men to Women	Ratio of Women to Men
Heart disease	90	74	1.22	0.82
Cancer	25	19	1.32	0.76
Cerebrovascular disease	23	21	1.10	0.91
Pneumonia	23	19	1.21	0.83
Fractures	7.8	21	0.37	2.69
Osteoarthritis	7.1	9.7	0.73	1.37
Diabetes mellitus	5.5	6.1	0.90	1.11

Source: Centers for Disease Control and Prevention, "Surveillance for Morbidity and Mortality among Older Adults—United States, 1995–1996," *MMWR, CDC Surveillance Summaries* 48, no. SS-8 (December 17, 1999): Table 2. Data from the National Hospital Discharge Survey.

TABLE 5.9
Elderly Death Rate (per 100 Discharges) from Short-Stay, Nonfederal
Hospitals: 1999

	Rate	Ratio to All Conditions
All conditions	5.2	1.00
Heart disease	5.3	1.02
Acute myocardial infarction	13	2.50
Congestive heart failure	6.0	1.15
All cancers	9.0	1.73
Cancer of the trachea, bronchus, or lung	16	3.08
Pneumonia	8.6	1.65
Cerebrovascular disease	7.6	1.46
Septicemia	20	3.85

Source: Jennifer Popovic, "1999 National Hospital Discharge Survey: Annual Summary with Detailed Diagnosis and Procedure Data," Vital and Health Statistics, series 13, no. 151 (Hyattsville, MD: National Center for Health Statistics, 2001): Table 23.

more likely to result in death than hospitalizations for other health problems (see Table 5.9).

Outpatient Hospital Services

■ The elderly account for 1 in 6 hospital visits

Compared with inpatient services, outpatient hospital services are less dramatically skewed toward the elderly. In 2000, the elderly accounted for 17 percent of all such visits, or an estimated 14.5 million outpatient visits—38 percent higher than in 1995.[20] The rate is not nearly as dramatic with age as it is for inpatient services (see Table 5.10). Women of all ages average more outpatient visits than men do, and blacks average more visits than whites.[21] Chronic problems are the major reason for an elderly person's outpatient visit. This occurs 53 percent of the time,[22] compared to 45 percent of the time for people aged 45 to 64 and 32 percent for people aged 25 to 44.

Emergency Department Hospital Services

■ The elderly account for 1 in 7 emergency room visits

During 2000, the elderly accounted for 15 percent of all hospital emergency department visits, or an estimated 16.2 million visits, 15 percent higher than in 1995.[23] One in five seniors report visiting the emergency room (ER) in a 12-month period (see Table 5.11).[24] Seniors aged 75+ are more likely to have had an ER visit

TABLE 5.10
Rate of Hospital Outpatient Department Visits (per 1,000 Persons) by Age, Sex, and Race: 2000

	Total	Men	Women	Ratio of Women to Men	White	Black	Ratio of Black to White
15–24 years	233	148	320	2.16	213	352	1.65
25–44	254	176	329	1.87	232	419	1.81
45–64	343	283	399	1.41	310	642	2.07
65–74	423	383	457	1.19	380	854	2.25
75+	467	424	494	1.17	437	853	1.95

Source: Nghi Ly and Linda F. McCaig, "National Hospital Ambulatory Medical Care Survey: 2000 Outpatient Department Summary," *Advance Data from Vital and Health Statistics*, no. 327 (Hyattsville, MD: National Center for Health Statistics, June 4, 2002): Table 1.

than their younger counterparts aged 65 to 74, but are just as likely as the youngest adults aged 18 to 24 to have visited an ER.

These older seniors are also the most intensive ER visitors, with 648 ER visits per 1,000 persons aged 75+ versus 369 visits per 1,000 seniors aged 65 to 74. Women aged 75+ have ER visit rates 15 percent higher than their male counterparts (685 per 1,000 versus 591 per 1,000).[25] Black seniors have substantially higher ER visit rates than their white counterparts do (see Table 5.12).

The elderly who visit ERs have a greater need for immediate care than younger people do. Twenty-eight percent of the elderly with an ER visit in 2000 needed to be

TABLE 5.11
Percent of Age Groups Visiting the Emergency Department within the Previous 12 Months: 1999

18–24 years	22%
25–44	17
45–54	14
55–64	15
65–74	17
75+	23

Source: National Center for Health Statistics, *Health, United States, 2001 with Urban and Rural Health Chartbook* (Hyattsville, MD, 2001), Table 79. Data from National Health Interview Survey.

TABLE 5.12
Rate (per 1,000 Persons) of Emergency Department Visits: 2000

	White	Black	Ratio of Black to White
65–74 years	349	587	1.68
75+	631	919	1.46

Source: Linda F. McCaig and Nghi Li, "National Hospital Ambulatory Medical Care Survey: 2000 Emergency Department Summary," *Advance Data from Vital and Health Statistics*, no. 326 (Hyattsville, MD: National Center for Health Statistics, April 22, 2002): Table 1.

seen within 15 minutes, compared with 19 percent of those aged 45 to 64 and 13 percent of those aged 15 to 44.[26] These statistics are partially reflected in the higher percentage of elderly who arrive via ambulance—23 percent of those aged 65 to 74 and 43 percent of those aged 75+ versus 16 percent of those aged 45 to 64 and 10 percent of those aged 15 to 44.[27]

PHYSICIAN AND OTHER PROFESSIONAL HEALTH CARE

■ Seniors see health care professionals more frequently than the general population does

In 1998, 93 percent of the elderly reported having any contact with a doctor or other health care professional within the prior 12 months; in contrast, 83 percent of the general population had contact with a physician.[28] These figures are substantially higher than comparable levels in 1964 (70 percent of seniors versus 67 percent of the general population).[29] Among the elderly who have seen a doctor or other health care professional in the prior year, 90 percent had contact within the previous 6 months.[30] This compares with 83 percent among people aged 45 to 64 and 76 percent among those aged 18 to 44.

Seniors had 200.3 million ambulatory care visits to physician offices in 2000, an increase of 19 percent since 1995.[31] On average, the elderly visit a physician's office about six times a year, compared with four or fewer times for younger Americans.

Except among those aged 75+, women of all ages average more physician office visits than men do, but the gap dramatically narrows among older people (see Table 5.13).[32] White people of all ages average more physician office visits than blacks do. Half of the time, the major reason for an office visit by a senior is related to a chronic problem; in contrast, this is true for 44 percent of the visits for adults aged 45 to 64 and 33 percent of the visits for those aged 25 to 44.[33]

TABLE 5.13
Rate of Physician Office Visits (per 1,000 Persons) by Age and Sex: 2000

	Total	Men	Women	Ratio of Women to Men	White	Black	Ratio of White to Black
15–24 years	1,744	1,179	2,317	1.97	1,897	1,110	1.71
25–44	2,400	1,644	3,128	1.90	2,542	1,655	1.54
45–64	3,579	3,011	4,115	1.37	3,639	3,071	1.18
65–74	5,771	5,387	6,089	1.13	5,681	5,118	1.11
75+	6,544	6,697	6,446	0.96	6,576	5,682	1.16

Source: Donald K. Cherry and David A. Woodwell, "National Ambulatory Medical Care Survey: 2000 Summary," *Advance Data from Vital and Health Statistics*, no. 328 (Hyattsville, MD: National Center for Health Statistics, June 5, 2000): Table 3.

■ Seniors usually visit physicians in their offices

Fifty-five percent of physician contacts among seniors aged 65 to 74 occurred in doctors' offices in 1996.[34] However, the figure declines to 44 percent among seniors aged 75+, who are more likely than their younger counterparts to have home-based contact (29 percent of contacts versus 10 percent). Overall, elderly home-based doctor contacts increased from 12 percent to 19 percent of all physician contacts between 1990 and 1996, which may reflect the increased use of home health care services by seniors.

Among those visiting some type of health care professional (excluding dentists or eye doctors) in the past year, 66 percent saw a general family practitioner.[35] Internists (20 percent) and cardiologists (18 percent) are the next most common types of health care professionals the elderly visited.

■ The elderly visit eye doctors more frequently than younger people do

Among all age groups, the elderly are the most likely to visit an eye doctor. According to Mediamark Research, one-third of the elderly report visiting an eye doctor in the previous 12 months, making them twice as likely as younger adults to have done so (see Chart 5.6 and detailed data in Table 5.14). People of all ages who wear prescription eyewear (eyeglasses and/or contact lenses) are substantially more likely than those who don't to see an eye doctor. According to Mediamark Research,

CHART 5.6   Percentage Who Visited Eye Doctor in Previous 12 Months, by Age and Corrective Eyewear Status: 2000

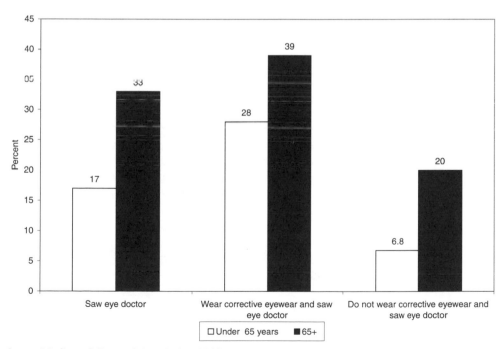

Source: Mediamark Research Inc. Spring 2000.

TABLE 5.14
Detailed Data for Chart 5.6: Percentage Who Visited
Eye Doctor in Previous 12 Months, by Age and
Corrective Eyewear Status: 2000

	Total	Those Wearing Corrective Eyewear	Those Not Wearing Corrective Eyewear
Under 65 years	17%	28%	6.8%
18–24	16	35	5.0
25–34	14	29	5.4
35–44	16	29	6.0
45–54	19	26	9.4
55–64	22	27	13
65+	33	39	20

Source: Mediamark Research Inc. Spring 2000.

71 percent of the elderly wear prescription lenses, and they are twice as likely as the elderly who do not wear prescription eyewear to have seen an eye doctor in the past year (39 percent versus 20 percent). Chapter 8 (Chronic Conditions and Common Health Problems) presents more information on vision impairment and corrective eyewear usage.

■ More than one-half of seniors have seen a dentist in the previous 12 months

Most elderly do not have dental insurance because it is typically an employee-provided benefit and Medicare does not usually cover dental care services. In fact, only 22 percent of the elderly were covered by private dental insurance in 1995.[36] Nonetheless, 55 percent of the elderly had at least one dental visit in the previous 12 months in 1999.[37] Among the elderly who still had their own teeth, 70 percent visited the dentist. Seniors' visits to the dentist are about the same as for other age groups. (In 1999, 65 percent of adults aged 18 to 64, as well as 73 percent of children aged 2 to 17, visited the dentist in the 12 months prior to the survey.) These figures for the elderly correspond closely with the 63 percent of older adults (aged 60+) who believe that a regular dental care routine is very important in helping to look one's best.[38]

Dental visits are more predominant among seniors who:[39]

- are white rather than black (57 percent versus 40 percent);
- are white non-Hispanic (57 percent) or Hispanic (44 percent), rather than black non-Hispanic (39 percent);
- are not poor rather than poor (64 percent versus 32 percent);

- live in urban rather than rural areas (58 percent of those who live within a Metropolitan Statistical Area versus 48 percent of those who do not); and
- live in the West (62 percent).

For 15 percent of the elderly, their last dental visit was more than a year ago but less than 3 years ago; 30 percent last saw a dentist more than 3 years ago.[40] Among seniors who had no dental visit in the past year, one-half stated it was because they had no teeth.[41] Whites gave that reason more often than blacks (51 percent versus 39 percent) and non-Hispanics more so than Hispanics (50 percent versus 32 percent). Thirty-one percent of all elderly mentioned that they had no dental problem. Only 4 percent of seniors who had no dental visits mentioned cost as a reason.

ATTITUDES ABOUT HEALTH CARE PROVIDERS

■ The elderly give doctors high approval ratings

According to RoperASW, older adults find doctors and pharmacists the most believable sources of information about health care problems and issues (see Table 5.15).[42] Doctors are a more frequent source of information than pharmacists are, probably due to the broader range of issues doctors can address. Friends and family, product packaging information, and advertising are less believable information sources and subsequently are used less often.

Greater believability translates into greater trust, with older adults expressing more trust in their doctor than in their health insurer. Two-thirds of older adults strongly agree that their doctor is someone they can trust, whereas only 37 percent

TABLE 5.15
Believability of Sources for Information about Health Care Problems or Issues and Frequency of Use among Adults Aged 60+: 1998

Source of Information	Very Believable	Consult Very Often
Doctor	57%	42%
Pharmacist	54	29
Nurse or nurse practitioner	39	19
Friends or family	21	12
Insurance or health care company	16	7
Books	14	10
Information on product packaging	12	11
Advertising	6	3
Alternative medicine providers	5	4

Source: RoperASW, 1998.

TABLE 5.16

Rating of Value for Various Services by Adults Aged 60+: 1997

Service	Excellent	Good	Excellent + Good
Doctors' services	13%	47%	60%
Hospital care	15	36	51
Health insurance	14	33	47

Source: RoperASW, 1997.

say they place trust in their health insurers. Some of this difference is due to older adults' beliefs that insurers are more motivated than doctors by cost containment.

Older adults' more positive views of doctors are also reflected in the greater value for the dollar they place on doctors' services relative to hospital care or health insurance (see Table 5.16).[43] Six in ten older adults feel that doctors' services are an excellent or good value, in contrast to less than one-half rating health insurance as an excellent or good value.

■ Seniors have better physician-related experiences than younger people do

According to a 1998 survey, seniors were less likely than younger age groups to think their doctors are too rushed to see them (20 percent of seniors versus 35 percent among those aged 18 to 29).[44] Additionally, only 8 percent of seniors felt that a doctor's office gatekeeper kept them from seeing the doctor, compared with 18 percent of all survey respondents. The same survey reported that only 3 percent of seniors were denied doctor-recommended treatment by their insurance provider versus 12 percent of all survey respondents.

Forecasts indicate the need for more doctors trained in geriatric medicine. In the United States, fewer than 9,000 geriatricians are in practice.[45] By 2030, with a projected population of about 65 million elderly Americans, more than 36,000 geriatricians will be needed.

USE OF PREVENTIVE HEALTH CARE SERVICES

Vaccinations

■ Two-thirds of seniors had a flu shot within the past year

In 1999, 90 percent of all U.S. deaths due to pneumonia or flu occurred among seniors, making these illnesses the fifth leading cause of death among seniors.[46] To reduce morbidity and mortality from these illnesses, annual vaccinations are recommended for seniors. During 1999, 67 percent of noninstitutionalized seniors reported receiving a flu shot during the previous 12 months—an increase of 1.5 percentage points in a 2-year period.[47]

Higher vaccination rates are noted for older seniors (aged 75+), those who are white or Hispanic, those with more education, those with more contact with the health care system, and those who have diabetes (see Table 5.17). Geographic differences are noticeable, with seniors in Washington, DC, substantially less likely to be inoculated than seniors in Rhode Island (56 percent versus 76 percent).

TABLE 5.17
Percentage of Noninstitutionalized Seniors Who Reported Receiving Influenza or Pneumococcal Vaccines: 1999

	Influenza Vaccine (Received in Previous Year)	Pneumococcal Vaccine (Ever Received)
Age		
65+ years	67%	54%
65–74	63	50
75+	73	61
Race/ethnicity		
Non-Hispanic white	69	57
Non-Hispanic black	48	36
Hispanic	59	35
Sex		
Men	68	54
Women	66	55
Education level		
Less than high school	61	47
High school	66	54
Beyond high school	71	59
Time since last checkup		
1–12 months	70	57
More than a year	48	36
Self-reported health status		
Poor	69	58
Fair	69	57
Good	67	55
Very good or excellent	66	51
Diabetes		
Yes	73	59
No	66	53

Source: Centers for Disease Control and Prevention, "Influenza and Pneumococcal Vaccination Levels among Adults Aged 65 Years," *Morbidity and Mortality Weekly Report* 50, no. 25 (June 29, 2001): 532–537. Data from the Behavioral Risk Factor Surveillance System.

■ More than one-half of seniors have been vaccinated against pneumonia

During 1999, 54 percent of noninstitutionalized seniors reported ever having received a pneumonia vaccination—an increase of 9 percentage points in a 2-year period.[48] Pneumococcal vaccination rates are higher among older seniors (aged 75+), whites, those who are more educated, those who have had more contact with the health care system and those who have diabetes (see Table 5.16). Significant geographic differences are also evident, with seniors in Washington, DC, once again having the lowest vaccination rates (35 percent). Delaware seniors are the most likely to be vaccinated against pneumonia (67 percent).

A 2002 study analyzing the 1998–1999 medical records of 107,311 elderly hospitalized patients found that doctors were not following recommended vaccination guidelines. Among the elderly patients who were unvaccinated prior to admission, 97 percent did not receive a flu vaccine and 99 percent did not receive a pneumonia vaccine before their discharge.[49]

■ Most nursing home residents have been vaccinated for flu in the last 12 months

Data from the 1999 National Nursing Home Survey indicated that among those residents with known vaccination status, 82 percent received a flu vaccination within the past 12 months.[50] This figure is unchanged from 1997.[51] In contrast, 64 percent had received a pneumonia vaccination at some time—a substantial increase from 51 percent in 1997.

CANCER SCREENING

■ Two-thirds of elderly women have had a recent mammogram

Sixty-four percent of elderly women reported in 1998 that they had had a mammogram in the past 2 years.[52] This is nearly three times the 23 percent level reported in 1987. However, elderly women are still less likely to have had a mammogram than the next youngest cohort (aged 50–64, of whom 74 percent had a mammogram). Mammogram use is less likely among senior women who:

- are below the poverty level (52 percent versus 66 percent among those at or above the poverty level);
- are less educated (55 percent among elderly women with less than a high school education versus 67 percent among those with a high school degree and 71 percent among those with at least some college); or
- are Hispanic (59 percent versus 61 percent for black non-Hispanics and 64 percent for white non-Hispanics).

■ Older men have higher rates of colon cancer screening than older women

Only 24 percent of senior women and 41 percent of men have had regular colon cancer screening.[53] Among men and women aged 60+, 22 percent report having had a fecal occult blood test during the previous year, and 34 percent had a sigmoidoscopy or proctoscopy during the preceding 5 years.[54] These rates are higher than those for adults aged 50 to 59 (16 percent and 24 percent, respectively).

■ Most elderly men have had a recent prostate exam

More than three-quarters (77 percent) of elderly male Medicare patients have had a prostate exam in the last 2 years, compared with 68 percent of privately insured men aged 50 to 64.[55] Only 10 percent of elderly male Medicare patients have never had a prostate exam.

■ Elderly women are less likely than younger women to have had a Pap smear

A 1998 study indicates that 42 percent of senior woman have had a Pap smear in the previous year compared with 65 percent of women aged 50 to 64.[56]

NOTES

1. Health Care Financing Administration, "The Characteristics and Perceptions of the Medicare Population (1998)," *Medicare Current Beneficiary Survey* (2001), Section 2. Available online at www.hcfa.gov/surveys/mcbs/PubCNP98.htm.
2. National Center for Health Statistics, *Health, United States, 2001, with Urban and Rural Health Chartbook* (Hyattsville, MD, 2001), Table 58. Data from the National Health Interview Survey.
3. Centers for Disease Control and Prevention, "Surveillance for Sensory Impairment, Activity Limitation, and Health-Related Quality of Life among Older Adults—United States, 1993–1997," *MMWR, CDC Surveillance Summaries* 48, no. SS-8 (December 17, 1999): Table 5. Data from the Behavioral Risk Factor Surveillance System.
4. Ibid.
5. Ibid., Table 7.
6. National Center for Health Statistics, "Summary Health Statistics for U.S. Adults: National Health Interview Survey, 1997," *Vital and Health Statistics,* series 10, no. 205 (Hyattsville, MD, May 2002): Table 17.
7. Ibid., Tables 18 and 19.
8. Health Care Financing Administration, "Characteristics and Perceptions."
9. Bureau of the Census, *Census 2000 Supplementary Survey Summary Tables*, Table P059. Available online at http://factfinder.census.gov.
10. Centers for Disease Control, "Prevalence of Disabilities and Associated Health Conditions among Adults—United States, 1999," *MMWR Weekly* 50, no. 7 (March 2, 2001): 120–125. Data from the Survey of Income and Program Participation.
11. Kenneth G. Manton and XiLiang Gu, "Changes in the Prevalence of Chronic Disability in the United States Black and Nonblack Population above Age 65 from 1982 to 1999," *Proceedings of the National Academy of Sciences* 98, no. 11 (May 22, 2001): 6354–6359.

12. B. Jackson and P. Doty, *Unmet and Undermet Need for Functional Assistance among the U.S. Disabled Elderly.* Paper presented at the 1997 annual meeting of the Gerontological Society of America, Cincinnati. Reported in *Long-Term Care for the Elderly with Disabilities: Current Policy, Emerging Trends, and Implications for the Twenty-First Century* by Robyn I. Stone, Milbank Memorial Fund (2000).

13. Margaret J. Hall and Maria F. Owings, "2000 National Hospital Discharge Survey," *Advance Data from Vital and Health Statistics*, no. 329 (Hyattsville, MD: National Center for Health Statistics, June 19, 2002).

14. Jennifer Popovic, "1999 National Hospital Discharge Survey: Annual Summary with Detailed Diagnosis and Procedure Data," *Vital and Health Statistics*, series 13, no. 151 (Hyattsville, MD: National Center for Health Statistics, 2001): Table 1.

15. Ibid., Table 2.

16. Ibid., Table 9.

17. Centers for Disease Control and Prevention, "Surveillance for Morbidity and Mortality among Older Adults—United States, 1995–1996," *MMWR, CDC Surveillance Summaries* 48, no. SS-8 (December 17, 1999): Table 2. Data from the National Hospital Discharge Survey.

18. Ibid.

19. Popovic, "1999 National Hospital Discharge Survey: Annual Summary," Table 23.

20. Nghi Ly and Linda McCaig, "National Hospital Ambulatory Medical Care Survey: 2000 Outpatient Department Summary," *Advance Data from Vital and Health Statistics*, no. 327 (Hyattsville, MD: National Center for Health Statistics, June 24, 2002): Table 1; National Center for Health Statistics, *Health, United States, 2001*, Table 83.

21. Ibid.

22. Ibid., Table 8.

23. Linda F. McCaig and Nghi Ly, "National Hospital Ambulatory Medical Care Survey: 2000 Emergency Department Summary," *Advance Data from Vital and Health Statistics*, no. 326 (Hyattsville, MD: National Center for Health Statistics, April 22, 2002): Table 1; National Center for Health Statistics, *Health, United States, 2001*, Table 83.

24. National Center for Health Statistics, *Health, United States, 2001*, Table 79. Data from the National Health Interview Survey.

25. McCaig and Ly, "National Hospital Ambulatory Medical Care Survey: 2000," Table 1.

26. Ibid., Table 4.

27. Ibid., Table 2.

28. National Center for Health Statistics. *Health, United States, 2000 with Adolescent Chartbook* (Hyattsville, MD, 2000), Table 72. Data from the National Health Interview Survey.

29. National Center for Health Statistics, *Health, United States, 1999*, Table 78. Data from the National Health Interview Survey.

30. National Center for Health Statistics, "Summary Health Statistics, 1997," Table 36.

31. National Center for Health Statistics, *Health, United States, 2001*, Table 83.

32. Donald K. Cherry and David A. Woodwell, "National Ambulatory Medical Care Survey: 2000 Summary," *Advance Data from Vital and Health Statistics*, no. 328 (Hyattsville, MD: National Center for Health Statistics, June 5, 2002), Table 3. National Center for Health Statistics, *Health, United States, 2001*, Table 83. Data from the National Ambulatory Medical Care Survey.

33. Cherry, Burt, and Woodwell, "National Ambulatory Medical Care Survey: 1999 Summary," Table 9.

34. National Center for Health Statistics, *Health, United States, 1999*, Table 76. Data from the National Health Interview Survey.

35. Mediamark Research Inc. Spring 2000.

36. Clemencia M. Vargas, Ellen A. Kramarow, and Janet A. Yellowitz, "The Oral Health of Older Americans," *Aging Trends*, no. 3. (Hyattsville, MD: National Center for Health Statistics, March 2001).
37. National Center for Health Statistics, *Health, United States, 2001*, Table 80. Data from the National Health Interview Survey.
38. RoperASW, 1999.
39. National Center for Health Statistics, *Health, United States, 2001*, Table 80. Data from the National Health Interview Survey.
40. National Center for Health Statistics, "Summary Health Statistics, 1997," Table 38.
41. U.S. Department of Health and Human Services, National Institute of Dental and Craniofacial Research, *Oral Health in America: A Report of the Surgeon General* (Rockville, MD: National Institutes of Health, 2000), Table 4.6. 1989 data.
42. RoperASW, 1998.
43. RoperASW, 1997.
44. Kemba Dunham, "Concern for Health Cuts across Social Boundaries," *The Wall Street Journal*, June 25, 1998, page A10.
45. Christine K. Cassel, Richard W. Besdine, and Lydia C. Siegel, "Restructuring Medicare for the Next Century: What Will Beneficiaries Really Need?" *Health Affairs* 18, no. 1 (January/February 1999): 118–131.
46. Donna L. Hoyert and Sherry L. Murphy, "Deaths: Final Data for 1999," *National Vital Statistics Reports* 49, no. 8 (Hyattsville, MD: National Health Statistics, September 21, 2001): Table 9.
47. Centers for Disease Control and Prevention, "Influenza and Pneumococcal Vaccination Levels among Adults Aged 65 Years," *Morbidity and Mortality Weekly Report* 50, no. 25 (June 29, 2001): 532–537. Data from the Behavioral Risk Factor Surveillance System.
48. Ibid.
49. Dale W. Bratzler et al., "Failure to Vaccinate Medicare Inpatients: A Missed Opportunity," *Archives of Internal Medicine* 162, no. 20 (2002): 2349–2356.
50. National Center for Health Statistics, *1999 National Nursing Home Survey*, CD-ROM series 13, no. 28 (Hyattsville, MD, November 2001).
51. National Center for Health Statistics, *1997 National Nursing Home Survey*, CD-ROM series 13, no. 23 (Hyattsville, MD, May 2000).
52. National Center for Health Statistics, *Health, United States, 2000*, Table 82.
53. Karen Davis, "Health and Aging in the 21st Century," *The Commonwealth Fund: 1999 Annual Report, President's Message.* Available online at www.cmf.org/annrcprt/1999/president99.asp.
54. "Screening for Colorectal Cancer—United States, 1997," *MMWR Weekly* 48, no. 6 (February 19, 1999): 116–121. Data from the Behavioral Risk Factor Surveillance System.
55. Center on an Aging Society, "Screening for Chronic Conditions: Underused Services," *Challenges for the 21st Century: Chronic and Disabling Conditions*, no. 1 (January 2002). Available online at www.aging-society.org.
56. Davis, "Health and Aging."

CHAPTER 6

Health Risks and Practices

Habit with him was all the test of truth, "It must be right: I've done it from my youth."

—George Crabbe

It seems, in fact, as though the second half of a man's life is made up of nothing but the habits he has accumulated during the first half.

—Fyodor Dostoevski

Ill habits gather unseen degrees, as brooks make rivers, rivers run to seas.

—John Dryden

This chapter covers information on alcohol and substance use among the elderly. It also covers the elderly's health practices, answering questions that ask, for example, how frequently the average older person exercises (they are less sedentary than in the past) and whether they spend enough time in social activities to benefit their health (they maintain relatively high levels of social activity.)

Highlights of this chapter include:

- Alcohol is the most commonly abused substance among seniors.

- Although seniors are less likely than younger age groups to smoke, they can be just as addicted to tobacco.

- More than half of the elderly weigh more than is deemed healthy, with elderly black women the most likely to be overweight or obese.

- Forty-one percent of seniors are controlling their diets in some manner, although few make efforts to actually reduce their weight.

- Fitness, not fatness, appears more important to longevity.

- At age 75+, physical inactivity becomes the norm. Most seniors exercise, although not for long enough periods, and some still exercise vigorously.

- Social interaction wanes with age.
- One in ten elderly has been tested for HIV infection.

HEALTH RISKS

Alcohol Use and Abuse

■ Seniors are the least likely age group to consume alcohol

The elderly are the least likely age cohort to drink alcohol; in 2000, 42 percent of seniors reported that they were current drinkers (see Chart 6.1 and detailed data in Table 6.1).[1] At all ages, drinking is more prevalent among men than women, but the differential is greatest among those aged 75+ (see Table 6.1). Among the elderly, 50 percent of men drink alcohol versus 36 percent of women.

■ White, non-Hispanic males are the most likely seniors to drink alcohol

In the elderly population, white, non-Hispanic men are the most likely to consume alcohol, with more than one-half reporting in 1999 that they were current drinkers (see Table 6.2). Black, non-Hispanic men and women are the least likely of

CHART 6.1   Percent of Adults Who Are Current Drinkers, by Age: 2000

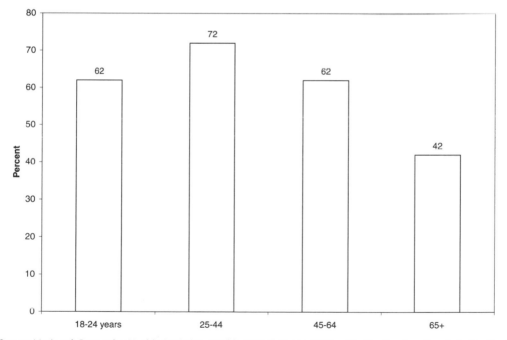

Source: National Center for Health Statistics, *Health, United States, 2002 with Chartbook on Trends in the Health of Americans* (Hyattsville, MD, 2002), Table 67. Data from the National Health Interview Survey.

TABLE 6.1
Detailed Data for Chart 6.1: Percent of Adults Who Are Current Drinkers, by Age and Sex: 2000

	Men	Women	Ratio of Men to Women
18–24 years	64%	55%	1.17
25–44	76	64	1.19
45–54	70	60	1.17
55–64	65	51	1.28
65–74	53	42	1.25
75+	47	30	1.57
65+	50	36	1.38

Source: National Center for Health Statistics, *Health, United States, 2002 with Chartbook on Trends in the Health of Americans* (Hyattsville, MD, 2002), Table 67. Data from the National Health Interview Survey.

their genders to drink. However, the gender differential is greatest among this group with black, non-Hispanic men more than twice as likely to drink as their female counterparts.

Other than the youngest adults, the elderly are the most likely cohort to be lifetime abstainers of alcohol (see Table 6.3).[2] Nearly one-half of women aged 75 and older are lifetime abstainers. Women of all ages are more likely than men to be lifetime abstainers.

DEFINITION: Lifetime abstainer means fewer than 12 drinks are consumed in a lifetime; former drinker means 12 or more drinks consumed in a lifetime but none in past year; current drinker means 12 or more drinks consumed in a lifetime and 1 or more drinks in past year.

TABLE 6.2
Percent of Elderly Who Are Current Drinkers, by Sex, Race, and Hispanic Origin: 1999

	Total	Men	Women	Ratio of Men to Women
White, non-Hispanic	44%	55%	37%	1.49
Hispanic	37	49	29	1.69
Black, non-Hispanic	22	33	15	2.20

Source: National Center for Health Statistics, *Health, United States, 2001 with Urban and Rural Health Chartbook* (Hyattsville, MD, 2001), Table 66. Data from the National Health Interview Survey.

TABLE 6.3

Percent Distribution of Current Alcohol Drinking Status, by Age and Sex: 1997–1998

	Total			Men			Women		
	Lifetime Abstainer	Former Drinker	Current Drinker	Lifetime Abstainer	Former Drinker	Current Drinker	Lifetime Abstainer	Former Drinker	Current Drinker
18–24 years	32%	6%	61%	28%	5%	67%	37%	7%	56%
25–44	16	12	71	12	12	77	21	13	66
45–64	19	19	62	11	20	70	26	18	56
65–74	27	25	48	15	29	57	36	23	41
75+	36	29	36	20	35	45	45	25	30

Source: Charlotte A. Schoenborn and Patricia Adams, "Alcohol Use among Adults: United States, 1997–98," *Advance Data from Vital and Health Statistics*, no. 324 (Hyattsville, MD: National Center for Health Statistics, September 14, 2001): Table 1.

■ Hard liquor, beer, and wine are equally preferred among older adults

About one-half of people aged 60+ drank hard liquor, beer, and/or wine during 1999.[3] Older adults who drink are less likely than their younger counterparts (aged 18 to 59) to consume beer (50 percent versus 71 percent) or hard liquor (48 percent versus 59 percent), but about equally as likely to drink wine (48 percent versus 44 percent).

■ Seniors spend less than younger adults on alcohol

Because the elderly are less likely to drink alcohol, it follows that their total alcoholic beverage expenditures are less than those of younger adults (see Chart 6.2 and detailed data in Table 6.4).[4] Elderly households, on average, spend one-half the amount that younger households spend on alcoholic beverages ($173 versus $355 annually).

Even though the elderly are the least likely group to drink alcohol, senior households increased their spending on alcoholic beverages between 1990 and 1999. In contrast, younger households decreased their spending during that time period. Specifically, between 1990 and 1999, average annual household spending (inflation-adjusted) on alcoholic beverages increased 6.8 percent among elderly households but decreased 17 percent among households under age 65.[5]

■ Alcohol is the most commonly abused substance among seniors

Alcohol is the most commonly abused substance among older adults.[6] Studies have found that alcoholism affects 2 to 15 percent of noninstitutionalized older adults, but increases to 18 to 44 percent among those who have been admitted to medical or psychiatric inpatient facilities.[7]

CHART 6.2   Average Annual Household Spending on Alcoholic Beverages (at Home and away from Home), by Age of Householder: 1999

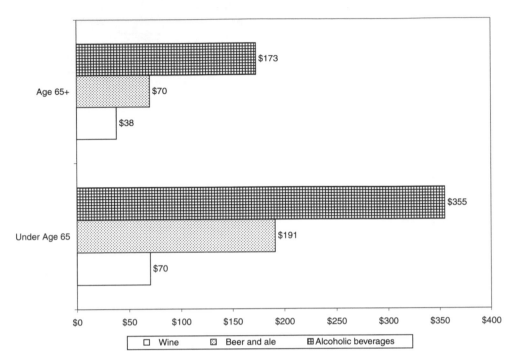

Sources: Sharon Yntema, ed., *Americans 55 and Older: A Changing Market*, 3rd ed. (Ithaca, NY: New Strategist Publications, 2001), 387, 416. 1999 Consumer Expenditure Survey data. Additional calculations made by authors.

Among current drinkers, seniors are substantially less likely than younger adults to be heavy drinkers (see Table 6.5). Men of all ages are more likely than women to be heavy drinkers. However, the gender differential is greatest among the elderly, with elderly men more than four times as likely as elderly women to be heavy drinkers.

TABLE 6.4
Detailed Data for Chart 6.2: Average Annual Household Spending (in dollars) on Alcoholic Beverages (at Home and away from Home), by Age of Householder: 1999

	Under 65 Years	65+ Years	65–74 Years	75+ Years
Alcoholic beverages	$355	$173	$219	$122
Beer and ale	191	70	94	44
Wine	70	38	45	30

Sources: Sharon Yntema, ed., *Americans 55 and Older: A Changing Market*, 3rd ed. (Ithaca, NY: New Strategist Publications, 2001), 387, 416. 1999 Consumer Expenditure Survey data. Additional calculations made by authors.

TABLE 6.5

Percent of Current Drinkers Who Drink Heavily (at least Five Drinks on at Least 1 Day in the Past Year), by Age and Sex: 2000

	Total	Men	Women	Ratio of Men to Women
18–24 years	52%	61%	42%	1.43
25–44	37	50	23	2.18
45–54	26	38	12	3.16
55–64	20	30	8.7	3.44
65+	9.1	15	3.4	4.35

Source: National Center for Health Statistics, *Health, United States, 2002 with Chartbook on Trends in the Health of Americans* (Hyattsville, MD, 2002), Table 67. Data from the National Health Interview Survey.

DEFINITION: Heavy drinkers are defined as those who had five or more drinks in 1 day in the past year.

■ About 1 in 25 elderly men excessively consumes alcohol

Self-reported data from the 2000 National Health Interview Survey indicated that 1.8 percent of the elderly consumed five or more drinks on one occasion at least 12 times during the past 12 months, with 3.7 percent of elderly men exhibiting such excessive consumption (see Table 6.6).[8] Men of all ages are substantially more likely

TABLE 6.6

Percent of Adults Excessively Consuming Alcohol, by Age and Sex: 2000

	Total	Men	Women	Ratio of Men to Women
18–24 years	16%	23%	8.4%	2.74
25–44	11	18	4.2	4.29
45–64	6.4	11	1.8	6.11
65+	1.8	3.7	0.4	9.25

Source: National Center for Health Statistics, *Early Release of Selected Estimates from the 2000 and Early 2001 National Health Interview Surveys* (Hyattsville, MD, September 20, 2001), Figure 9.2. Available online at www.cdc.gov/nchs/nhis.

than women to overimbibe, especially among the elderly. Excessive alcohol consumption is substantially less prevalent among the elderly than younger adults.

DEFINITION: Excessive consumption of alcohol is defined as consuming five or more drinks on one occasion at least 12 times during the past 12 months.

A strong relationship exists between a substance abuse disorder earlier in life and recurrences later in life.[9] The majority of older adults who receive alcohol abuse treatment are early-onset drinkers, defined as those who started drinking in their twenties or thirties. Older adults who are early-onset drinkers are more like younger abusers in that they use alcohol to cope with a wide range of psychosocial or medical problems.

About 1 in 3 older adults with drinking problems is thought to be a late-onset drinker (experiencing first alcohol-related problems after age 40 or 50). Women experience more late-onset alcoholism than men do.[10]

Late-onset drinkers are generally both physically and mentally healthier than their early-onset counterparts. Their late-onset drinking is more in response to a sudden change in their lives (death of a spouse, divorce, or a change in health or lifestyle status).[11] In fact, older white men who experience depression and begin drinking heavily after the death of a spouse have the highest suicide rates.

Chronic illnesses make seniors more sensitive to alcohol, as do age-related changes such as decreased body water and decreased alcohol metabolism. Alcohol-related hospital admission rates among older people are about equal to those for heart attacks.

■ Driving under the influence of alcohol is rare among seniors

Only 0.4 percent of seniors aged 65 to 74, and 0.2 percent of those aged 75+, report drinking and driving during the past 30 days.[12]

Other Substance Abuse

■ Nicotine and psychoactive drugs are other commonly abused substances

Aside from alcohol, older adults are most likely to abuse nicotine and psychoactive prescription medications.[13] Older adults who also abuse alcohol are more likely to abuse these substances.

The combination of psychoactive drugs and alcohol can be dangerous. Seniors account for more than one-half of all reported adverse drug reactions that lead to hospitalization.[14] A recent study found that the combination of alcohol and over-the-counter pain medications was the most common source of adverse drug reactions among older patients.[15]

Females are more at risk for abusing prescription medications because older women are more likely than men to visit physicians and receive prescriptions for psychoactive drugs.[16]

According to the Substance Abuse and Mental Health Services Administration, in 2000, the lifetime prevalence of illicit drug use was 6.4 percent among seniors, the lowest of any age group monitored.[17] This compares with 14 percent among those aged 60 to 64 and 29 percent among those aged 55 to 59. Past year usage was 0.7 percent among seniors, 1.8 percent among those aged 60 to 64, and 4.2 percent among those aged 55 to 59.

DEFINITION: Illicit drugs include marijuana/hashish, cocaine, crack cocaine, heroin, hallucinogens, inhalants or any prescription-type psychotherapeutic used nonmedically.

■ Seniors are less likely than younger age groups to smoke

Among all age groups, smoking is least prevalent among seniors; in 2000, 9.7 percent of seniors reported smoking versus 24 percent of those aged 45 to 64 and 27 percent of those aged 18 to 44.[18] Detailed age, sex, and race data for 2000 showed that elderly men are as likely to smoke as elderly women (see Chart 6.3 and detailed data in Table 6.7).[19] However, racial differences exist among the elderly, with blacks more likely than whites to smoke, and black men somewhat more likely than black women to smoke.

CHART 6.3   Percent of Adults Who Currently Smoke, by Age and Sex: 2000

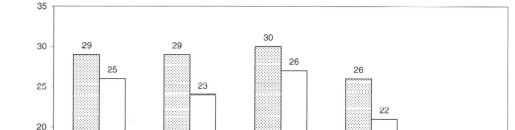

Source: National Center for Health Statistics, *Health, United States, 2002 with Chartbook on Trends in the Health of Americans* (Hyattsville, MD, 2001), Table 61. Data from the National Health Interview Survey.

TABLE 6.7

Detailed Data for Chart 6.3: Percent of Adults Who Currently
Smoke, by Age, Sex, and Race: 2000

	Men	Women	Ratio of Men to Women
Age			
18–24 years	29%	25%	1.14
25–34	29	23	1.29
35–44	30	26	1.15
45–64	26	22	1.22
65+	9.8	9.3	1.10
Race			
White, 65+ years	9.8	9.1	1.08
Black, 65+	14	10	1.39

Source: National Center for Health Statistics, *Health, United States, 2002
with Chartbook on Trends in the Health of Americans* (Hyattsville, MD,
2002), Table 61. Data from the National Health Interview Survey.

■ Desire and ability to quit smoking is lowest among the elderly

According to the 2000 National Health Interview Survey, nearly 6 in 10 elderly
smokers (57 percent) wanted to quit smoking compared with 68 percent of those
smokers aged 45 to 64 and 72 percent of those aged 18 to 44.[20] Elderly smokers were
less successful than younger adults at quitting smoking for 1 day; 32 percent of elderly smokers succeeded compared with 39 percent of those smokers aged 45 to 64,
42 percent of those aged 25 to 44 and 53 percent of those aged 18 to 24. According
to RoperASW, 2 percent of older adults (aged 60+) gave up smoking in 1999.[21]

■ Elderly smokers appear to be as addicted as younger smokers to tobacco

Mediamark Research data indicate that elderly smokers are about as dependent
upon tobacco as are younger smokers. Elderly smokers smoke an average of 9 packs
of cigarettes in a 7-day period versus 10 packs for younger smokers.[22]

Three percent of elderly men smoke cigars in a 6-month period, a considerably
lower proportion than the 10 percent of younger male adults who smoke cigars.
However, elderly male cigar smokers are much heavier users, having smoked an average of 12 cigars in a 7-day period compared with 8 cigars in a 7-day period for
younger male smokers.

■ Elderly households spend less than younger households on tobacco

Elderly households spend substantially less than younger households for tobacco
and smoking supplies, paralleling the overall smoking rate differences between these
two age groups. According to the 1999 Consumer Expenditure Survey, average an-

CHART 6.4   Average Annual Household Spending on Tobacco-Related Products, by Age of Householder: 1999

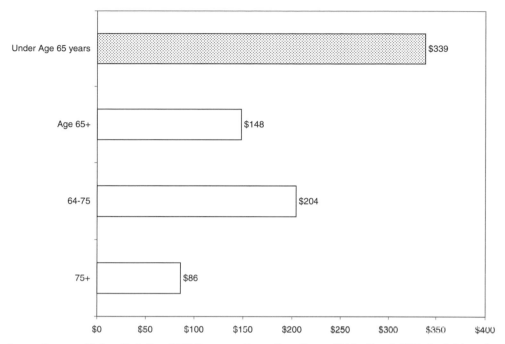

Source: Bureau of Labor Statistics, *1999 Consumer Expenditure Survey*, Tables 3 and 4500. Available online at www.bls.gov.

nual spending for tobacco-related products in households headed by the elderly is less than one-half that of households headed by those under age 65 ($148 versus $339; see Chart 6.4).[23] Households headed by persons aged 75+ spend less than one-half as much on tobacco-related products as do those headed by persons aged 65 to 74.[24]

Declines in smoking are also evident in reduced spending on tobacco and smoking supplies. Between 1990 and 1999, average annual per household, inflation-adjusted spending for tobacco-related products declined 26 percent among elderly households and 13 percent among younger households.[25]

Attitudes about Substance Use and Abuse

Similar to younger generations, the majority of older adults (aged 60+) view drug addiction, drunk driving, and alcoholism as major problems in today's society; in fact, more than three-quarters of all adults feel this way (see Table 6.9).[26] Social drinking and abuse of over-the-counter drugs are perceived to be less of a problem.

Generational differences are evident in the acceptance of marijuana and tranquilizer use and social drinking, with older adults substantially more likely than younger adults to view these as major problems in today's society.

One in ten elderly has been tested for HIV infection

According to self-reported data from the 2000 National Health Interview Survey, 9 percent of the elderly have ever been tested for human immunodeficiency virus (HIV) (12 percent of elderly men and 6.5 percent of elderly women; see Table 6.8). Not surprisingly, these are the lowest levels for any age group. Elderly women, along with their younger cohort aged 45 to 64, are less likely than similarly aged men to have been tested. This is in contrast to younger cohorts in which women outpace men in HIV testing.

Source: National Center for Health Statistics, *Early Release*, Figure 10.2.

TABLE 6.8
Percent of Adults Who Have Ever Been Tested for HIV, by Age and Sex: 2000

	Total	Men	Women	Ratio of Men to Women	Ratio of Women to Men
18–24 years	34%	25%	44%	0.57	1.76
25–34	51	43	59	0.73	1.37
35–44	42	41	44	0.93	1.07
45–64	25	27	22	1.23	0.81
65+	8.9	12	6.5	1.85	0.54

Source: National Center for Health Statistics, *Early Release of Selected Estimates from the 2000 and Early 2001 National Health Interview Surveys* (Hyattsville, MD, September 20, 2001), Figure 10.2. Available online at www.cdc.gov/nchs/nhis.

TABLE 6.9
Percent Saying a Particular Situation Is a Major Problem in Today's Society: 1999

Social Problem	Younger Adults (18–59 Years)	Older Adults (60+ Years)	Ratio of Older to Younger Adults
Drug addiction	86%	90%	1.05
Drunk driving	86	85	0.99
Alcoholism	77	80	1.04
Marijuana	56	68	1.21
Cigarette smoking	59	64	1.08
Tranquilizers/pep pills	47	57	1.21
Abuse of over-the-counter drugs	45	50	1.11
Social drinking	30	42	1.40

Source: RoperASW, 1999.

■ One in three older adults believes alcohol consumption is harmful

One-third (35 percent) of older adults feel that alcohol in any amount is harmful to one's health, and 60 percent feel it is harmful only in excess.[27] Only 27 percent of younger adults feel that alcohol in any amount is harmful.

■ Adults use alcohol because they enjoy the taste

As with younger adults aged 18 to 59, older adults who drink do so mostly because they enjoy the taste (see Table 6.10). Celebrating is the second most commonly stated reason, and health reasons are among the least commonly stated reasons. Older adults' reasons for drinking are weaker than those stated by younger adults, except for health-related reasons.

■ Most elderly believe smoking in any amount is harmful

Three-quarters (76 percent) of older adults believe that smoking in any amount is harmful, while 22 percent feel it is harmful only in excess. Being around people who smoke, though, is perceived to be less harmful, with 48 percent feeling the behavior is harmful in any amount.[28]

Body Weight

■ Most seniors weigh more than is recommended

More than 6 in 10 elderly men and women weigh more than what is considered healthy (see Chart 6.5). Between 22 and 37 percent of elderly men and women are of healthy weight, and 3 percent or less are underweight.

TABLE 6.10
Percent Stating Major Reason for Drinking an Alcoholic Beverage (among Those Who Ever Drink): 2000

Reason for Drinking	Younger Adults (18–59 Years)	Older Adults (60+ Years)	Ratio of Older to Younger Adults
Enjoy the taste	57%	50%	0.88
To celebrate	44	32	0.73
Helps to relax or relieve stress	34	23	0.68
Goes well with meals	26	22	0.85
It's something I do with friends	27	17	0.63
It's good for my health	9	11	1.22
It's part of a routine	9	10	1.11
I like the way it makes me feel	18	8	0.44

Source: RoperASW, 2000.

Important note to readers:

For the statistical purposes of this book, the authors have defined the various weight classifications into four mutually exclusive categories according to body-mass index (BMI), defined as weight in kilograms divided by the square of height in meters:

Underweight (BMI less than 18.5 kg/m2)
Healthy weight (BMI of 18.5 to <25)
Overweight (BMI of 25 to <30)
Obese (BMI of 30 or higher)

Please note that the National Center for Health Statistics defines overweight as a BMI of 25 or more, such that the data include those who are obese. In those instances, the authors have recalculated the data into these four mutually exclusive categories. Additionally, unless otherwise specified, weight data are based on physical exam rather than self-reports.

Want to calculate your BMI? Multiply your weight in pounds by 703, then divide the result by your height in inches. Divide that result by your height in inches a second time to arrive at your BMI. Or, use the calculator at www.nhlbisupport.com/bmi/bmi-calc.htm.

Source: National Center for Health Statistics, *Health, United States, 2001*, Table 69. Data from the National Health and Nutrition Examination Survey.

CHART 6.5   Weight Distribution among the Elderly, by Age and Sex: 1999–2000

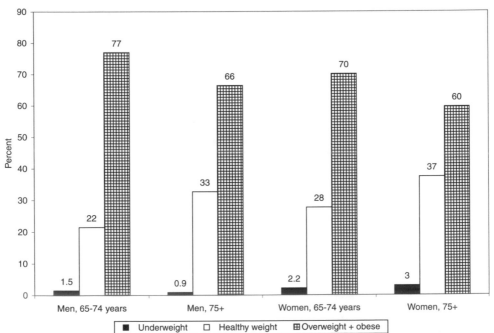

Source: National Center for Health Statistics, *Health, United States, 2002 with Chartbook on Trends in the Health of Americans* (Hyattsville, MD, 2002), Table 70. Data from the National Health and Nutrition Examination Survey. Additional calculations made by authors.

TABLE 6.11
Percent Overweight or Obese (Self-Reported), by Age, Race, and Sex: 1996–1997

	Men			Women		
	White	Black	Ratio of Black to White Men	White	Black	Ratio of Black to White Women
65–74 years	65%	66%	1.02	53%	74%	1.40
75+	51	56	1.10	43	58	1.35

Sources: Centers for Disease Control and Prevention, "Surveillance for Five Health Risks among Older Adults— United States, 1993–1997," *MMWR, CDC Surveillance Summaries* 48, no. SS-8 (December 17, 1999): Table 4. Data from the Behavioral Risk Factor Surveillance System.

■ Elderly black women are most likely to be overweight or obese

Being overweight or obese is equally likely among elderly black men as elderly white men (see Table 6.11). However, black women, are about 40 percent more likely than white women to be overweight or obese, and are even more likely than men to be heavier than is deemed healthy.

■ Men and women have different propensities toward unhealthy weight

The occurrence of unhealthy weight (overweight or obesity) among the U.S. adult population increases with age, peaking at age 65 to 74 for men and age 55 to 64 for women (see Chart 6.6A).

Men of all ages are more likely to be overweight than obese (see Chart 6.6B). The greatest differential is among men aged 75+, who are the least likely group, in age and gender, to be obese (20 percent are obese) but the most likely to be overweight (46 percent are overweight). Among women, the overweight and obesity patterns are more variable. Between the ages of 35 and 74, women are more likely to be obese than overweight. In fact, among similar age groups, women are more likely than men to be obese, whereas men are more likely to be overweight.

■ Obesity has become substantially more prevalent among all age groups

Trend data from the National Health and Nutrition Examination Survey indicate that people in 1999–2000 were generally heavier than their same-aged counterparts were in 1988–1994 (see Table 6.12). The major differences were in the proportion that are obese, as overweight proportions remained relatively stable. Between 1988– 1994 and 1999–2000, the prevalence of obesity among the elderly increased more than 30 percent.

CHART 6.6A Percent Who Weigh More Than Recommended Levels (Are Overweight or Obese), by Age and Sex: 1999–2000

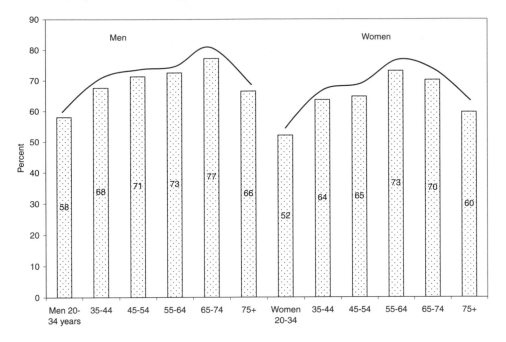

CHART 6.6B Percent Who Are Overweight or Obese, by Age and Sex: 1999–2000

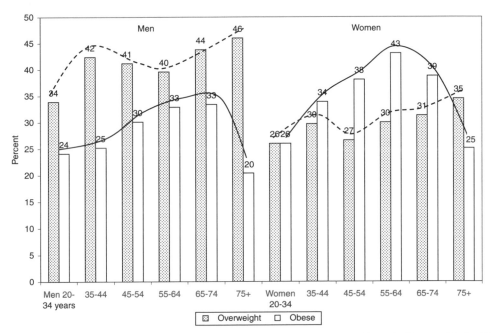

Sources for Charts 6.6A and 6.6B: National Center for Health Statistics, *Health, United States, 2002 with Chart-book on Trends in the Health of Americans* (Hyattsville, MD, 2002), Table 70. Data from the National Health and Nutrition Examination Survey. Additional calculations made by authors.

TABLE 6.12

Trends in Percent of Overweight and Obese Adults, by Age and Sex: 1988–1994 versus 1999–2000

	Men			Women		
	1988–1994	1999–2000	Percent Change	1988–1994	1999–2000	Percent Change
Overweight						
20–34 years	33%	34%	1.5%	19%	26%	39%
35–44	44	42	–3.6	24	30	23
45–54	43	41	–4.0	28	27	–4.7
55–64	43	40	–8.5	33	30	–8.0
65–74	44	44	–1.4	33	31	–6.3
75+	43	46	6.2	33	35	4.2
Obese						
20–34 years	14	24	71	19	26	39
35–44	22	25	17	26	34	33
45–54	23	30	30	32	38	18
55–64	27	33	21	34	43	28
65–74	24	33	39	27	39	44
75+	13	20	55	19	25	31

Source: National Center for Health Statistics, *Health, United States, 2002 with Chartbook on Trends in the Health of Americans* (Hyattsville, MD, 2002), Table 70. Additional calculations made by authors.

Body Weight and Mortality

■ Obesity may be beneficial

Interestingly, despite progressively increasing BMIs among all groups of Americans since 1960, mortality rates have declined.[29] As well, no consensus has been reached on the optimal weight for older people, and no clear epidemiological evidence exists as to what constitutes the best body weight for longevity.[30] However, most studies indicate that people who are excessively thin or fat die earlier, but that obesity may actually confer benefits later in life. Current recommendations advise that people aged 50+ maintain their current weight.[31]

Research indicates that the net negative impact of obesity on median life expectancy is minimal to nonexistent. Specifically, obese people are 2 percent more likely to die between ages 44 and 54 than lean individuals, but are 6 percent less likely to die between ages 64 and 74.[32] In another study, Yale University researchers recently presented evidence that moderately overweight older people do not exhibit a greater risk of death.[33] Specifically, a wide range of increasing BMI is related to minimal excessive mortality in the elderly. In fact, higher BMI values in the elderly are consistent with a smaller relative morality risk compared to young and middle-aged populations. Thus, the optimum BMI for the elderly tends to be higher than that for younger adults.

Another study assessed BMI with the risk of dying in the hospital. The study (which controlled for disease severity) found that, up to a point, mortality declined with increasing weight and, in fact, was highest among those with a BMI of less than 20.[34] Specifically, for patients aged 50 to 79, the lowest risk of dying was among those with a BMI of 40 (morbidly obese). Among patients aged 80+, the optimum BMI was 32 (severely obese).

Numerous possible explanations surround these findings. For one, overweight people who survive to old age may have characteristics that insulate them from the adverse effects of excessive weight.[35] The risks of being underweight might actually outweigh those of being overweight. In fact, it is believed that fat reserves can assist survival when a person is challenged with illness or aging.[36] It is also possible that various risk factors might change with increased age. The Yale researchers pointed out studies that indicated declining, or even no, relationship between cholesterol levels and mortality with increasing age.[37]

Various studies also have found that obese people are less likely to develop cancer and are protected against such other health problems as infectious diseases, chronic obstructive pulmonary disease, osteoporosis, and renovascular hypertension.[38] Even though hypertension is one of the greatest health risks among obese people, today's improved treatments can minimize the risk.

Weight gain in excessively thin patients may actually be beneficial. A weight gain program among elderly patients found that those who increased their weight by at least 5 percent showed reduced mortality and extended longevity.[39]

HEALTH PRACTICES

Weight and Diet Control

Fewer than 1 in 5 adults aged 60 and older (17 percent) has ever lied about their weight compared with 25 percent of younger adults.[40]

■ Four in ten seniors are controlling their diets

According to Mediamark Research, 41 percent of seniors are presently controlling their diets in some manner, compared to slightly more than the 36 percent of younger adults. The elderly are more likely than younger adults to be controlling their cholesterol or blood sugar levels and salt intake through diet,[41] but less likely to be using their diet to lose weight or to pursue physical fitness (see Table 6.13).

■ Few seniors make efforts to reduce their weight

Relatively few elderly appear to be making efforts to reduce their weight (see Table 6.13), and in light of the previously discussed information on the possible longevity benefits to the elderly of being overweight, perhaps they are making the right decision. Even though more than 50 percent of the elderly are overweight or obese, only

TABLE 6.13
Percent of Adults Stating Reasons for Diet Control (among
Those Controlling Their Diets): 2000

Reason for Diet Control	18–64 Years	65+ Years	Ratio of Seniors to Younger Adults
Cholesterol level	19%	43%	2.26
Maintain weight	30	29	0.97
Blood sugar level	13	29	2.23
Weight loss	44	22	0.50
Physical fitness	30	19	0.63
Salt restriction	6	16	2.67
Regularity	4	5	1.25

Source: Mediamark Research Inc. Spring 2000.

9 percent are presently trying to lose weight by controlling their diets. This may be related to skepticism about weight reduction diets; RoperASW reports that 48 percent of older adults (aged 60+) believe that weight reduction diets result in only temporary weight loss, and 27 percent believe that such diets are usually not successful.[42] Similar views are held by adults of all ages.

Additionally, being overweight is tolerated by most older adults, with 55 percent stating that being overweight is harmful only in excess; however, 41 percent state that being overweight in any amount is harmful.[43]

Pairing individuals' attitudes about being overweight with the individuals' actual weight measurements further indicates an acceptance of weight, or a lack of understanding about what constitutes being overweight. According to the USDA's most recently available Diet and Health Knowledge Survey (DHKS), more than 70 percent of older adults aged 60+ (72 percent of men and 79 percent of women) believe that maintaining a healthy weight is very important.[44] However, on average, these more motivated older adults are technically heavier than what is deemed healthy, with an average BMI of 26.

■ More than 1 in 4 older adults is overconfident of caloric intake

The DHKS data also indicated that older adults are very confident about their caloric intake, with about 60 percent stating their caloric intake as "about right" compared with what is healthy. However, further analysis conducted by Kris Hodges showed that among these "calorie confident" individuals, nearly 60 percent of the older men and 40 percent of the older women are actually heavier than what is deemed healthy. The net result is that 37 percent of older men and 26 percent of older women are overconfident of their caloric intake; they think it is appropriate,

TABLE 6.14

Percent of the Dieting Elderly Giving Various Reasons for Controlling Their Diets: 2000

Control diet for cholesterol level and buy foods labeled low-cholesterol and/or low-fat	78%
Low-cholesterol	66
Low-fat	49
Control diet for weight loss and buy foods labeled fat free, low-fat, and/or low-calorie	84
Fat free	67
Low-fat	49
Low-calorie	42
Control diet to maintain weight and buy foods labeled fat free, low-fat, and/or low-calorie	76
Fat free	58
Low-fat	49
Low-calorie	37
Control diet for blood sugar and buy foods labeled sugar-free	74
Control diet for salt and buy food labeled low-sodium	56

Source: Mediamark Research Inc. Spring 2000.

yet they are overweight or obese. Older adults are more likely than younger adults to be overconfident, perhaps reflecting greater acceptance of weight or less knowledge of what constitutes being overweight.

■ Dieting seniors read food labels

The elderly who are controlling their diets appear to be paying attention to food labels (see Table 6.14).[45] Specifically:

- Among the elderly who are controlling their cholesterol levels through diet, two-thirds buy food specifically labeled "low-cholesterol" and one-half buy food labeled "low-fat."

- Among the elderly who control their diet for weight reasons (maintenance or loss), the use of foods labeled "fat free" edge out those labeled "low-fat" or "low-calorie."

- Three-quarters of the elderly who are controlling their blood sugar through diet seek out sugar-free products.

- The elderly who are on salt-restricted diets are least likely to seek out specially labeled products, with slightly more than one-half buying food labeled "low-sodium."

PERSONAL HEALTH HABITS

Exercise

■ Fitness, not fatness, appears more important to longevity

Fitness appears to be a better predictor of longevity than body weight, with the lowest death rates observed in people with the highest fitness levels regardless of their BMI.[46] In fact, increased physical activity and aerobic fitness (independent of weight loss) have been shown to reduce mortality rates more than intentional weight loss alone.

■ Exercise confers numerous benefits

Physical activity confers many health-related benefits, such as reducing the risk of some chronic diseases; relieving depression; improving weight management; and controlling blood pressure, glucose levels, and cholesterol. Furthermore, physical activity is of benefit in maintaining independent living and enhancing overall quality of life. Evidence also exists that exercise can enhance memory. A recent study of nearly 6,000 women aged 65+ showed that those who walked the most were the least likely to show a cognitive decline over the 6- to 8-year test period.[47] The study found a 13 percent lower chance of cognitive decline for every mile walked per week. In another study of 120 men and women aged 60 to 75, half were given a program of aerobic exercise (1 hour of walking, three times a week) and half were given strength and flexibility training. After 6 months, those on the aerobic program showed improvements of 15 to 20 percent on memory tests, while those on the strength program showed no improvements.

Even among frail and very old adults, physical activity improves mobility and functioning.[48] Older people who exercise daily have better balance and are less likely to fall than those who do not exercise.[49] In contrast, physical inactivity is found to be associated with bone loss and osteoporosis, and aging itself is associated with loss of muscle mass and strength.[50]

■ The elderly aged 75+ are likely to be physically inactive

According to the National Health Interview Survey, up until age 75, people are more likely to be physically active than inactive during their leisure time, although the tendency diminishes as age increases (see Chart 6.7).[51] Among people aged 75+, inactivity is more prevalent. Women of all ages are more physically inactive than men (see Table 6.15).

DEFINITION: The government defines physical inactivity as never engaging in any light-moderate or vigorous leisure-time physical activity lasting 10 minutes or longer, and can include strengthening activities without any other type of physical activity.

CHART 6.7   Leisure-Time Physical Activity Levels of Adults, by Age: 1997–1998

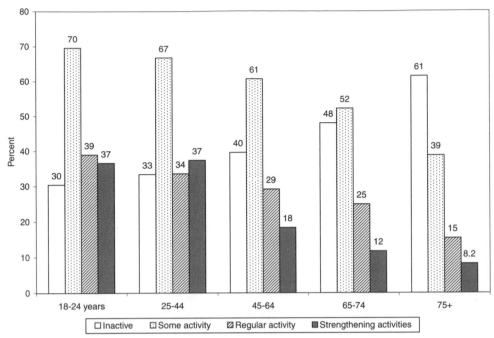

Source: Charlotte A. Schoenborn and Patricia M. Barnes, "Leisure-Time Physical Activity among Adults: United States, 1997–98," *Advance Data from Vital and Health Statistics,* no. 325 (Centers for Disease Control and Prevention, April 7, 2002): Tables 1, 4, and 5.

TABLE 6.15
Leisure-Time Physical Activity Level of Adults, by Age and Sex: 1997–1998

	Inactive			At Least Some Physical Activity		
	Men	Women	Ratio of Women to Men	Men	Women	Ratio of Men to Women
18–24 years	25%	36%	1.43	75%	64%	1.17
25–44	31	35	1.14	69	65	1.06
45–64	38	41	1.08	62	59	1.05
65–74	44	51	1.15	56	49	1.14
75+	54	66	1.22	46	34	1.36

Source: Charlotte A. Schoenborn and Patricia M. Barnes, "Leisure-Time Physical Activity among Adults: United States, 1997–98," *Advance Data from Vital and Health Statistics,* no. 325 (Centers for Disease Control and Prevention, April 7, 2002): Table 1.

TABLE 6.16
Percent Who Are Physically Inactive, by Age, Sex, and
Race: 1994–1996

	White	Black	Ratio of Black to White
Total			
55–64 years	33%	48%	1.45
65–74	34	51	1.50
75+	44	60	1.36
Men			
55–64 years	34	48	1.41
65–74	31	47	1.52
75+	37	59	1.59
Women			
55–64 years	33	49	1.48
65–74	36	53	1.47
75+	47	61	1.30

Sources: Centers for Disease Control and Prevention, "Surveillance for Five Health Risks among Older Adults—United States, 1993–1997," *MMWR, CDC Surveillance Summaries*, 48, no. SS-8 (December 17, 1999): Table 12. Data from the 1994–1996 Behavioral Risk Factor Surveillance System.

Sixteen percent of health/fitness club members are aged 60 or older.[52]

Another study among the elderly showed that about one-third reported no leisure-time physical activity during the preceding month (see Table 6.16).[53] Inactivity levels are similar among those aged 55–64 and 65–74, but increase substantially among those aged 75+. Blacks are more inactive than whites at all age levels. White men are the least inactive followed by white women. Black men and women have comparable levels of inactivity and are the most physically inactive older adults.

About 1 in 5 elderly regularly participates in physical activity

As with younger adults, less than half of the physically active elderly *regularly* participate in leisure-time physical activity, which encompasses regular light-moderate activity (at least five times a week) and/or regular vigorous activity (at least three times a week; see Chart 6.7).[54] Overall, about 1 in 5 elderly is regularly active (25 percent of those aged 65–74 and 15 percent of those aged 75+).[55]

Up until age 65, people are more likely to regularly engage in vigorous than light-moderate leisure-time physical activity, although the tendency diminishes as age increases (see Chart 6.8).

Among the elderly, vigorous activity takes a back seat in favor of light-moderate activity (see Chart 6.8). In fact, people aged 75+ are one-sixth as likely as adults aged 18 to 24 to engage in vigorous activity. The drop-off in light-moderate activity is

CHART 6.8   Degree of Regular Leisure-Time Activity of Adults, by Age: 1997–1998

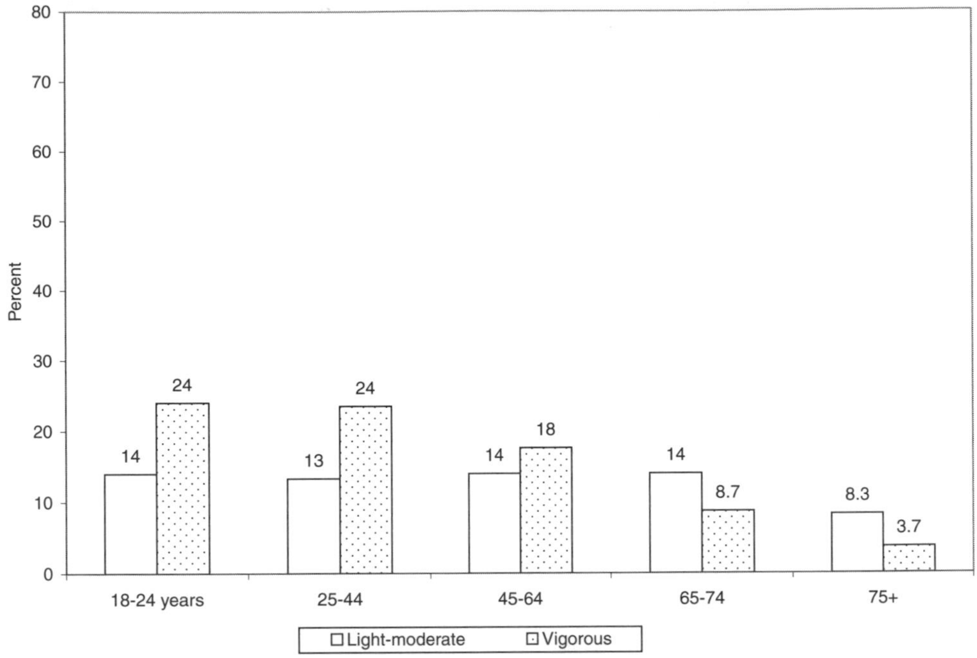

Source: Charlotte A. Schoenborn and Patricia M. Barnes, "Leisure-Time Physical Activity among Adults: United States, 1997–98," *Advance Data from Vital and Health Statistics,* no. 325 (Centers for Disease Control and Prevention, April 7, 2002): Table 4.

much less dramatic, with people aged 75+ about two-thirds as likely as the youngest adults to engage in such activity.

> **DEFINITION:** Light-moderate activity causes light sweating or a slight to moderate increase in breathing or heart rate; vigorous activity causes heavy sweating or large increases in breathing or heart rate.

Men of all ages are more likely than women to regularly participate in leisure-time physical activity, whether it be light-moderate or vigorous (see Table 6.17). Regular physical activity declines much more dramatically for women than for men with age. Women aged 75+ are one-third as likely to regularly participate in leisure-time physical activity as are the youngest women aged 18 to 24 (11 percent versus 32 percent); for men of the same ages, respectively, the differential is about one-half (22 percent versus 46 percent). Vigorous activity levels decline much more rapidly than light-moderate levels do with age.

■ Strengthening activities are not common with the elderly

About 1 in 10 elderly engages in leisure-time strengthening activities, such as weight lifting or calisthenics (see Chart 6.7).[56] Involvement with strengthening ac-

TABLE 6.17

Percent of Adults Who Participate in Regular Leisure-Time Physical Activity: 1997–1998

	Any			Light-Moderate			Vigorous		
	Men	Women	Ratio of Men to Women	Men	Women	Ratio of Men to Women	Men	Women	Ratio of Men to Women
18–24 years	46%	32%	1.44	19%	14%	1.31	39%	24%	1.64
25–44	36	31	1.16	15	13	1.09	30	24	1.26
45–64	32	27	1.18	15	14	1.10	23	18	1.32
65–74	31	20	1.51	19	14	1.40	17	8.7	1.99
75+	22	11	1.96	16	8.3	1.88	8.6	3.7	2.32

Source: Charlotte A. Schoenborn and Patricia M. Barnes, "Leisure-Time Physical Activity among Adults: United States, 1997–98," *Advance Data from Vital and Health Statistics,* no. 325 (Centers for Disease Control and Prevention, April 7, 2002): Table 4.

tivities diminishes with age. Men of all ages are substantially more likely than women to engage in strengthening activities (see Table 6.18).

■ Enjoyment of activity is an Important motivator for physical activity

Among older adults who engage in physical activity fairly regularly, 42 percent exercise for both enjoyment and the physical benefits of the activity.[57] Keeping physically fit is a primary reason stated by 36 percent of older adults, and the enjoyment of the activity is a motivating reason for 22 percent. Forty-four percent feel that regular exercise is very important in helping to look one's best.[58]

TABLE 6.18

Percent of Adults Who Engage in Any Strengthening Activities, by Age: 1997–1998

	Men	Women	Ratio of Men to Women
18–24 years	47%	26%	1.78
25–44	32	23	1.37
45–64	21	16	1.32
65–74	14	10	1.45
75+	11	6.4	1.73

Source: Charlotte A. Schoenborn and Patricia M. Barnes, "Leisure-Time Physical Activity among Adults: United States, 1997–98," *Advance Data from Vital and Health Statistics,* no. 325 (Centers for Disease Control and Prevention, April 7, 2002): Table 5.

■ Walking is the most common form of exercise among the elderly

Walking is the most common form of exercise, noted by 65 percent of the elderly who are not sedentary.[59] Other common forms of exercise are gardening (54 percent of men and 38 percent of women) and stretching (25 percent of men and 32 percent of women). Less than 10 percent of the elderly report strenuous exercise, such as swimming, aerobics, and stair climbing, in a 2-week period.

Social Activity

■ Seniors remain socially active

Social interactions provide emotional and physical support that helps seniors remain active in the community and reduces the likelihood of needing formal health care services.

Virtually all noninstitutionalized seniors aged 70+ reported some social activity during a 2-week period in 1994, and two-thirds were satisfied with their level of activity.[60] Even the oldest-old were socially active, with only 4 percent reporting no involvement with any of seven common social events.

■ Older people are less socially active than younger people are

Social activity declines across increasing age groups; 64 percent of seniors aged 70 to 74 participated in five to seven different social activities in a 2-week period compared with 38 percent of seniors aged 85+.[61] Participation in out-of-home activities (religious events, group events, eating out, and volunteer work) is less common among those in older age groups (see Table 6.19).[62]

TABLE 6.19
Percent of Seniors 70+ Engaging in Various Social Activities: 1995

Social Activity	70+ Years	70–74 Years	75–79 Years	80–84 Years	85+ Years
Contact with relatives with whom they do not live	92%	93%	92%	91%	89%
Contact with friends or neighbors	88	91	88	86	81
Go out to a restaurant	64	70	66	58	47
Attend church, temple, other religious event	50	54	51	48	39
Attend movie, sports event, club, group event	27	33	28	24	14
Volunteer work (past 12 months)	16	20	17	13	7

Source: Federal Interagency Forum on Aging Related Statistics, Older Americans 2000: Key Indicators of Well-Being (Hyattsville, MD, 2000), Table 19a. Data from the National Health Interview Survey.

■ Disability reduces social interaction

Seniors who have difficulty with at least one activity of daily living (ADL) are less socially involved than their nondisabled counterparts.[63] The greatest effect of disability is reduced participation in out-of-home activities. For example, nondisabled seniors are 1.7 times more likely to have attended a religious ceremony and are 1.5 times more likely to have eaten in a restaurant than their disabled counterparts during a 2-week period.

NOTES

1. National Center for Health Statistics, *Health, United States, 2002 with Chartbook on Trends and Health of Americans* (Hyattsville, MD, 2001), Table 67. Data from the National Health Interview Survey.
2. Charlotte A. Schoenborn and Patricia Adams, "Alcohol Use among Adults: United States, 1997–98," *Advance Data from Vital and Health Statistics*, no. 324 (National Center for Health Statistics, September 14, 2001): Table 1.
3. RoperASW, 2000.
4. Sharon Yntema, ed., *Americans 55 and Older: A Changing Market*, 3rd ed. (Ithaca, NY: New Strategist Publications, 2001), 387, 416. 1999 Consumer Expenditure Survey data. Additional calculations made by authors.
5. Ibid., 340. Additional calculations made by authors.
6. U.S. Department of Health and Human Services, "Chapter 5, Older Adults and Mental Health" in *Mental Health: A Report of the Surgeon General* (Rockville, MD: U.S. Department of Health and Human Services, 1999).
7. National Council on the Aging, "Substance Abuse among Older Americans." Available online at www.ncoa.org/news/subabuse.
8. National Center for Health Statistics, *Early Release of Selected Estimates from the 2000 and Early 2001 National Health Interview Surveys* (September 20, 2001), Figure 9.2. Available online at www.cdc.gov/nchs/nhis.
9. National Council on the Aging, "Substance Abuse."
10. National Council on the Aging, "Let's Face the Geriatric Substance Abuse Problem; A Conversation with Nelba R. Chavez, Ph.D." Available online at www.ncoa/news/archives.
11. National Council on the Aging, "Substance Abuse."
12. Centers for Disease Control and Prevention, "Surveillance for Five Health Risks among Older Adults—United States, 1993–1997," *MMWR, CDC Surveillance Summaries*, 48, no. SS-8 (December 17, 1999). Data from the Behavioral Risk Factor Surveillance System.
13. National Council on the Aging, "Substance Abuse."
14. National Council on the Aging, "Let's Face."
15. National Council on the Aging, "Substance Abuse."
16. U.S. Department of Health and Human Services, "Chapter 5."
17. Substance Abuse and Mental Health Services Administration, *Summary of Findings from the 2000 National Household Survey on Drug Abuse*, NHSDA series H-13, DHHS Publication no. (SMA) 01-3549 (Rockville, MD: U.S. Department of Health and Human Services, 2001). Available online at www.DrugAbuseStatistics.SAMHSA.gov.
18. National Center for Health Statistics, *Early Release*, Figure 8.3.
19. National Center for Health Statistics, *Health, United States, 2001*, Table 60. Data from the National Health Interview Survey.

20. Centers for Disease Control and Prevention, "Cigarette Smoking among Adults—United States, 2000," *MMWR* 51, no. 29 (July 26, 2002): 642–645. Available online at www.cdc.gov/mmwr.
21. RoperASW, 2000.
22. Mediamark Research Inc. Spring 2000.
23. Bureau of Labor Statistics, *1999 Consumer Expenditure Survey*, Table 4500. Available online at www.bls.gov.
24. Ibid., Table 3.
25. Sharon Yntema, ed., *Americans 55 and Older*, 344. 1999 Consumer Expenditure Survey data. Additional calculations made by authors.
26. RoperASW, 1999.
27. RoperASW, 2000.
28. Ibid.
29. Paul Ernsberger and Richard J. Koletsy, "Biomedical Rationale for a Wellness Approach to Obesity: An Alternative to a Focus on Weight Loss," *Journal of Social Issues* 55, no. 2 (1999): 221–260.
30. Glenn A. Gaesser, "Thinness and Weight Loss: Beneficial or Detrimental to Longevity?" *Medicine & Science in Sports & Exercise* (1999): 1118–1128.
31. National Center for Health Statistics, *Health, United States, 1999 with Health and Aging Chartbook* (Hyattsville, MD, 1999).
32. Ernsberger and Koletsy, "Biomedical Rationale."
33. Asefeh Heiat, Viola Vaccarino, and Harlan M. Krumholz, "An Evidence-Based Assessment of Federal Guidelines for Overweight and Obesity as They Apply to Elderly Persons," *Archives of Internal Medicine* 161, no. 9 (May 14, 2001): 1194–1203.
34. Ernsberger and Koletsy, "Biomedical Rationale."
35. Heiat, Vaccarino, and Krumholz, "An Evidence-Based Assessment."
36. Ernsberger and Koletsy, "Biomedical Rationale."
37. Heiat, Vaccarino, and Krumholz, "An Evidence-Based Assessment."
38. Ernsberger and Koletsy, "Biomedical Rationale."
39. Ibid.
40. RoperASW, 1997.
41. Mediamark Research Inc. Spring 2000.
42. RoperASW, 1998.
43. RoperASW, 2000.
44. U.S. Department of Agriculture, Food Surveys Research Group, Table Set 19, "Results from USDA's 1994–96 Diet and Health Knowledge Survey" (Beltsville, MD, 2000). Available online at www.barc.usda.gov/bhnrc/foodsurvey/home.htm.
45. Mediamark Research Inc. Spring 2000.
46. Gaesser, "Thinness and Weight Loss."
47. Jerry Adler and Joan Raymond, "Fighting Back, with Sweat," *Newsweek—Health for Life* (Fall/Winter 2001): 35–41.
48. Federal Interagency Forum on Aging Related Statistics. *Older Americans 2000: Key Indicators of Well-Being* (Hyattsville, MD, 2000).
49. Chris Parkhurst, "Getting Older, Feeling Better," *WebMD Health* (January 2000). Available online at http://my.webmd.com/content/article/1738.50051.
50. Centers for Disease Control and Prevention, "Surveillance for Five Health Risks," Table 5. Data from the Behavioral Risk Factor Surveillance System.
51. Charlotte A. Schoenborn and Patricia M. Barnes, "Leisure-Time Physical Activity among Adults: United States, 1997–98," *Advance Data from Vital and Health Statistics*, no. 325 (Centers for Disease Control and Prevention, April 7, 2002): Table 1.
52. "Grandpa Gets Fit," *American Demographics* (November 2001): 13. Data from the International Health, Racquet and Sportsclub Association 2001 survey.

53. Centers for Disease Control and Prevention, "Surveillance for Five Health Risks," Table 12. Data from the 1994–1996 Behavioral Risk Factor Surveillance System.
54. Schoenborn and Barnes, "Leisure-Time Physical Activity among Adults," Tables 1 and 4.
55. Ibid., Table 4.
56. Ibid., Table 5.
57. RoperASW, 2000.
58. RoperASW, 1999.
59. National Center for Health Statistics, *Health, United States, 1999.* Data from the National Health Interview Survey.
60. National Center for Health Statistics, *Health, United States, 1999.* Data from the National Health Interview Second Supplement on Aging. Federal Interagency Forum on Aging Related Statistics, *Older Americans 2000*, Table 19b. Data from the National Health Interview Second Supplement on Aging.
61. National Center for Health Statistics, *Health, United States, 1999.* Data from the National Health Interview Second Supplement on Aging.
62. Federal Interagency Forum on Aging Related Statistics, *Older Americans 2000*, Table 19a. Data from the National Health Interview Survey.
63. National Center for Health Statistics, *Health, United States, 1999.* Data from the National Health Interview Second Supplement on Aging.

CHAPTER 7

Nutrition

There is no more sincere love than the love of food.

—George Bernard Shaw

Food is the most primitive form of comfort.

—Sheila Graham

What is food to one man is bitter poison to another.

—Lucretius

Nutrition plays an important role in longevity and the quality of life. In a 1998 report on health and nutrition, the U.S. Surgeon General wrote, "If you are among the 2 out of 3 Americans who do not smoke or drink excessively, your choice of diet can influence your long-term health prospects more than any other action you might take."[1]

This chapter reports on and analyzes the nutritional status of seniors. Included is a special analysis conducted by Kris Hodges based on data from the U.S. Department of Agriculture (USDA) Diet and Health Knowledge Survey (DHKS). This analysis provides unique findings on how older adults perceive the adequacy of their diets versus how well those diets actually measure up to dietary guidelines.

Highlights of this chapter include:

- Many physiological changes occur with aging that impact nutrition. Additionally, illness, chronic conditions, and social isolation affect the nutrition of the elderly.

- Elderly Nutrition Programs provide an important safety net for nutritionally at-risk elders. During fiscal year 1995, Elderly Nutrition Programs provided more than 100 million meals to more than 3 million older adults.

- Today's seniors have healthier diets than their elderly predecessors did. For example, they eat less red meat and drink more lower-fat milks. Nonetheless, nutritional concerns still exist.

- Vitamin and mineral supplement use is highest among seniors; they are nearly twice as likely as adults aged 18 to 24 to use supplements.

- Older adults are more confident than younger adults that their diets are healthy relative to various nutritional aspects, but this greater confidence does not necessarily translate to better diets.

NUTRITION AND AGING

Diet has an impact on the top three leading causes of death among the elderly—heart disease, cancer, and stroke. The links between high saturated-fat intake and coronary heart disease are well established. Sodium consumption contributes to hypertension, which is a leading risk factor for heart and cerebrovascular disease. Additionally, poor diet may account for one-third of all cancer deaths.[2]

Many chronic diseases that develop late in life have nutrition-related beginnings earlier in life. For example, insufficient calcium intake and lack of exercise earlier in life contribute to osteoporosis later in life, and obesity contributes to diabetes. Dietary aspects are suspected in Alzheimer's disease as well.

All is not lost, however, when adults reach their elderly years. Studies show that good nutrition in the senior years is important in keeping bodies strong and healthy and aids in warding off and minimizing the effects of disease. In fact, many vitamins and minerals have been associated with health benefits. Antioxidants, such as vitamins C and E, may lower risks of cancer, heart disease, and even Alzheimer's disease, and the B vitamins have been linked to cardiovascular health.

Proper nutrition helps keep the elderly healthy by improving their disease resistance, decreasing recovery time when ill, and aiding tolerance to surgical and medical interventions and trauma.[3] A study of older hospitalized patients found that those who were malnourished at the time of hospital admission stayed in the hospital 5.6 days longer and had hospital charges twice that of their well-nourished counterparts.

Several other studies reflect the costs of poor nutrition and the benefits of good nutrition. One recent analysis of adults aged 55+ with diabetes and/or cardiovascular disease found that those who received medical nutrition therapy (nutrition status assessment and diet modification, enteral nutrition, or parenteral nutrition) had fewer hospital admissions and physician visits.[4]

A small-scale study found that home-delivered meal programs appear beneficial in reducing costs by shortening the length of hospitalization. Elderly patients who received home-delivered meals spent an average of about 9 days in the hospital in contrast to 16 days for those who had not received meals at home.[5]

The cost of 1 day of hospitalization is enough to pay for a whole year of home-delivered meals to an older person.[6]

TOURO COLLEGE LIBRARY

■ Physiological changes challenge the elderly's nutrition

The elderly have unique challenges that can dramatically affect their nutritional status. As people age, physiological changes have an impact on their nutritional requirements:[7]

- The ability to taste and smell diminishes, and this impacts appetite.
- The gastrointestinal system becomes more sluggish, contributing to constipation and a feeling of fullness.
- Lean body mass diminishes while body fat increases, contributing to the use of less energy and a tendency to gain weight.
- The ability to concentrate urine decreases, causing a subsequent decline in the thirst response and contributing to dehydration.
- Bone mass decreases, which can result in bone fractures and osteoporosis.

■ Social isolation impacts nutritional status

Social isolation, caused by the loss of a spouse or prolonged years of living alone, affects appetite and is a common problem for seniors. One study found that newly widowed people are less likely to report enjoyment of mealtimes, good eating behavior, and good appetites than their married counterparts are.[8] In addition, nearly 85 percent of widows and widowers reported a weight change during the 2 years following their spouse's death, compared with 30 percent of people whose spouses were still alive.

The study also found that most women enjoyed cooking when they were married, but once widowed, the activity was a "chore" because there was no one to appreciate their efforts. In contrast, widowed men who are not used to cooking for themselves may be likely to snack, eat out, or eat highly processed foods that are not as nutritionally well balanced.

■ Chronic conditions and illness challenge nutritional status

Chronic conditions that afflict the elderly (e.g., hypertension, diabetes, and heart disease) often require special diets, which may require extra effort in meal preparation. Lack of motivation, knowledge, and skill on the part of the elderly can prevent them from making the proper dietary changes.

Disease, illness, and many medications can also affect appetite and the ability to eat. Depression and cancer treatments can greatly affect appetite and subsequently impact weight and well being. At least 10 to 20 percent of widows and widowers have clinically significant depression during the first year of bereavement.[9]

In addition,

- Parkinson's disease, stroke, and other neuromuscular conditions can affect the elderly's ability to feed themselves and swallow.
- Certain mental impairments can affect the ability of seniors to remember what, and when, they have eaten and can keep them from shopping or preparing food for themselves.

- Medications may alter taste, cause gastrointestinal discomfort, or interfere or interact with various nutrients.

- Poor oral health can result in chewing difficulties.

- Financial well-being also affects nutrition, with those of meager means less able to afford healthy food or even to afford food at all. Poverty can cause the elderly to delay medical and dental treatments that could alleviate problems that interfere with good nutrition.

According to the Census 2000 Supplementary Survey, 4.9 percent of older noninstitutionalized adult households (those having at least one person aged 60+) received food stamps. This is less than the 6.6 percent of younger adult households that received food stamps.[10]

Caloric intake declines by as much as 500 calories between the ages of 65 and 85 years.[11] Additionally, studies show that body fat usually doubles between the ages of 20 and 60 years.[12] Recent studies suggest that reduced ability to oxidize fat may play a role in this increase. One small-scale study found that women in their sixties and seventies, compared with those in their twenties, have lower rates of fat oxidation after a large meal.[13] There are no differences after a smaller, less caloric meal. Earlier studies with men find that resting metabolism does not increase in older men after overeating, as it does in younger men.[14] These findings suggest that smaller, more frequent meals could reduce the risk of weight gain in the elderly.

ELDERLY NUTRITION PROGRAMS

■ Elderly Nutrition Programs have waiting lists

The first home-delivered meal program in the United States began in 1954 in Philadelphia.[15] Nearly 20 years later, in 1972, the Elderly Nutrition Program (ENP) of the Older Americans Act was signed into law, creating services (among them home-delivered meals and congregate dining programs) that provide nourishing meals and companionship for older people. ENPs promote good health among the elderly, decrease malnutrition, maintain social interactions, and link older adults with community services to help them stay at home, as opposed to being institutionalized.

The Administration on Aging administers the ENP and provides grants to support nutrition services to 3.1 million elderly participants (under Title III) as well as Native Americans (under Title VI).[16] During fiscal year 1995, the ENP provided 123 million meals to 2.4 million people at congregate meal sites, and 119 million home-delivered meals to 989,000 homebound older adults. In fiscal year 1998, funding for the Title III congregate and home-delivered meal program was $486 million, 56 percent of the Administration on Aging's budget.

Participant contributions account for 20 percent of the cost of both congregate and home-delivered meals. Local donations and volunteer time account for 14 percent of the costs.

Forty-one percent of Title III ENP service providers have a waiting list for home-delivered meals, suggesting a significant unmet need for the service. The average waiting period is 2.6 months. Only 9 percent of the congregate meal programs have waiting lists, with an average waiting period of 2.1 months.

■ Elderly Nutrition Programs are reaching at-risk older Americans

A congressionally mandated evaluation of the ENP found that 80 to 90 percent of Title III participants have incomes below 200 percent of the Department of Health and Human Services' poverty level index (twice the rate for the overall elderly population).[17] Title III participants were also more than twice as likely as the overall elderly population to live alone, and about 60 percent were either over or under their desired weight. Title III home-delivered meal participants had more than twice as many physical impairments as the overall elderly population. Additionally, 63 percent of Title III home-delivered participants rated their health as fair or poor—more than twice the rate of the general elderly Medicare population (26 percent).[18]

Title III home-delivered participants are more disabled than their congregate dining counterparts. Specifically, home-delivered participants are more likely to have had:

- a hospital or nursing home stay in the previous year (43 percent versus 26 percent of congregate diners),
- difficulty doing one or more everyday tasks (77 percent versus 23 percent), and
- greater inability to prepare meals or difficulty with it (41 percent versus 8 percent).

The congressional study also found that ENP recipients, when compared with similar nonparticipants, had higher daily intakes of key nutrients and nearly 20 percent more social contacts per month.[19] Thus, the availability of nutritious home-delivered meals is very likely crucial to maintaining participant independence.

DIETARY ATTITUDES AND KNOWLEDGE

■ Diet and nutrition are more important to women than men

According to the USDA's 1994–1996 Diet and Health Knowledge Survey (DKHS), women aged 60+, as well as those who are younger, place higher importance on various dietary aspects than do comparably aged men (see Table 7.1).[20] For women, importance peaks among those aged 40 to 59 and remains relatively stable among older women aged 60+. In contrast, among men, importance does not peak until age 60, at which point they have almost caught up to the levels stated by women.

TABLE 7.1

Percent Reporting Dietary Aspect as Being "Very Important," by Age and Sex: 1994–1996

Very Important Dietary Aspect	Men			Women			Ratio of Women Aged 60+ to Men Aged 60+ Years
	20–39 Years	40–59 Years	60+ Years	20–39 Years	40–59 Years	60+ Years	
Choosing diet with plenty of fruits and vegetables	55%	61%	68%	72%	79%	79%	1.16
Maintaining healthy weight	65	70	72	78	78	74	1.03
Eating variety of foods	50	58	66	61	71	71	1.08
Choosing diet low in fat	43	53	62	60	67	70	1.13
Choosing diet low in cholesterol	44	55	62	53	65	69	1.11
Using salt and sodium only in moderation	37	52	60	47	62	67	1.12
Choosing diet low in saturated fat	40	50	60	54	64	65	1.08
Choosing diet with adequate fiber	35	50	57	46	64	62	1.09
Eating at least two servings of dairy products daily	33	24	25	47	39	42	1.68
Choosing diet with plenty of breads, cereals, rice, or pasta	30	26	30	33	37	34	1.13

Source: U.S. Department of Agriculture, Food Surveys Research Group, Table Set 19, "Results from USDA's 1994–96 Diet and Health Knowledge Survey" (Beltsville, MD, 2000). Available online at www.barc.usda.gov/bhnrd/foodsurvey/home.htm.

Two-thirds of older adults (aged 60+) feel that eating healthy foods is very important in helping look one's best.[21]

■ Older adults are aware of the connection between diet and health

Older men and women are quite aware of the health problems related to various dietary issues (see Table 7.2).[22] Virtually all older adults recognize health problems associated with being overweight or eating too much salt or sodium. At least three-quarters of older men and women recognize health problems related to consuming too much cholesterol, fat, or sugar, or not enough calcium. Older adults least recognize the problems caused by eating too little fiber; nevertheless, two-thirds are aware of the associated problems.

Eighty-one percent of the elderly think they are more knowledgeable about nutrition today than they were in the past.[23]

TABLE 7.2

Percent of Adults Aged 60+ Who Are Aware of Related Health Problems:
1994–1996

Heard of Health Problem Associated with:	Men	Women	Ratio of Women to Men
Being overweight	89%	91%	1.02
Eating too much salt or sodium	86	91	1.06
Eating too much cholesterol	84	83	0.99
Eating too much fat	83	86	1.04
Not eating enough calcium	75	80	1.07
Not eating enough fiber	66	70	1.06

Source: U.S. Department of Agriculture, Food Surveys Research Group, Table Set 19,
"Results from USDA's 1994–96 Diet and Health Knowledge Survey" (Beltsville, MD, 2000).
Available online at www.barc.usda.gov/bhnrc/foodsurvey/home.htm.

■ Most older adults are aware of the connection between vitamins and health

Nearly all older adults (92 percent) are aware of taking vitamins for improved health, and most (76 percent) believe that vitamins are effective (32 percent, very effective; 44 percent, moderately effective).[24] Not surprisingly, almost all (91 percent) of those who have taken vitamins for improved health believe in a positive outcome (43 percent, very effective; 48 percent, moderately effective).

Forty-four percent of older adults believe that vitamins or nutritional supplements are very important in helping to look one's best.

■ More than 6 in 10 elderly take supplements

Vitamin and mineral supplement usage is higher among older people, with more than 6 in 10 elderly using such a product over a 6-month period, compared with 1 in 3 of the youngest adults (see Table 7.3). Women of all ages are more likely than men to use supplements.

The elderly most commonly take multivitamin or mineral supplements or vitamin E; about one-third of the supplement-taking seniors do so (see Table 7.4). Vitamin C and calcium supplements are used by about one-quarter of supplement-taking seniors.

The primary gender difference is for calcium supplementation. Senior women who take supplements are twice as likely as elderly men to take a calcium supplement (33 percent versus 16 percent), in all likelihood due to their concern about osteoporosis. Overall, 23 percent of all senior women have used calcium supplements over a 6-month period—a proportion four times greater than women aged 18 to 34, twice that of women aged 35 to 44, and comparable to women aged 45 to 64.

TABLE 7.3
Percent Using Vitamin or Mineral Supplements in a 6-Month Period: 2000

	Total	Men	Women	Ratio of Women to Men
18–24 years	35%	33%	37%	1.12
25–34	38	34	42	1.24
35–44	48	42	53	1.26
45–54	54	48	60	1.25
55–64	63	59	66	1.12
65+	63	56	68	1.21
Under age 65	47	42	51	1.21

Source: Mediamark Research Inc. Spring 2000.

TABLE 7.4
Profile of Vitamin and Mineral Supplement Use by the Elderly in a 6-Month Period: 2000

Supplement	All Elderly			Elderly Who Use Supplements		
	Total	Men	Women	Total	Men	Women
Vitamin and mineral supplements	63%	56%	68%	100%	100%	100%
Multivitamin/mineral supplements	23	21	24	36	38	35
Vitamin E	20	19	21	32	34	31
Calcium	17	9	23	27	16	33
Vitamin C	15	14	16	24	24	24

Source: Mediamark Research Inc. Spring 2000.

DIETARY STATUS OF THE ELDERLY

■ Seniors have better diets than do middle-aged adults

According to the government's Healthy Eating Index, the diets of more three-quarters of seniors are poor or need improvement (see Chart 7.1). Nevertheless, seniors' diets are better than those of their middle-aged counterparts (see Table 7.5). Specifically, 21 percent of seniors have good diets (based on the Healthy Eating Index) compared with 13 percent of adults aged 45 to 64.[25] Poverty also plays a significant role in nutrition, with seniors in poverty twice as likely to have poor diets as those who are above the poverty level (see Table 7.5).

■ Today's seniors have healthier diets than their elderly predecessors did

A recent study comparing elderly consumption patterns from three nationwide surveys found that seniors' diets in 1994–1996 were substantially improved over

CHART 7.1 Dietary Quality Ratings among the Elderly, Based on the Healthy Eating Index: 1994–1996

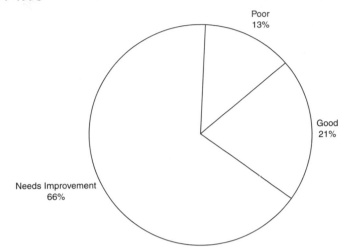

Note: The Healthy Eating Index is the sum of 10 components, each of which can have a score ranging from 0 to 10. A "good" score is 81+, "needs improvement" is 51–80, and "poor" is 50 or less.

Source: Federal Interagency Forum on Aging Related Statistics, *Older Americans 2000: Key Indicators of Well-Being* (Hyattsville, MD, 2000), Table 23a.

TABLE 7.5
Percent of Seniors with Various Dietary Quality Ratings, by Age and Poverty Levels: 1994–1996

Healthy Eating Index Score	45–64 Years	65+ Years	65+ Years, below Poverty Level	65+ Years, above Poverty Level
Good	13%	21%	13%	22%
Needs improvement	70	67	66	67
Poor	18	12	21	11

Source: Federal Interagency Forum on Aging Related Statistics, *Older Americans 2000: Key Indicators of Well-Being* (Hyattsville, MD, 2000), Table 23a.

those of people in the same age group in the late 1970s.[26] Beneficial changes include lower consumption of red meat, whole milk, eggs, and table fats and an increased intake of nutritious foods such as grains, tomatoes, deep-green vegetables, legumes, nuts, seeds, and fruit (see Table 7.6). Specifically:

- The average elderly person in 1994 to 1996 ate less than half the amount of red meat that their counterparts did nearly two decades earlier (1977–1978).

- Egg consumption declined 29 percent for the average elderly woman and 46 percent for the average elderly man.

TABLE 7.6
Average Daily Intake among Adults Aged 65+ in 1994–1996 and Percentage
Change versus Similar Adults in 1977–1978

	Men		Women	
	Intake (grams)	Percent Change	Intake (grams)	Percent Change
Total meat	204	–9%	151	–3%
Red meat	39	–52	24	–53
Luncheon meats	21	0	13	18
Poultry	22	–19	22	–8
Fish	15	50	12	33
Mixtures	102	52	77	67
Total dairy products	260	3	211	–2
Total fluid milk	185	–12	148	–6
Whole milk	43	–60	29	–61
Reduced-fat milks	93	65	70	37
Cheese	15	8	13	–24
Milk desserts	37	54	28	40
Eggs	21	–46	15	–29
Legumes, nuts, and seeds	42	50	26	63
Total grains	301	30	232	27
Breads and rolls	61	6	48	–2
Other baked goods	48	–26	35	–22
Cereals and pasta	102	52	71	29
Grain snacks	8	167	6	100
Mixtures	64	106	57	84
Total vegetables	252	2	210	–4
White potatoes	66	–8	47	–18
Tomatoes	35	21	30	3
Dark-green vegetables	16	45	18	50
Deep-yellow vegetables	15	25	11	–27
Other vegetables	120	–2	104	–2
Total fruits	214	27	195	10
Citrus	79	20	78	6
Other fruits	130	26	113	10
Fats and oils	17	13	14	17
Table fats	7	–22	5	–17
Salad dressing	9	50	9	125
Sugars and sweets	23	–23	18	–10
Nonalcoholic beverages, excluding milk	717	16	629	10
Coffee	419	–5	344	–8
Tea	131	12	147	4
Carbonated soft drinks	121	195	93	127
Fruit drinks	44	165	39	129

Source: Shirley Gerrior, "Dietary Changes in Older Americans from 1977 to 1996:
Implications for Dietary Quality," *Family Economics and Nutrition Review* 12, no. 2
(1999): 3–14.

- Whole milk consumption declined 60 percent, and consumption of reduced-fat milks increased substantially to the point that the latter now account for nearly one-half of the fluid milk that the elderly drink (versus about 30 percent in 1977–1978). However, the diets of today's elderly still contain about the same amount of dairy products as seniors consumed in the late 1970s.

- Today's seniors eat nearly one-third more grains and 50 percent more dark-green vegetables than their counterparts did in the late 1970s. Elderly women consume 10 percent more fruit, and men consume 27 percent more.

- Table fat consumption declined by about 20 percent for seniors in 1994–1996 compared to seniors in the late 1970s.

These changes are reflected in the fact that the diets of today's elderly (men and women alike) have higher intakes of calcium and vitamins A, C, and B$_6$ (see Table 7.7). Today's seniors are also generally receiving more than adequate intakes of vitamins A and C, folate, and iron. Average cholesterol intakes are at lower-than-the-maximum recommended levels, especially for elderly women.

■ Not all dietary changes have been beneficial

Not all dietary changes among the elderly have been beneficial. Comparisons from food consumption surveys reveal a more than doubling of carbonated soft drink consumption (see Table 7.6).[27] Carbonated soft drinks now account for about 12 percent of the elderly's nonalcoholic beverage consumption compared with 5 percent in 1977–1979 (see Table 7.15). Low-calorie sodas account for about 40 percent of the carbonated beverages the elderly consume.

In addition, total fat and oil consumption by the elderly increased by more than 10 percent due to a significant increase in fats consumed in salad dressing; 50 percent among men and 125 percent among women (see Table 7.6). However, this downside may be partially offset by a presumable increase in fresh vegetable consumption.

■ There is still room for improvement

Despite healthier diets among today's elders, there is still room for improvement (see Table 7.7). On average, today's elders have:

- fat intakes that exceed the recommended level for total fat and saturated fat,

- dietary fiber levels that are below recommended levels, with only 11 percent of women and 20 percent of men achieving the recommended levels,[28] and

- vitamin E intakes significantly lower than recommended.

Additionally, elderly women are still struggling to achieve their recommended calcium intake levels, and elderly men still have sodium intakes at higher than recommended maximum levels.

TABLE 7.7
Average Intake as a Percent of Recommended Values for Adults Aged 65+: 1977,
1989–1991, and 1994–1996

	Men			Women		
	1977	1989–1991	1994–1996	1977	1989–1991	1994–1996
Vitamin A	127%	170%	181%	150%	191%	183%
Vitamin C	144	182	172	146	169	160
Iron	127	163	167	94	120	125
Folate	—	154	143	—	133	128
Sodium	—	136	132	—	94	98
Total fat	129	112	111	129	112	107
Saturated fat	—	118	110	—	113	103
Vitamin B_6	82	96	99	81	93	95
Calcium	89	92	96	69	74	75
Vitamin E	—	87	88	—	89	82
Cholesterol	—	95	85	—	65	62
Dietary fiber	—	70	74	—	54	56

Source: Shirley Gerrior, "Dietary Changes in Older Americans from 1977 to 1996: Implications for Dietary Quality," *Family Economics and Nutrition Review* 12, no. 2 (1999): 3–14.

DIETARY PERCEPTIONS

■ Most seniors feel their diets are "about right"

More than 16,000 people participated in the USDA's nationwide Continuing Survey of Food Intakes by Individuals in 1994–1996. Approximately one-third of the respondents were subsequently surveyed on their attitudes and knowledge about dietary guidance and health in the follow-up DHKS.[29] Kris Hodges analyzed the data from the most recent DHKS to determine how older adults (aged 60+) perceive the adequacy of their diets and how well those diets actually meet dietary guidelines.

DHKS respondents were asked their impressions of their diet on various dietary practices ranging from fat, sodium, and cholesterol intake to fiber and calcium consumption. Specifically, respondents were asked: "Compared to what is healthy, do you think your diet is too low, too high, or about right in . . ." These perceptions form the basis for what Hodges characterizes as "confidence"; the higher the "about right" response among a group of respondents, the higher that group's confidence in their diet with respect to the characteristic.

The analysis finds that older adults are quite confident about the quality of their diets, with 60 percent or more feeling their diets are "about right" relative to various key dietary practices (see Charts 7.2 and 7.3). Older men and women are quite similar in their dietary self-assessments, and are more confident than younger adults.

CHART 7.2 Percent of Men Reporting Their Diet Is "about Right" on Various Dietary Aspects: 1994–1996

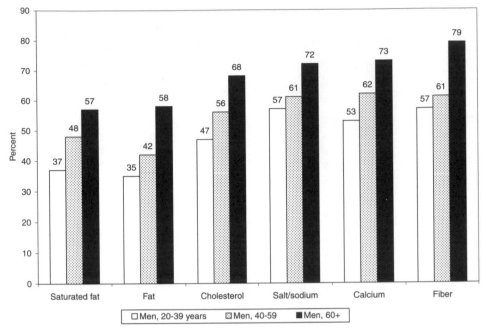

☐ Men, 20-39 years   ☒ Men, 40-59   ■ Men, 60+

CHART 7.3 Percent of Women Reporting Their Diet Is "about Right" on Various Dietary Aspects: 1994–1996

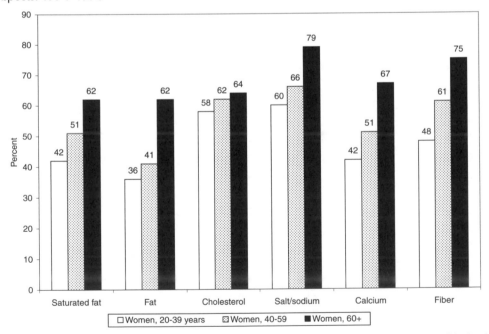

☐ Women, 20-39 years   ☒ Women, 40-59   ■ Women, 60+

Source for Charts 7.2 and 7.3: U.S. Department of Agriculture, Food Surveys Research Group, Table Set 19, "Results from USDA's 1994–96 Diet and Health Knowledge Survey" (Beltsville, MD, 2000). Available online at www.barc.usda.gov/bhnrc/foodsurvey/home.htm.

DIETARY REALITY

■ Older adults are often overconfident about their diets

A key question concerns how the actual diets of "confident" older adults compare with their perceptions. By assessing the actual dietary intake of these "confident" respondents from the DHKS data, Hodges' analysis finds that a significant percentage of older men and women are actually *over*confident about their dietary self-assessment (see Charts 7.4 and 7.5). That is, they believe they are consuming appropriately healthy levels of nutrients but actually are not achieving recommended levels. Specifically:

- Older adults are generally more overconfident than younger adults about dietary intakes.

- Older men are most overconfident of their sodium and fiber intakes.

- Older women are most overconfident of their fiber and calcium intakes.

- Older men are more overconfident than older women about their sodium and cholesterol intakes (see Chart 7.6).

- Older women are more overconfident than older men about their fiber and calcium intakes.

CHART 7.4   Nutrient Overconfidence in Men: Percent of Men Who State Their Diet Is "about Right" but Have Intakes Different Than Recommended, 1994–1996

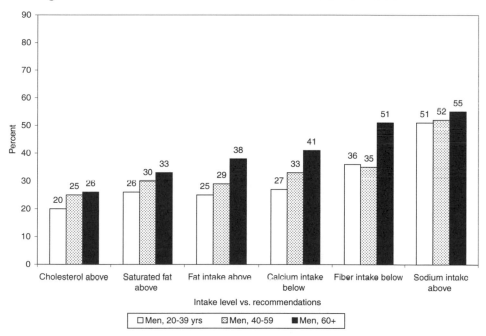

Source: Special analysis conducted by Kris Hodges based on data from U.S. Department of Agriculture, Food Surveys Research Group, Table Set 19, "Results from USDA's 1994–96 Diet and Health Knowledge Survey" (Beltsville, MD, 2000). Available online at www.barc.usda.gov/bhnrc/foodsurvey/home.htm.

CHART 7.5   Nutrient Overconfidence in Women: Percent of Women Who State Their Diet Is "about Right" but Have Intakes Different Than Recommended, 1994–1996

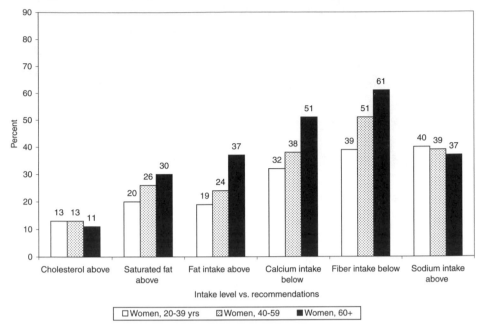

CHART 7.6   Nutrient Overconfidence in Older Adults: Percent of Older Adults Who State Their Diet Is "about Right" but Have Intakes Different Than Recommended, by Sex, 1994–1996

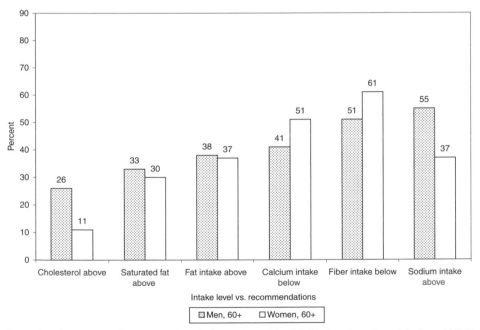

Source for Charts 7.5 and 7.6: Special analysis conducted by Kris Hodges based on data from U.S. Department of Agriculture, Food Surveys Research Group, Table Set 19, "Results from USDA's 1994–96 Diet and Health Knowledge Survey" (Beltsville, MD, 2000). Available online at www.barc.usda.gov/bhnrc/foodsurvey/home.htm.

The thrust of this analysis is to point out potential areas of concern. Recommended intakes for fiber, fat, saturated fat, cholesterol, and sodium are based on guidelines established by various government agencies. Calcium intake is based on the recommended daily allowance (RDA), which provides an appropriate safety factor. This safety factor exceeds the actual requirements of most people. Thus, people with intakes below the RDA do not necessarily have inadequate intakes. Additionally, intakes that qualify as "below" the RDA can range widely from 0 to just below 100 percent of the RDA. The dietary component of this analysis also does not account for vitamin or mineral supplement usage.

SPECIFIC NUTRITIONAL CONCERNS

Sodium

■ Sodium levels are a particular problem for older men

Sixty percent of older men believe it is very important to use salt or sodium in moderation (see Chart 7.7). However, regardless of the level of motivation, older men have sodium intakes that are more than 1.3 times higher, on average, than recommended levels (see Table 7.8).

CHART 7.7   Sodium-related Dietary Aspects, Men versus Women: 1994–1996

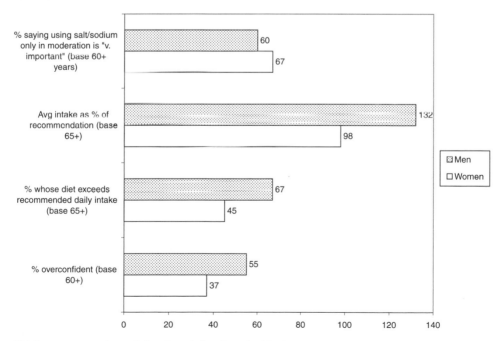

Note: This is a summary chart of data found elsewhere in this chapter.

TABLE 7.8

Average Sodium Intake among Adults Aged 60+ Years, by Perceived Importance of Using Salt or Sodium only in Moderation: 1994–1996

	Average Sodium Intake (milligrams per day; 2-day average)		
	Very Important	Somewhat Important	Not Too Important or Not at All Important
Men	3,405	3,464	3,482
Women	2,490	2,454	2,203

Note: Recommended sodium intake is 2,400 milligrams per day. Levels reported here exclude salt added at the table.

Source: U.S. Department of Agriculture, Food Surveys Research Group, Table Set 19, "Results from USDA's 1994–96 Diet and Health Knowledge Survey" (Beltsville, MD, 2000). Available online at www.barc.usda.gov/bhnrc/foodsurvey/home.htm.

Few improvements in sodium consumption have occurred since 1989 (see Table 7.7). In fact, two-thirds of elderly men exceed their recommended daily sodium intake (see Chart 7.7). Exacerbating the problem is that more than one-half (55 percent) of older men are overconfident of their salt intake, thinking their intake is "about right," but actually having intakes higher than recommended maximum levels.

Older women place somewhat greater importance than men on moderate salt use; 67 percent of women versus 60 percent of older men state that it is very important (see Chart 7.7). Although sodium content in women's diets is less of an issue (elderly women, on average, have intakes at recommended levels), 45 percent still exceed daily recommended maximum levels.

Women of all ages are less likely than men to be overconfident of their salt intake; about 40 percent of all women are overconfident compared with 55 percent of older men.

Fiber

■ More than half of older adults are overconfident of their fiber consumption

Adults aged 60+ place high importance on choosing a diet with adequate fiber; about 60 percent state that this is very important (see Chart 7.8). These more motivated adults have fiber intakes somewhat higher than their less motivated counterparts (see Table 7.9).

However, as a group, elderly adults are not achieving the recommended levels of fiber in their diets. Only 11 percent of elderly women and 20 percent of men achieve

CHART 7.8   Fiber-related Dietary Aspects, Men versus Women: 1994–1996

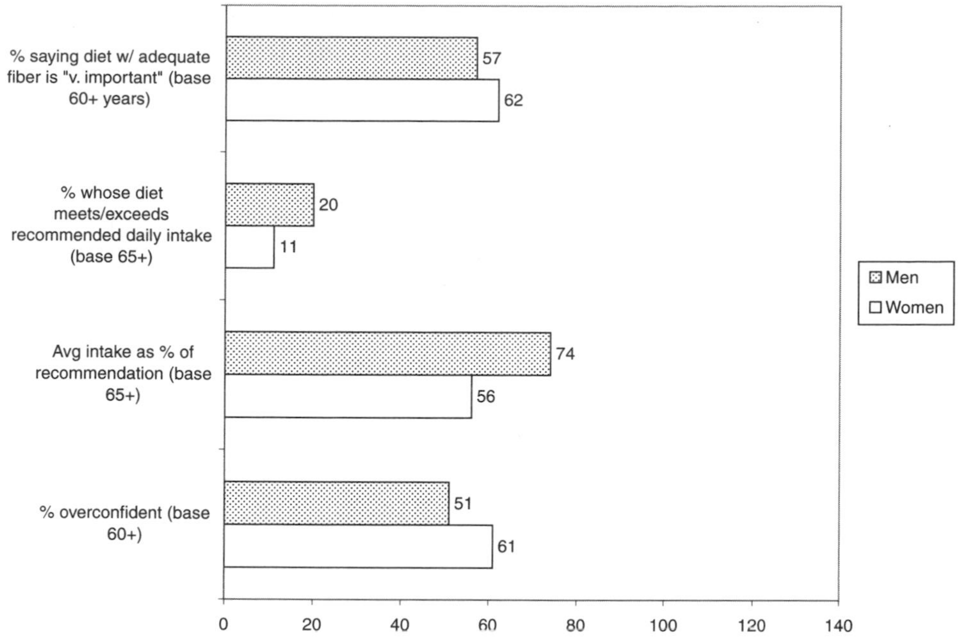

Note: This is a summary chart of data found elsewhere in this chapter.

100 percent or more of the recommended daily intake of fiber (see Chart 7.8). On average, elderly women consume only about one-half of the recommended fiber intake, and elderly men about three-quarters.

Hampering improvements, however, is the fact that more than one-half of older adults (51 percent of older men and 61 percent of older women) are overconfident about their fiber intake. That is, they believe their fiber intake to be adequate, but in

TABLE 7.9
Average Fiber Intake among Adults Aged 60+ Years, by Perceived Importance of Choosing a Diet with Adequate Fiber: 1994–1996

	Average Fiber Intake (grams per day; 2-day average)		
	Very Important	Somewhat Important	Not Too Important or Not at All Important
Men	20	17	16
Women	15	12	12

Note: Recommended fiber intake is 25 grams per day.
Source: U.S. Department of Agriculture, Food Surveys Research Group, Table Set 19, "Results from USDA's 1994–96 Diet and Health Knowledge Survey" (Beltsville, MD, 2000). Available online at www.barc.usda.gov/bhnrc/foodsurvey/home.htm.

fact it is below recommended levels. Older adults are substantially more overconfident than are younger adults. Another compounding factor is that older adults' knowledge about health problems associated with too little fiber is considerably weaker than for other dietary-related health problems (see Table 7.2).

Calcium

■ Many older people incorrectly believe their diet is adequate in calcium

Adequate calcium intake is important for older women, given their high rates of osteoporosis. One in five women aged 65 to 74 has osteoporosis in the hip, and this increases to one-half of all women aged 85 and older.[30] However, only 42 percent of women aged 60+ think it is very important to consume at least two servings of dairy products daily (see Chart 7.9). But even this more motivated group of older women consumes an average of only 1.3 servings of dairy products a day, which, although low, is twice the average of their least motivated counterparts (see Table 7.10).

Older men aged 60+ are not immune to osteoporosis, yet they place even less importance on consuming dairy products; only 25 percent state that it is very important (see Chart 7.9). This highly motivated group, however, consumes an average of only 1.6 servings of dairy products a day, but this is substantially higher than the 1.1 average servings among their least motivated counterparts (see Table 7.10).

CHART 7.9   Calcium-related Dietary Aspects, Men versus Women: 1994–1996

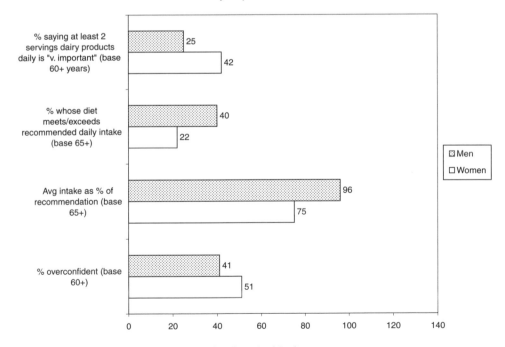

Note: This is a summary chart of data found elsewhere in this chapter.

TABLE 7.10
Average Dairy Intake among Adults Aged 60+ Years,
by Perceived Importance of Eating at Least Two Servings
of Dairy Products Daily: 1994–1996

	Average Number of Dairy Servings per Day (2-day average)		
	Very Important	Somewhat Important	Not Too Important or Not at All Important
Men	1.6	1.4	1.1
Women	1.3	1.0	0.7

Source: U.S. Department of Agriculture, Food Surveys Research Group,
Table Set 19, "Results from USDA's 1994–96 Diet and Health Knowledge
Survey" (Beltsville, MD, 2000). Available online at www.barc.usda.gov/
bhnrc/foodsurvey/home.htm.

Although calcium intake in elderly diets has increased somewhat since 1977 (see Table 7.7), only 1 in 5 older women aged 60+ is consuming at least 100 percent of the recommended daily allowance for calcium (see Chart 7.9). Older men are doing better, with 40 percent meeting or exceeding recommended daily calcium intakes. Subsequently, average calcium intakes for older men are nearly at recommended levels, whereas those for older women are three-quarters of recommended levels.

Compounding the problem is that 41 percent of older men and one-half of older women are overconfident of their calcium intake, believing it to be adequate while in reality failing to meet recommended levels (see Chart 7.9). Older adults are substantially more likely to be overconfident than younger adults of their calcium intake.

More than one-third (37 percent) of older adults, though, are making a special effort to get enough calcium, mostly through supplements.[31] However, as a group, their efforts are somewhat weaker than for adults aged 45 to 59 (44 percent).

Fat

Three in ten older adults feel that eating any amount of food that is high in fat is harmful, whereas two-thirds feel it is harmful only in excess.[32]

■ More than 3 in 10 older adults are overconfident of their fat intake

More than 60 percent of older adults state that choosing a diet low in fat and saturated fat is very important to them (see Chart 7.10). Although these more highly motivated adults have fat intakes that are at about recommended maximum levels, their intake is not substantially better than that of their less motivated counterparts (see Table 7.11).

CHART 7.10   Fat-related Dietary Aspects, Men versus Women: 1994–1996

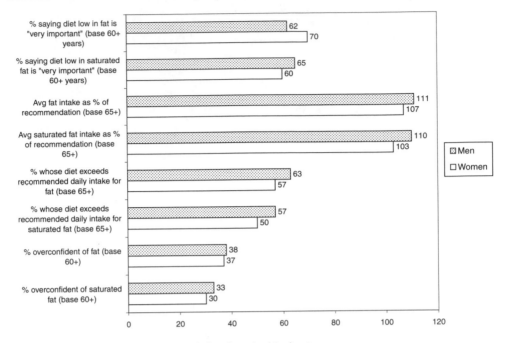

Note: This is a summary chart of data found elsewhere in this chapter.

TABLE 7.11

Average Fat Intakes among Adults Aged 60+ Years, by Perceived Importance of Choosing a Diet Low in Fat and Saturated Fat: 1994–1996

	Average Fat Intake (% of kilocalories per day; 2-day average)		
	Very Important	Somewhat Important	Not Too Important or Not at All Important
Fat			
Men	33	34	36
Women	32	34	36
Saturated Fat			
Men	11	12	12
Women	10	11	11

Note: Recommendations are for no more than 30 percent of total calories to be from total fat and less than 10 percent from saturated fat.

TABLE 7.12
Percent of Adults (Aged 60+) with Opinions about Various
Words or Phrases Used by Food Companies: 1999

Word or Phrase	Used in a Confusing Manner	Companies Abuse Meaning
Light	43%	24%
Low-fat	42	22
99% fat free	36	25
Fat free	33	25

Source: RoperASW, 1999.

Although average fat intakes among the elderly have declined since 1977, the average senior's diet still exceeds the recommended maximum level for total fat and saturated fat (see Table 7.11). From 50 to 63 percent of seniors exceed guidelines for the percent of calories they derive from fat or saturated fat (see Chart 7.10). More than 3 in 10 older adults think their fat intake is about right, whereas in reality it exceeds recommended guidelines. These figures are higher than for younger adults.

Exacerbating the problem is older adults' confusion about the use of terms to describe foods. More than one-third of older adults think that the terms "low-fat," "light," and even "99% fat free" or "fat free" are used in a confusing manner by food companies, and about one-quarter think the terms are usually abused (see Table 7.12).[33]

Cholesterol

■ Cholesterol consumption is lower among older adults

Having a diet low in cholesterol is very important to more than 60 percent of older adults (see Chart 7.11). This motivation appears to have a particular effect upon older men, for whom a higher motivation is related to a 10 to 20 percent lower consumption of cholesterol (see Table 7.13).

Dietary trends indicate that cholesterol consumption has declined somewhat and remains below recommended maximum levels, especially for elderly women (see Table 7.7). The average cholesterol intake for women aged 65+ is, on average, 62 percent of recommended levels, and that for men is 85 percent (see Chart 7.11). Nonetheless, one-third of elderly men and one-fifth of elderly women exceed recommended maximum cholesterol intake levels.

Perception and reality are much more in line regarding cholesterol consumption than for other nutrients, with only 26 percent of older men and 11 percent of older women incorrectly thinking their cholesterol levels are about right (see Chart 7.11). These figures are comparable across age groups.

CHART 7.11   Cholesterol-related Dietary Aspects, Men versus Women: 1994–1996

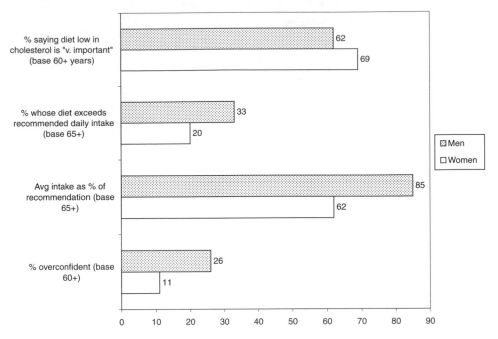

Note: This is a summary chart of data found elsewhere in this chapter.

TABLE 7.13

Cholesterol Intake among Adults 60+ Years, by Perceived Importance of Choosing a Diet Low in Cholesterol: 1994–1996

	Average Cholesterol Intake (milligrams per day; 2-day average)		
	Very Important	Somewhat Important	Not Too Important or Not at All Important
Men	285	312	349
Women	198	208	195

Note: Recommended daily cholesterol consumption is 300 milligrams or less per day.

Source: U.S. Department of Agriculture, Food Surveys Research Group, Table Set 19, "Results from USDA's 1994–96 Diet and Health Knowledge Survey" (Beltsville, MD, 2000). Available online at www.barc.usda.gov/ bhnrc/ foodsurvey/home.htm.

FOOD PREFERENCES

■ Older adults have specific food preferences

According to the United States Department of Agriculture data, older people (aged 60+) exhibit certain food preferences (see Table 7.14). Specifically, on any one day:

- Tomatoes are about as popular as potatoes, with each being eaten by about 4 in 10 older people.
- Bananas are substantially more popular than apples. About 25 percent of older people eat bananas compared with about 15 percent who eat apples.
- Hot dogs, sausages, and luncheon meats are the most popular meat source, followed by pork and beef.
- Eggs and cheese are popular non-meat protein sources, being eaten by about 1 in 4 older adults.

■ Coffee is the beverage of choice among older adults

Even though the amount of coffee the elderly consume is more than 5 percent lower than in the late 1970s (see Table 7.6) and accounts for less than half of all non-alcoholic beverages consumed (see Table 7.15), coffee still is the beverage of choice among older people. Three-quarters of older adults consume coffee on any one day (see Table 7.14). Milk is the next most popular beverage choice, chosen by about 6 in 10 older people. Among older people aged 60 to 69, carbonated soft drinks edge out fruit juices, while the opposite is true among those aged 70+.

Fruit drinks are a small but growing part of seniors' beverage choices. Today's elderly consume more than three times as much fruit drinks, on average, as seniors did nearly 20 years ago (see Table 7.6). Fruit drinks now account for about 5 percent of the elderly's nonalcoholic beverage consumption (see Table 7.15).

■ Food preferences among older men and women are quite similar

Food preferences among older people are relatively minor, with men somewhat more likely than women to consume fried white potatoes, hot dogs, sausages, and luncheon meats, eggs, beef, and beer or ale (see Table 7.14). Older women are more likely than older men to consume yogurt and tea.

■ Older adults have different food preferences from the general adult population

Older men and women are more likely than all adults to consume certain foods such as ready-to-eat cereals, bananas, citrus juices, dried fruits, milk products (especially low-fat milk), table fat, and coffee (see Table 7.14). Some of the most dramatic differences are in dried fruit, table fat, and coffee consumption. Specifically, men and women aged 70+ are two to three times more likely than adults in general

TABLE 7.14

Percent of People Consuming Various Types of Food in 1 Day: 1994–1996

	Men			Women		
	20+ Years	60–69 Years	70+ Years	20+ Years	60–69 Years	70+ Years
Breads						
Cakes, cookies, pastries, pies	39%	42%	48%	40%	42%	47%
Ready-to-eat cereals	22	28	38	24	27	35
Crackers, popcorn, pretzels, corn chips	26	25	24	27	29	23
Vegetables						
Total white potatoes	47	44	44	41	39	39
Fried white potatoes	28	20	14	20	13	10
Tomatoes	42	42	37	39	40	36
Lettuce, lettuce-based salads	28	29	25	29	32	24
Dark-green vegetables	11	13	13	12	14	16
Fruits						
Bananas	15	24	29	16	20	26
Apples	10	14	16	12	17	14
Dried fruits	2.1	3.2	7.1	2.6	3.4	5.4
Milk products						
Milk and milk products	74	80	86	77	79	83
Total fluid milk	50	60	68	51	58	64
Low-fat milk	24	28	36	23	25	31
Whole milk	15	15	18	15	14	17
Skim milk	10	15	16	14	19	17
Cheese	33	28	29	32	29	24
Milk desserts	17	21	26	16	20	22
Yogurt	2.8	2.2	2.1	5.4	5.1	3.4
Meats and proteins						
Hot dogs, sausages, luncheon meats	32	33	32	24	27	23
Beef	25	25	20	18	19	16

to consume dried fruit, and about one-third more likely to use table fats and drink coffee.

In contrast, older people are less likely than the average adult to consume fried white potatoes, cheese, carbonated soft drinks, and beer or ale. The most dramatic difference is in soft drink consumption where men and women aged 70+ are less than half as likely as adults in general to drink carbonated soft drinks.

■ Vegetarianism is less popular among older people but "light" foods are more popular

According to RoperASW, most older adults (69 percent of those aged 60+) eat meat often or regularly, and only 3 percent of older adults are vegetarians (compared with 5 percent of all adults).[34] Twenty-six percent are careful about how much meat they eat.

TABLE 7.14
Continued

	Men			Women		
	20+ Years	60–69 Years	70+ Years	20+ Years	60–69 Years	70+ Years
Meats and proteins (continued)						
Pork	18	22	25	17	19	21
Eggs	22	27	28	19	24	19
Chicken	19	17	17	19	19	20
Legumes	15	15	15	15	15	12
Fish and shellfish	10	12	12	8.4	10	10
Fats and sweets						
Table fats	32	45	47	34	42	45
Salad dressings	32	35	31	33	35	28
Sugars	34	45	45	36	39	38
Candy	12	12	7.4	12	8.3	8.5
Beverages (excluding milk)						
Coffee	56	78	75	54	71	71
Carbonated soft drinks	54	38	26	49	37	21
Regular	43	23	16	32	21	12
Low calorie	13	16	10	18	17	8.9
Tea	24	26	26	30	33	29
Fruit juices, citrus	20	23	28	21	25	31
Fruit juices, non-citrus	4.9	4	7.1	5.1	5.2	6.2
Wine	4.7	6.1	5.5	5.1	7.9	3.4
Beer and ale	17	10	5.7	4.5	1.7	0.7

Source: U.S. Department of Agriculture, Food Surveys Research Group, Table Set 10, "Results from USDA's 1994–96 Continuing Survey of Food Intakes by Individuals and 1994–96 Diet and Health Knowledge Survey" (Beltsville, MD, 1997). Available online at www.barc.usda.gov/bhnrc/foodsurvey/home.htm.

TABLE 7.15
Share of Nonalcoholic Beverage Consumption among Adults Aged 65+:
1977–1978 and 1994–1996

	Men		Women	
	1977–1978	1994–1996	1977–1978	1994–1996
Total nonalcoholic beverages	100	100	100	100
Coffee	54	47	51	45
Milk	25	21	22	19
Tea	14	15	19	19
Carbonated soft drinks	5	13	5.6	12
Fruit drinks	1.9	4.9	2.3	5.1

Source: Author calculations based on data from Shirley Gerrior, "Dietary Changes in Older Americans from 1977 to 1996: Implications for Dietary Quality," *Family Economics and Nutrition Review* 12, no. 2 (1999): 3–14.

TABLE 7.16
Percent Who Usually Use Lighter Version of Various
Products (among Those Using the Products), by Age: 1997

	18–59 Years	60+ Years	Ratio of 60+ Years to 18–59 Years
Milk	44%	54%	1.23
Mayonnaise	28	37	1.32
Salad dressing	27	36	1.33
Ice cream	17	25	1.47
Cheese	15	25	1.67
Cookies	12	22	1.83

Source: RoperASW, 1997.

Older adults are more likely users of "light" foods than are younger adults (see Table 7.16). Fat-reduced milk and nonfat milk are the most frequently used "light" foods among older adults; more than one-half use a light version of milk. Older adults still favor the regular version of sweets, with only 1 in 4 older adults usually using some lighter version of cookies or ice cream.

ATTITUDES ABOUT FOOD AND FOOD PURCHASING

■ Food safety and taste matter most

At least 80 percent of older adults say food safety and taste are the most important aspects of food buying (see Table 7.17). Additionally, more than half of older adults indicate nutrition and how well food keeps as being very important.

TABLE 7.17
Percent Reporting Various Aspects as Being "Very Important" When Buying Food: 1994–1996

Very Important Aspect of Food	Men			Women			Ratio of Women Aged 60+ to Men Aged 60+
	20–39 Years	40–59 Years	60+ Years	20–39 Years	40–59 Years	60+ Years	
Food safety	76%	81%	81%	86%	92%	90%	1.11
Taste	79	79	80	85	88	88	1.10
Nutrition	49	54	65	65	73	75	1.15
How well food keeps	48	55	57	58	58	74	1.30
Price	45	36	38	45	43	55	1.45
Ease of preparation	35	35	35	39	39	41	1.17

Source: U.S. Department of Agriculture, Food Surveys Research Group, Table Set 19, "Results from USDA's 1994–96 Diet and Health Knowledge Survey" (Beltsville, MD, 2000). Available online at www.barc.usda.gov/bhnrc/foodsurvey/home.htm.

TABLE 7.18
Percent Agreeing with the Statement "I Always Check the Ingredients and Nutritional Content of Food Products before I Buy Them": 1999

	Men		Women	
	18–64 Years	65+ Years	18–64 Years	65+ Years
Agree	43%	54%	54%	65%
Agree mostly	13	21	19	31
Agree somewhat	30	33	36	34

Source: Mediamark Research Inc. Fall 1999.

Older women place more importance than older men on all food buying aspects, probably because they are the ones most responsible for meals (90 percent of older women versus 25 percent of older men prepare meals). Older women are substantially more concerned than men about price and about how well food keeps.

■ More than half of seniors read food labels

Seniors are more likely than younger adults to check the ingredients and nutritional content of food products, and women are more likely than men to do so (see Table 7.18).

■ Older adults are more willing to forgo good taste for nutrition

A survey of 3,700 adults conducted by George P. Moschis and associates revealed that nearly one-half (48 percent) of elderly Americans sacrifice good taste for good nutrition, compared with 35 percent of baby boomers.[35] This may account, in part, for the fact that older adults are more likely than younger adults to use light versions of food products (see Table 7.16).[36]

NOTES

1. "Position of the American Dietetic Association: Cost-Effectiveness of Medical Nutrition Therapy," *Journal of the American Dietetic Association* 95 (1995): 88–91.
2. Ibid.
3. Ibid.
4. John F. Shils, Robert Rubin, and David Stapleton, "The Estimated Costs and Savings of Medical Nutrition Therapy: The Medicare Population," *Journal of American Dietetic Association* 99, no. 4 (1999): 426–435. As reprinted on www.healthandage.com.
5. T. L. Adams et al., "The Effect of Home-Delivered Meals on Length of Hospitalization for Elderly People," *Journal of American Dietetic Association* 98 (1998): page A-12 (supplement). Abstract.
6. "Position of the American Dietetic Association."
7. Deborah Adams, R.D, *Nutrition* (University of Maryland at Baltimore: n.d.). Available online at http://cpmcnet.columbia.edu/dept/dental/Dental_Educational_Software/Gerontology_and_Geriatric_Dentistry/nutrition/Nutrition-Phys_Changes.html.

8. Paula Kurtzweil, "Growing Older, Eating Better," *FDA Consumer*, publication no. (FDA) 97-2301 (Food and Drug Administration, December 1996). Available online at http://vm.cfsan.fda.gov.
9. U.S. Department of Health and Human Services, "Chapter 5, Older Adults and Mental Health," in *Mental Health: A Report of the Surgeon General* (Rockville, MD, 1999).
10. Bureau of the Census, *Census 2000 Supplementary Survey Summary Tables*, Table P094. Available online at http://factfinder.census.gov.
11. Center for Nutrition Policy and Promotion, USDA, "A Focus on Nutrition for the Elderly: It's Time to Take a Closer Look," *Nutrition Insights*, Insight 14 (July 1999). Available online at www.usda.gov/cnpp.
12. United States Department of Agriculture, "Big Meals May Contribute to Body Fat in Older People," USDA Release No. 0340-97. Available online at www.usda.gov/news/releases/1997/10/0340.
13. Ibid.
14. Ibid.
15. Administration on Aging, "More Than a Meal: Celebrating Older Americans Act Elderly Nutrition Programs." Available online at www.aoa.dhhs.gov/25th.
16. "Administration on Aging, The Elderly Nutrition Program." Available online at www.aoa.dhhs.gov/factsheets.enp.html.
17. Administration on Aging, "Executive Summary: Serving Elders at Risk; the Older Americans Act Nutrition Programs—National Evaluation of the Elderly Nutrition Program, 1993–1995." Available online at www.aoa.dhhs.gov/aoa/nutreval/execsum.html.
18. Health Care Financing Administration, "The Characteristics and Perceptions of the Medicare Population (1998)," *Medicare Current Beneficiary Survey* (2001): Section 2. Available online at www.hcfa.gov/surveys/mcbs/PubCNP98.htm.
19. Administration on Aging, "Executive Summary."
20. U.S. Department of Agriculture, Food Surveys Research Group, Table Set 19, "Results from USDA's 1994–96 Diet and Health Knowledge Survey" (Beltsville, MD, 2000). Available online at www.barc.usda.gov/bhnrc/foodsurvey/home.htm.
21. RoperASW, 1999.
22. U.S. Department of Agriculture, Food Surveys Research Group, Table Set 19.
23. George P. Moschis et al., *The Maturing Marketplace, Buying Habits of Baby Boomers and Their Parents* (Westport, CT: Quorum Books, 2000), 21.
24. RoperASW, 1999.
25. Federal Interagency Forum on Aging Related Statistics, *Older Americans 2000: Key Indicators of Well-Being* (Hyattsville, MD, 2000), Table 23a.
26. Shirley Gerrior, "Dietary Changes in Older Americans from 1977 to 1996: Implications for Dietary Quality," *Family Economics and Nutrition Review* 12, no. 2 (1999): 3–14.
27. Ibid.
28. Ibid.
29. U.S. Department of Agriculture, Food Surveys Research Group, Table Set 19, "Results from USDA's 1994–96 Diet and Health Knowledge Survey" (Beltsville, MD, 2000). Available online at www.barc.usda.gov/bhnrc/foodsurvey/home.htm.
30. National Center for Health Statistics, *Health, United States, 1999 with Health and Aging Chartbook* (Hyattsville, MD, 1999). Data from the 1988–1994 National Health and Nutrition Examination Survey.
31. RoperASW, 1999.
32. RoperASW, 2000.
33. RoperASW, 1999.
34. Ibid.
35. Moschis et al., *Maturing Marketplace*.
36. RoperASW, 1997.

CHAPTER 8

Chronic Conditions and Common Health Problems

Good health and good sense are two of life's greatest blessings.

—Publilius Syrus

Old age is not a disease—it is strength and survivorship, triumph over all kinds of vicissitudes and disappointments, trials, and illness.

—Maggie Kuhn

The middle period of life is the safest, for it is not disturbed by the heat of youth, nor by the chill of age. Old age is more exposed to chronic diseases, youth to acute ones.

—Celsus (Roman 25 B.C.E.–50 C.E.)[1]

Chronic conditions, those which usually persist over a long period of time and which have no cure, constitute the most prevalent health problem for seniors, often leading to activity limitation, the need for extensive caregiving, and significant spending for health care. This chapter provides information on the major chronic illnesses that strike the elderly and other common health problems such as urinary incontinence, dental and visual impairments, hypertension, osteoporosis, and medical injuries.

Highlights of this chapter include:

- Chronic health problems are prevalent among the elderly and 1 in 3 has activity limitations associated with these conditions.
- Cancer is a common chronic health condition of the elderly. Seniors account for 6 in 10 of all cancers diagnosed each year.
- One in three people aged 70+ has a hearing impairment, and 1 in 5 is visually impaired.
- Incontinence is a problem for 20 percent of noninstitutionalized seniors.
- Nearly 1 in 3 seniors has no natural teeth.

- Nearly three-fourths of senior women have reduced hip bone density, and one-half of all women aged 85+ have osteoporosis.

- One in sixteen hospitalized elderly experiences a medical injury while in the hospital.

CHRONIC CONDITIONS

▪ Chronic conditions are common among the elderly

A study released in late 2002, analyzing a random sample of more than 1.2 million elderly Medicare beneficiaries' claims, found that 82 percent were treated for one or more chronic conditions in 1999. Treatment rates declined to 65 percent for two or more chronic conditions, 43 percent for three or more, and 24 percent for four or more types of chronic conditions. Study participants, on average, had 2.34 types of chronic conditions ranging from 1.88 types among people aged 65 to 69 years to 2.71 types among those aged 85+.[2]

According to self-reported data from the 1997 National Health Interview Survey, hypertension, hearing difficulties, and arthritic symptoms are among the most commonly reported chronic health problems among the elderly; one-third to nearly one-half of the elderly suffer from at least one of these ailments (see Chart 8.1).[3]

CHART 8.1   Percent of Elderly Reporting Selected Chronic Conditions: 1997

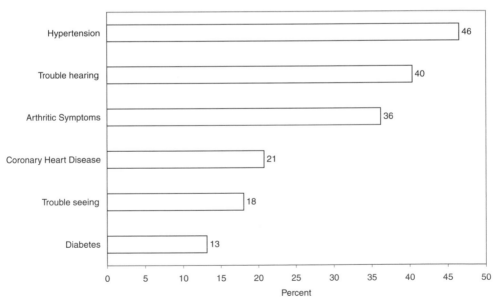

Source: Debra L. Blackwell, John Gary Collins, and Richard Coles, "Summary Health Statistics for U.S. Adults: National Health Interview Survey," series 10, no. 205 (National Center for Health Statistics, Vital and Health Statistics, May 2002). Additional calculations made by authors.

About 1 in 5 elderly has coronary heart disease or some trouble seeing and 13 percent of the elderly report having diabetes.

The likelihood of suffering from a chronic illness increases with age. For example, about one-quarter of people aged 45 to 64 report having hypertension compared with nearly one-half of those aged 75+. This trend is similar for most chronic conditions.

◼ Chronic conditions are more debilitating for the elderly than for younger adults

One-third (36 percent) of seniors report at least some activity limitation associated with chronic conditions, compared with 21 percent of adults aged 55 to 64, 13 percent of those aged 45 to 54, and 6 percent of those aged 18 to 44.[4] Among seniors, those aged 75+ are much more likely than those aged 65 to 74 to have activity limitations (46 percent versus 28 percent).

Senior men and women report similar levels of activity limitation. Younger black seniors aged 65 to 69, however, are 1.5 times more likely than younger white seniors to report activity limitations from chronic conditions (47 percent versus 32 percent).[5] In addition, less affluent seniors (those with annual incomes less than $10,000) are nearly twice as likely as those with annual incomes of $35,000 or more to report activity limitations (50 percent versus 28 percent, respectively).

Hypertension

◼ Hypertension affects 4 in 10 seniors

Hypertension (high blood pressure) affects 46 percent of the elderly and is a leading risk factor for heart and cerebrovascular disease (see Chart 8.1).[6] Data suggest that treating hypertension in people aged 60+ reduces mortality from all causes and reduces morbidity and mortality from stroke and coronary heart disease.[7] Unfortunately, only about one-half of people with hypertension have their condition controlled.[8]

Hypertension is most prevalent among older adults. Seniors are 1.7 times more likely than younger adults aged 45 to 64 to report they have the condition (see Chart 8.2).[9] Hypertension in the elderly is more common among women than men and among non-Hispanic blacks than non-Hispanic whites or Hispanics.

When based on physical examination, hypertension is more prevalent at all ages, but age and gender differences remain comparable to self-reported cases (see Table 8.1). Examination-based measures indicate that more than one-half of the elderly have hypertension.

◼ Nearly one-half of adults aged 50+ do not know their blood pressure

A recent survey among adults aged 50+ indicated that among those that have had their blood pressure taken, 45 percent did not know their own blood pressure measurements.[10] For those with high blood pressure, the figure was somewhat better, 35 percent. Forty-nine percent of all respondents said they had their blood pressure

CHART 8.2   Percent Reporting Hypertension, by Age, Sex, and Race/Ethnicity: 1997

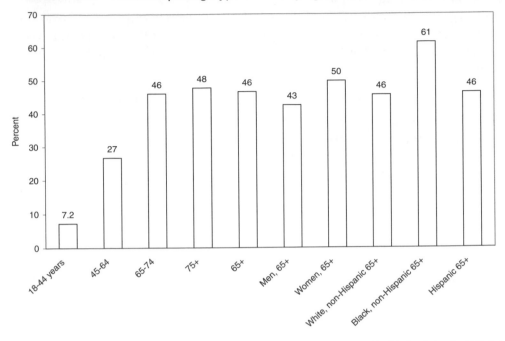

Source: Debra L. Blackwell, John Gary Collins, and Richard Coles, "Summary Health Statistics for U.S. Adults: National Health Interview Survey," series 10, no. 205 (National Center for Health Statistics, Vital and Health Statistics, May 2002). Additional calculations made by authors.

TABLE 8.1
Percent of Population with Hypertension, by Age and Sex: 1988–1994

	Men	Women	Ratio of Men to Women	Ratio of Women to Men
20–34 years	8.6%	3.4%	2.53	0.40
35–44	21	13	1.65	0.61
45–54	34	25	1.36	0.74
55–64	43	44	0.97	1.03
65–74	57	61	0.94	1.06
75+	64	77	0.83	1.20

Note: Data are based on physical examination in which blood pressure is at least 140/90, or the person is taking antihypertensive medication.
Source: National Center for Health Statistics, *Health, United States, 2002 with Chartbook on Trends in the Health of Americans* (Hyattsville, MD, 2002), Table 68. Data from the National Health and Nutrition Examination Survey.

checked in the past month, and 80 percent said it was checked in the past 4 months. Additionally, most were reasonably well informed about lifestyle and dietary changes that can help control blood pressure. People with high blood pressure had their blood pressure checked quite frequently; over a 12-month period, 5 percent have checked it daily, 15 percent at least weekly (but not daily), and 35 percent at least monthly (but not weekly).

Hearing Impairments

■ Four in ten older seniors are hearing impaired

Forty percent of seniors report trouble hearing (without a hearing aid), with men more likely than women to report such conditions (see Chart 8.3).[11] About equal numbers of adults aged 70+ experience either deafness in both ears (7 percent) or deafness in one ear (8 percent).[12]

Hearing impairments are more common at older ages. Seniors aged 75+ are 1.4 times more likely to have a chronic hearing impairment than younger seniors aged 65 to 74 (see Chart 8.3). These younger seniors are, in turn, 1.6 times as likely as to have a chronic hearing impairment as are younger adults aged 45 to 64. Non-Hispanic white seniors report a chronic hearing impairment 1.7 times as often as do non-Hispanic black seniors.

CHART 8.3   Percent Reporting Trouble Hearing, by Age, Sex, and Race/Ethnicity: 1997

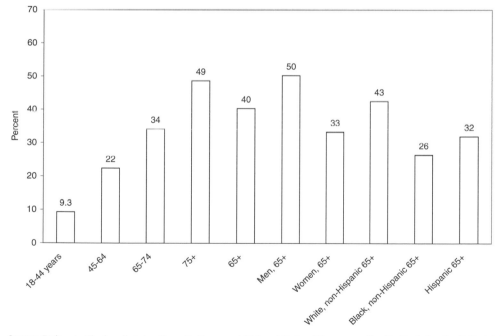

Source: Debra L. Blackwell, John Gary Collins, and Richard Coles, "Summary Health Statistics for U.S. Adults: National Health Interview Survey," series 10, no. 205 (National Center for Health Statistics, Vital and Health Statistics, May 2002). Additional calculations made by authors.

According to the 1999 National Nursing Home Survey, almost one-quarter (23 percent) of elderly nursing home residents of known status have any difficulty in hearing, even when wearing a hearing aid.[13] Three-quarters of hearing-impaired residents are partially impaired, 23 percent are severely impaired, and 2 percent are deaf.

■ Hearing impairments affect seniors' quality of life

Hearing impairment is a deterrent to activity (see Table 8.2). Adults aged 70+ who are hearing-impaired are more likely than their nonimpaired peers to report difficulty with various daily activities and to experience more medical conditions. Hearing impairment does not diminish social activities, however, such as restaurant attendance or getting together with friends or family.

■ Most hearing-impaired seniors do not use hearing aids

Unfortunately, only one-third of hearing-impaired adults aged 70+ report using a hearing aid during the previous 12 months.[14] Overall, 11 percent of elderly nursing home patients use a hearing aid.[15] This proportion rises to 26 percent among those who have difficulty hearing (even with a hearing aid) and varies from 21 percent of those who are partially impaired, 42 percent of those who are severely impaired, and 25 percent of those who are deaf.

A 1999 study of hearing-impaired adults aged 50+ indicated that the most common reason given for not using a hearing aid, even among those with severe hearing

TABLE 8.2
Percent of Elderly Aged 70+ Reporting Various Conditions, by Hearing Status: 1994

	Hearing Impaired	Nonimpaired	Ratio of Impaired to Nonimpaired
Getting together with relatives	77%	75%	1.03
Getting together with friends	69	72	0.96
Going out to eat at a restaurant	63	64	0.98
Difficulty walking	31	21	1.48
Difficulty getting outside	17	12	1.42
Difficulty getting into or out of a bed or chair	15	10	1.50
Difficulty preparing meals	12	7.6	1.58
Heart disease	28	19	1.47
A fall	28	18	1.56
Stroke	12	7.8	1.54
Frequently depressed or anxious	9.9	7.2	1.38

Source: Centers for Disease Control and Prevention, "Surveillance for Sensory Impairment, Activity Limitation, and Health Related Quality of Life among Older Adults—United States, 1993–1997," *MMWR, CDC Surveillance Summaries* 48, no. SS-8 (December 17, 1999): Table 3. Data from the National Health Interview Second Supplement on Aging.

TABLE 8.3

Percent of Hearing-Impaired Adults Aged 50+ Giving Various Reasons for Not Using Hearing Aids: 1999

	All Respondents	Milder Hearing Loss	More Severe Hearing Loss
Denial			
My hearing isn't bad enough	69%	73%	64%
I can get along without one	68	78	55
Consumer concerns			
They are too expensive	55	48	64
They won't help my specific problem	33	31	36
I've heard they don't work well	28	26	31
I don't trust hearing specialists	25	22	29
I tried one and it didn't work	17	15	20
Stigma or vanity			
It would make me feel old	20	18	22
I don't like the way they look	19	18	21
I'm too embarrassed to wear one	18	16	21
I don't like what others will think about me.	16	15	19

Source: The National Council on the Aging, "The Consequences of Untreated Hearing Loss in Older Persons" (May 1999). Available online at www.ncoa.org.

loss, is their belief that they do not need hearing aids (see Table 8.3).[16] Expense is the second most prevalent reason for nonuse, followed by a lack of belief that hearing aids will help. Stigma and vanity-related reasons are among the least stated reasons, but are still noted by about 1 in 5 hearing-impaired people who do not use hearing aids.

Hearing aids improve quality of life

Older adults who do not use hearing aids are more likely than those who do to report diminished quality of life. They report feeling sadness or depression, worry, anxiety, or paranoia, and they experience emotional turmoil and insecurity and less social activity.[17]

Conversely, when hearing loss is treated, adults often report improvements in many areas of their lives including better relationships with their families, better feelings about themselves, improved mental health, greater independence and security, and more social interaction. Improvements are greatest among those whose hearing loss was more severe. Family members of the hearing impaired report even greater lifestyle improvements when hearing aids are used by their hearing-impaired relatives.

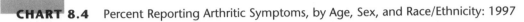

CHART 8.4   Percent Reporting Arthritic Symptoms, by Age, Sex, and Race/Ethnicity: 1997

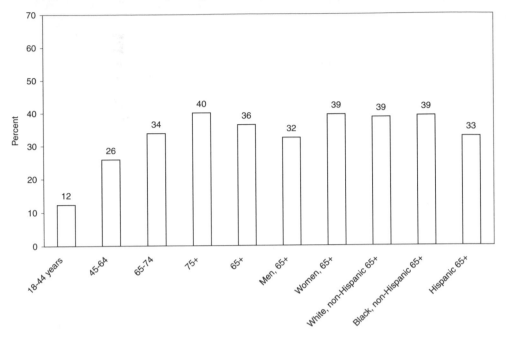

Source: Debra L. Blackwell, John Gary Collins, and Richard Coles, "Summary Health Statistics for U.S. Adults: National Health Interview Survey," series 10, no. 205 (National Center for Health Statistics, Vital and Health Statistics, May 2002). Additional calculations made by authors.

Arthritic Symptoms

■ Nearly 1 in 2 seniors suffers from arthritic symptoms

Forty-six percent of seniors experience arthritic symptoms (see Chart 8.1).[18] Arthritis is 1.4 times as common among seniors as among younger adults aged 45 to 64 and is somewhat more likely among older seniors than younger seniors (see Chart 8.4). Chronic arthritis is also more prevalent among elderly women than among elderly men, and elderly non-Hispanics than elderly Hispanics.

Coronary Heart Disease

■ Coronary heart disease is reported by 1 in 5 seniors

Twenty-one percent of seniors report having coronary heart disease, including heart attack and angina but not hypertension.[19] Coronary heart disease is three times as common in the elderly as in younger adults aged 45 to 64 (see Chart 8.5). Among the elderly, it is also more common among older than younger seniors, men than women, and non-Hispanic whites than Hispanics.

CHART 8.5   Percent Reporting Coronary Heart Disease, by Age, Sex, and Race/Ethnicity: 1997

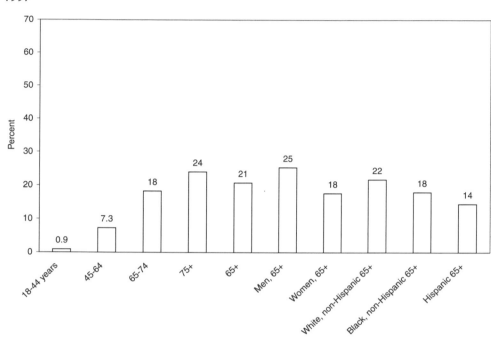

Source: Debra L. Blackwell, John Gary Collins, and Richard Coles, "Summary Health Statistics for U.S. Adults: National Health Interview Survey," series 10, no. 205 (National Center for Health Statistics, Vital and Health Statistics, May 2002). Additional calculations made by authors.

Vision Impairments

Six percent of adults aged 60+ purchased a large-print book in 1998.[20]

■ About 1 in 5 American seniors is visually impaired

Nearly 1 in 5 seniors (18 percent) reports trouble seeing even when wearing glasses or contact lenses.[21] The elderly are 1.5 times more likely than younger adults aged 45 to 64 to be visually impaired (see Chart 8.6). Among the elderly, vision impairments vary by age but do not vary considerably by gender or race/ethnicity. Vision impairments are 1.6 times more common in the elderly aged 75+ than in those aged 65–74.

A 1995 study, the Lighthouse National Survey on Vision Loss, reported that 21 percent of the elderly said they have some form of vision impairment.[22] Specifically, 17 percent of people aged 65 to 74 and 26 percent of those aged 75+ reported some form of vision impairment. Eleven percent of the elderly (or half of all vision-impaired elderly) reported severe vision impairment. This group included those who are blind in both eyes.

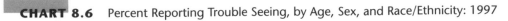

CHART 8.6   Percent Reporting Trouble Seeing, by Age, Sex, and Race/Ethnicity: 1997

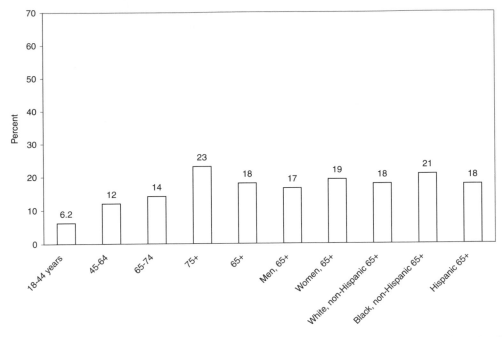

Source: Debra L. Blackwell, John Gary Collins, and Richard Coles, "Summary Health Statistics for U.S. Adults: National Health Interview Survey," series 10, no. 205 (National Center for Health Statistics, Vital and Health Statistics, May 2002). Additional calculations made by authors.

DEFINITION: Severe vision impairment is defined as the inability to see to read ordinary newspaper print even when wearing corrective lenses.

The vast majority of vision impairments entail partial sightedness rather than to-tal blindness.[23] Only 2 percent of seniors aged 70+ report blindness in both eyes; 4 percent are blind in one eye.

According to the 1999 National Nursing Home Survey, 29 percent of elderly nurs-ing home residents of known status have difficulty seeing, even if they wear glasses.[24] Two-thirds (67 percent) of vision-impaired residents are partially vision im-paired, one-quarter are severely vision impaired, and 8 percent are blind.

Age-related macular degeneration is the leading cause of irreversible visual im-pairment among people aged 75+, and it is the most common cause of new cases of visual impairment among all elderly.[25] An estimated 5 percent of the elderly have some visual impairment as a result of macular degeneration. More than one-third of people aged 75+ have macular degeneration, and about 3 percent are in the late stages of the disease.

Six percent of the elderly have glaucoma.[26] Clinical data indicate that half of the population aged 65 to 74 have cataracts, and this increases to about 70 percent among those aged 75+. Self-reported data from the National Health Interview Survey indicated that 15 percent of the elderly aged 65 to 74 and 20 percent of those aged 75+ have cataracts.[27]

To aid their vision, 92 percent of adults aged 70+ report wearing glasses, 17 percent use a magnifier, and 15 percent had a lens implant to treat a cataract.[28]

■ Vision impaired seniors are less active

Vision impairments are far more detrimental to activities and medical outcomes than are hearing impairments. Vision-impaired adults aged 70+ report substantially more activity limitations and medical problems than their nonimpaired counterparts.[29] They are more than twice as likely as their nonimpaired counterparts to report difficulty with various activities and to have a higher occurrence of certain medical conditions (see Table 8.4). Vision-impaired older adults are also less likely to get together with friends and less likely to go out to eat at a restaurant.

■ Few elderly wear contact lenses

According to Mediamark Research, 7 in 10 elderly wear prescription eyeglasses or contact lenses (see Table 8.5).[30] Eyeglasses are by far the preferred method for correcting vision problems, with 69 percent of the elderly wearing prescription eyeglasses and only 3 percent wearing contact lenses. Contact lens use falls dramatically and prescription eyeglass usage rises among older age groups. (See Chapter 5, "Health Status, Use of Health Services, and Attitudes toward Health Care Providers," for information on eye care.)

TABLE 8.4
Percent of Elderly Aged 70+ Reporting Various Conditions, by Vision Status: 1994

	Vision Impaired	Nonimpaired	Ratio of Impaired to Nonimpaired
Getting together with relatives	74%	76%	0.97
Getting together with friends	65	73	0.89
Going out to eat at a restaurant	56	65	0.86
Difficulty walking	43	20	2.15
Difficulty getting outside	29	10	2.90
Difficulty getting into or out of a bed or chair	22	9.3	2.37
Difficulty preparing meals	19	6.7	2.84
Difficulty managing medication	12	4.4	2.73
Hypertension	54	43	1.26
A fall	31	19	1.63
Heart disease	30	20	1.50
Stroke	17	7.3	2.33
Frequently depressed or anxious	13	7.0	1.86

Source: Centers for Disease Control and Prevention, "Surveillance for Sensory Impairment, Activity Limitation, and Health Related Quality of Life among Older Adults—United States, 1993–1997," *MMWR, CDC Surveillance Summaries* 48, no. SS-8 (December 17, 1999): Table 3.

TABLE 8.5
Percent of Elderly Who Wear Prescription Eyeglasses or Contacts: 2000

	18–24 Years	25–34 Years	35–44 Years	45–54 Years	55–64 Years	65+ Years	Under 65 Years
Wear prescription eyeglasses and/or contacts	37%	36%	43%	59%	66%	71%	47%
Eyeglasses or bifocals	26	27	35	54	62	69	39
Contact lenses	19	19	15	11	7	3	15

Source: Mediamark Research Inc. Spring 2000.

According to the 1999 National Nursing Home Survey, 65 percent of elderly nursing home residents wear eyeglasses or contacts.[31] The likelihood of wearing corrective eyewear is 70 percent among those with partial sight impairments, 62 percent among those with severe vision impairments, and 29 percent among those who are blind.

■ About 1 in 10 seniors has both hearing and vision impairments

About 9 percent of those aged 70+ report both a hearing and vision impairment with no measurable difference by sex.[32] The effect of dual impairments upon activities and medical outcomes is virtually the same as for those who have visual impairments only.

Diabetes

■ Diabetes afflicts 1 in 10 seniors

Diabetes mellitus is a group of diseases characterized by high levels of blood glucose resulting from defects in insulin secretion, insulin action, or both. Diabetes can be associated with serious complications and premature death, but people with diabetes can take measures to reduce the likelihood of such occurrences.

According to the National Health Interview Survey, slightly more than 1 in 10 elderly are afflicted with diabetes with elderly men and women equally afflicted (see Chart 8.7).[33] Diabetes is 1.7 times as common among seniors as among younger adults aged 45 to 64. Elderly non-Hispanic blacks and Hispanics are twice as likely as non-Hispanic whites to have diabetes.

According to data from the 1998 Behavioral Risk Factor Surveillance System, diabetes prevalence increases with age, with older Americans eight times more likely than the youngest adults to report diabetes (see Table 8.6).[34] Diabetes has become more prevalent among all age groups since 1990.

CHART 8.7   Percent Reporting Diabetes, by Age, Sex, and Race/Ethnicity: 1997

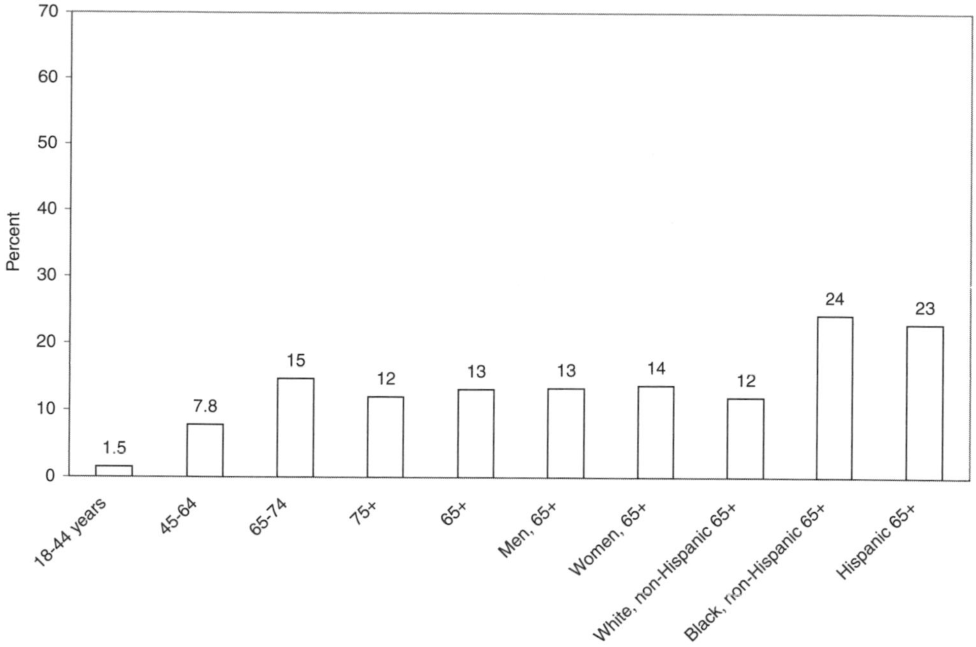

Source: Debra L. Blackwell, John Gary Collins, and Richard Coles, "Summary Health Statistics for U.S. Adults: National Health Interview Survey," series 10, no. 205 (National Center for Health Statistics, Vital and Health Statistics, May 2002). Additional calculations made by authors.

TABLE 8.6
Percent Reporting Diabetes, by Age: 1990 and 1998

	1990	1998	Percent Difference 1998 versus 1990
18–29 years	1.5%	1.6%	9.1%
30–39	2.1	3.7	70
40–49	3.6	5.1	40
50–59	7.5	9.8	31
60–69	11	13	17
70+	12	13	10

Source: Ali H. Mokdad et al., "Diabetes Trends in the U.S.: 1990–1998," *Diabetes Care* 23, no. 9 (September 2000): 1278–1283, Table 3.

TABLE 8.7
Incidence (per 100,000 Persons) of New Cancers,
by Age and Sex: 1994–1998

	Men	Women	Ratio of Men to Women
65+ years	2,833	1,665	1.70
65–69	2,275	1,351	1.68
70–74	2,931	1,691	1.73
75–79	3,213	1,889	1.70
80–84	3,393	2,015	1.68
85+	3,254	1,920	1.69

Source: National Cancer Institute, *SEER Cancer Statistics Review 1973–1998* (Bethesda, MD, 2001), Table II-3.

Cancer

All cancer statistics in this section as well as the following sections on breast, prostate, lung, and colorectal cancers, come from the National Cancer Institute's *SEER Cancer Statistics Review*, covering data from 1973 to 1996.[35]

■ Senior men are more likely than senior women to be diagnosed with cancer

Cancer is the second leading cause of death for the elderly and a major chronic condition for this age group. Seniors account for 59 percent of all cancers diagnosed annually. Senior men are 1.7 times as likely as their female counterparts to be diagnosed with cancer (see Table 8.7).

Among the elderly, white women are more likely than black women to be diagnosed with cancer and black men, except those aged 85+, are more likely than white men to be diagnosed with cancer (see Table 8.8). Although senior black women are the least likely to be diagnosed with cancer, they have the lowest 5-year survival rate (only 40 percent are still alive 5 years after their cancer diagnosis).

Men who are diagnosed with cancer during their senior years have a 5-year relative survival rate of 63 percent compared with 53 percent for women. Between 1973 and 1996, the annual incidence of newly diagnosed cancers among the elderly increased about 25 percent.

Breast Cancer

■ Breast cancer is the most commonly diagnosed cancer among senior women

Senior women account for 46 percent of all breast cancers diagnosed annually. Breast cancer is the most commonly diagnosed cancer among senior women and is

TABLE 8.8

Incidence (per 100,000 Persons) of New Cancers, by Age, Sex, and Race: 1994–1998

	White	Black	Ratio of White to Black	Ratio of Black to White
Men, 65+ years	2,828	3,348	0.84	1.18
65–69	2,271	2,791	0.81	1.23
70–74	2,907	3,739	0.78	1.29
75–79	3,206	3,731	0.86	1.16
80–84	3,401	3,680	0.92	1.08
85+	3,293	3,039	1.08	0.92
Women, 65+ years	1,705	1,616	1.06	0.95
65–69	1,396	1,311	1.06	0.94
70–74	1,735	1,667	1.04	0.96
75–79	1,932	1,817	1.06	0.94
80–84	2,045	1,942	1.05	0.95
85+	1,940	1,848	1.05	0.95

Source: National Cancer Institute, *SEER Cancer Statistics Review 1973–1998* (Bethesda, MD, 2001), Table II-3.

diagnosed nearly twice as often as lung cancer. White women are more likely than black women to be diagnosed with breast cancers (see Table 8.9). From 1973 to 1996, breast cancer incidence among elderly women increased about 40 percent.

Women who are diagnosed with breast cancer in their senior years have an overall 5-year survival rate of 86 percent: 87 percent for white women and 73 percent for black women. These survival rates are the same as those for nonelderly women.

TABLE 8.9

Incidence (per 100,000 Persons) of New Breast Cancers among Elderly Women, by Age and Race: 1994–1998

	Total	White	Black	Ratio of White to Black
65+ years	449	468	383	1.22
65–69	410	428	352	1.22
70–74	471	492	398	1.24
75–79	490	510	418	1.22
80–84	482	497	413	1.20
85+	397	411	340	1.21

Source: National Cancer Institute, *SEER Cancer Statistics Review 1973–1998* (Bethesda, MD, 2001), Table IV-2.

TABLE 8.10
Incidence (per 100,000 Persons) of New Prostate Cancers
among Elderly Men, by Age and Race: 1994–1998

	Total	White	Black	Ratio of Black to White
65+ years	966	932	1,458	1.56
65–69	860	838	1,304	1.56
70–74	1,084	1,046	1,748	1.67
75–79	1,057	1,010	1,562	1.55
80–84	937	895	1,293	1.44
85+	852	822	1,108	1.35

Source: National Cancer Institute, *SEER Cancer Statistics Review
1973–1998* (Bethesda, MD, 2001), Table XXII-2.

Prostate Cancer

■ Prostate cancer is the most commonly diagnosed cancer among senior men

Senior men account for 71 percent of all prostate cancers diagnosed annually. About 1 percent of senior men are diagnosed with prostate cancer each year, with black men about 1.6 times more likely than white men to be diagnosed (see Table 8.10).

Between 1973 and 1996, prostate cancer incidence among elderly men increased about 70 percent. Men who are diagnosed with prostate cancer in their senior years have a 5-year survival rate of 97 percent.

Lung Cancer

■ Lung cancer is more common among senior men than senior women

More than two-thirds (68 percent) of diagnosed lung cancers are among seniors. Elderly men are substantially more likely to be diagnosed with lung cancer than are women, and black men more so than white men (see Tables 8.11 and 8.12). From 1973 to 1998, however, the incidence of lung cancer dramatically increased among senior women. Elderly women in 1998 were 3.5 times as likely to be diagnosed with lung cancer than their counterparts in 1973. In contrast, senior men were only 11 percent more likely.

Men who are diagnosed with lung cancer during their senior years have a 5-year relative survival rate of 12 percent, compared with 14 percent for women.

TABLE 8.11
Incidence (per 100,000 Persons) of New Lung and
Bronchus Cancers, by Age and Sex: 1994–1998

	Men	Women	Ratio of Men to Women
65+ years	477	260	1.83
65–69	389	235	1.66
70–74	508	287	1.77
75–79	556	295	1.88
80–84	554	268	2.07
85+	448	172	2.60

Source: National Cancer Institute, SEER Cancer Statistics
Review 1973–1998 (Bethesda, MD, 2001), Table XV-3.

Colorectal Cancer

Seniors account for 71 percent of the colorectal cancers diagnosed annually. Elderly
men are more likely than women to be diagnosed with colorectal cancer (see Table
8.13). Elderly black women are more likely than elderly white women to be diag-

TABLE 8.12
Incidence (per 100,000 Persons) of New Lung and Bronchus Cancers,
by Age, Sex, and Race: 1994–1998

	White	Black	Ratio of White to Black	Ratio of Black to White
Men, 65+ years	476	621	0.77	1.30
65–69	388	515	0.75	1.33
70–74	502	713	0.70	1.42
75–79	560	709	0.79	1.27
80–84	561	696	0.81	1.24
85+	452	439	1.03	0.97
Women, 65+ years	271	245	1.11	0.90
65–69	249	230	1.08	0.92
70–74	300	280	1.07	0.93
75–79	305	265	1.15	0.87
80–84	275	228	1.21	0.83
85+	171	171	1.00	1.00

Source: National Cancer Institute, SEER Cancer Statistics Review 1973–1998
(Bethesda, MD, 2001), Table XV-3.

TABLE 8.13

Incidence (per 100,000 Persons) of New Colorectal Cancers, by Age and Sex: 1994–1998

	Men	Women	Ratio of Men to Women
65+ years	345	246	1.40
65–69	240	155	1.55
70–74	319	227	1.41
75–79	406	290	1.40
80–84	513	382	1.34
85+	523	421	1.24

Source: National Cancer Institute, SEER Cancer Statistics Review 1973–1998 (Bethesda, MD, 2001), Table VI-3.

nosed with colorectal cancer, except in the 85+ age category (see Table 8.14). Generally, elderly black men tend to have slightly lower colorectal cancer diagnosis rates than do elderly white men.

From 1973 to 1996, the incidence of new colorectal cancers among seniors overall declined about 8 percent. However, blacks have seen a 14 percent increase compared with a 9 percent decrease for whites.

TABLE 8.14

Incidence (per 100,000 Persons) of New Colorectal Cancers, by Age, Sex, and Race: 1994–1998

	White	Black	Ratio of White to Black	Ratio of Black to White
Men, 65+ years	349	342	1.02	0.98
65–69	241	224	1.08	0.93
70–74	320	344	0.93	1.08
75–79	412	411	1.00	1.00
80–84	520	523	0.99	1.01
85+	542	430	1.26	0.79
Women, 65+ years	248	274	0.91	1.10
65–69	154	190	0.81	1.23
70–74	227	267	0.85	1.18
75–79	293	326	0.90	1.11
80–84	384	401	0.96	1.04
85+	433	363	1.19	0.84

Source: National Cancer Institute, SEER Cancer Statistics Review 1973–1998 (Bethesda, MD, 2001), Table VI-3.

Seniors who are diagnosed with colorectal cancer during their senior years have a 5-year relative survival rate of 61 percent. However, survival rates for blacks are significantly lower than for whites (49 percent versus 62 percent).

OTHER COMMON HEALTH PROBLEMS

Urinary Incontinence

When you get to my age, life seems little more than one long march to and from the lavatory.

—John Mortimer

Mediamark Research data indicate that 7 percent of the elderly used incontinence products in a 6-month period (10 percent of elderly women and 4 percent of elderly men).[36] Product usage is heavily skewed toward the elderly because only 1 percent of younger adults have used the products.

■ Urinary incontinence is higher among institutionalized seniors

According to the 1998 Medicare Current Beneficiary Survey, 23 percent of elderly Medicare beneficiaries suffer urinary incontinence (see Table 8.15). Urinary incontinence is more prevalent among older seniors, afflicting 4 in 10 of the oldest-old. Women are more likely than men to suffer from incontinence, although this gap narrows at the oldest age categories.

DEFINITION: Incontinence is defined as losing urine beyond one's control at least once during the last 12 months.

Predictably, incontinence is substantially more prevalent among the institutionalized elderly Medicare population—64 percent versus 20 percent of elderly community residents. The earlier figure is relatively comparable to the 1999 National Nurs-

TABLE 8.15
Percent of Elderly Medicare Beneficiaries Who Have Urinary Incontinence: 1998

	Total	Men	Women	Ratio of Women to Men
65+ years	23%	13%	29%	2.14
64–74	17	8.9	23	2.56
75–84	25	16	30	1.83
85+	41	32	44	1.42

Source: Health Care Financing Administration, Medicare Current Beneficiary Survey, "The Characteristics and Perceptions of the Medicare Population (1998)," (2001).

TABLE 8.16
Percent of Elderly Medicare Beneficiaries Who Have Urinary
Incontinence, by Residence: 1998

	Community Residents	Institutionalized	Ratio of Institutionalized to Community Residents
65+ years	20%	64%	3.20
64–74	16	54	3.38
75–84	23	63	2.74
85+	34	66	1.94

Source: Health Care Financing Administration, Medicare Current Beneficiary Survey, "The Characteristics and Perceptions of the Medicare Population (1998)," (2001).

ing Home Survey figure of 56 percent of elderly residents (of known status) having difficulty controlling their bladders.[37] Urinary incontinence ranges from 54 percent of the youngest institutionalized elderly Medicare beneficiaries to 66 percent of the oldest (see Table 8.16).

The total cost of urinary incontinence in 1995 is estimated at $26.3 billion.[38] Of that, $23.6 billion is for diagnosis, treatment, and routine care. An additional $2 billion is spent on other related care requirements, such as skin conditions and longer periods of inpatient care, and $704 million is spent on indirect costs, such as home health care services.

Dental Problems

■ About 1 in 3 seniors has untreated dental caries

Older adults are at higher risk for various oral conditions and diseases due to underlying chronic conditions, medications, and age-related physiological changes. Older adults who do not receive regular dental care are at risk for oral diseases that can significantly impact their quality of life.[39]

Dental decay is a major cause of tooth loss in the elderly. Between 1988 and 1994, nearly 1 in 3 seniors with natural teeth had untreated dental caries in the roots or crowns of their teeth.[40] Elderly men are more likely than elderly women to have at least one untreated dental carie (35 percent versus 27 percent). Elderly black people are twice as likely as elderly white people to have untreated dental caries (47 percent versus 23 percent).[41] Poor elderly people of both races are more likely to have dental caries than are those who are not poor. One study of nursing home residents found that 70 percent had untreated dental decay.[42]

TABLE 8.17
Percent of Adults with Severe Periodontal Disease: 1996

	Total	Men	Women	Socioeconomic Status		
				Low	Middle	High
25–34 years	3%	4%	2%	4%	3%	1%
35–44	7	10	4	12	7	4
45–54	14	18	10	26	17	8
55–64	19	25	14	22	18	18
65–74	23	30	18	38	19	17
75+	30	35	26	36	26	23

Source: U.S. Department of Health and Human Services, *Oral Health in America: A Report of the Surgeon General* (Rockville, MD: U.S. Department of Health and Human Services, National Institute of Dental and Craniofacial Research, National Institutes of Health, 2000), Figures 4.7, 4.9–4.11.

■ One in four seniors has severe periodontal disease

Periodontal disease is more prevalent among older people than younger adults.[43] Severe periodontal disease occurs in about 1 in 4 seniors aged 65 to 74 and in 30 percent of those aged 75+ (see Table 8.17). The disease is more than twice as likely in adults aged 75+ as it is in those aged 45 to 54.

> **DEFINITION:** Severe periodontal disease is defined as having 6 millimeters or more of detached gum tissue at one or more sites.

Among seniors aged 70+, non-Hispanic blacks are twice as likely as non-Hispanic whites to have severe periodontal disease (47 percent versus 24 percent). At every age, severe periodontal disease is more prevalent in men and people of lower socioeconomic status (see Table 8.17).

■ Nearly 1 in 3 seniors has no natural teeth

Total tooth loss is most prevalent among the elderly with 30 percent of seniors having no natural teeth (see Chart 8.8).[44] An additional 13 percent are missing either their upper or lower teeth. Forty-nine percent of elderly nursing home residents have no permanent teeth,[45] and at least 80 percent of nursing home residents have some tooth loss.[46]

According to the National Health Interview Survey, up until age 75, people are more likely to have all their natural teeth, although the tendency diminishes as age increases (see Chart 8.8).[47] People aged 75+ are just as likely to have some tooth loss as they are to have all their natural teeth. Among the elderly, non-Hispanic blacks are the most likely race/ethnic group to be missing all their teeth.

Seniors in West Virginia, Kentucky, and Louisiana are the most likely to be toothless: 48 percent, 44 percent, and 43 percent of seniors in these states, respectively,

CHART 8.8   Tooth Loss Status by Age, Sex, and Race/Ethnicity: 1997

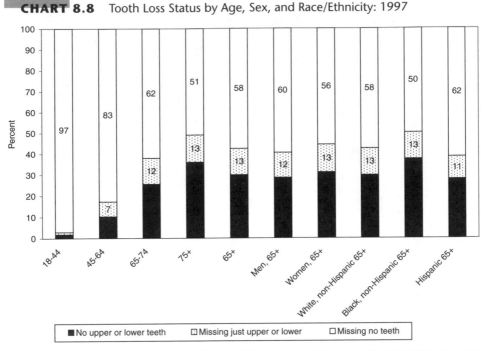

■ No upper or lower teeth   ▨ Missing just upper or lower   ☐ Missing no teeth

Source: Debra L. Blackwell, John Gary Collins, and Richard Coles, "Summary Health Statistics for U.S. Adults: National Health Interview Survey," series 10, no. 205 (National Center for Health Statistics, Vital and Health Statistics, May 2002). Additional calculations made by authors.

have no teeth.[48] In contrast, fewer than 20 percent of seniors in Hawaii, California, Oregon, Arizona, and Wisconsin have no teeth.

Between 1983 and 1993, the prevalence of total tooth loss among the elderly declined 23 percent from (38 percent to 30 percent); improvements occurred for all racial and socioeconomic groups.[49]

Thirty-eight percent of the elderly are apparent denture wearers, having used denture adhesive, fixatives, or cleaners in a 6-month period.[50] Forty-five percent of elderly nursing home residents wear dentures,[51] and one-half of nursing home residents who wear dentures need to have them replaced or relined.[52]

According to Mediamark Research, nearly half of seniors use dental floss and, on average, do so on a daily basis.[53] Due at least in part to higher rates of total tooth loss, the elderly are substantially less likely than younger adults to use dental floss (47 percent versus 62 percent).

Falls, Fractures, and Osteoporosis

■ One in three elderly falls each year

Although data are limited, available statistics indicate that unintentional falls accounted for 87 percent of the fractures for which seniors were treated in emergency rooms in 1977.[54] On average, 1 in 3 seniors falls each year, with 20 to 30 percent of

those who fall suffering moderate to severe injuries that reduce mobility and independence and increase the risk of premature death.[55]

In 1997, 8.6 percent of seniors received medical attention for fall-related injuries
compared with 3.2 percent of younger adults aged 45 to 64.[56] Elderly women are
more than twice as likely as elderly men to be treated for a fall-related injury (11 percent versus 4.7 percent). The total direct cost of fall-related injuries for seniors in the
United States was $20.2 billion in 1994 and is expected to reach $32.4 billion by
2020.[57]

■ Hip fractures are extremely disabling

Hip fractures are one of the most serious consequences of falls among the elderly.
Ninety-five percent of hip fractures result from falls.[58] One-half of all older adults
who suffer hip fractures never regain their former level of functioning.[59] In fact, 1 in
4 elderly people who incur an osteoporotic hip fracture will require long-term nursing home care, and one-half will need assistance walking. Additionally, the mortality risk increases up to 24 percent within the first year following the fracture.[60]

Women account for three-quarters of fall-related hip fractures among the elderly
and are about two to three times more likely than men to be hospitalized due to a
hip fracture (see Table 8.18).[61] Hip fractures accounted for more than 300,000 hospitalizations among seniors in 1996, 80 percent of whom were elderly women.[62]

Elderly white women are hospitalized for hip fractures at five times the rate of
black women, in part because the prevalence and severity of osteoporosis is greatest
among white women. There are 1,174 hospitalizations for hip fracture among every
100,000 white women, compared to 230 hospitalizations for every 100,000 black
women.[63, 64] Other risk factors include low body mass index, a previous history of
osteoporosis, and having had a previous hip fracture.[65]

From 1988 to 1996, hip fracture hospitalization rates increased for women but remained unchanged for men. Hospitalization rates for hip fractures also increase dramatically with age: men aged 85+ are 13 times, and women 8 times, more likely

TABLE 8.18
Rate (per 100,000 Persons) of Hospitalizations for
Hip Fractures, by Age and Sex: 1996

	Men	Women	Ratio of Women to Men
65–74 years	168	501	2.98
75–84	682	1,620	2.38
85	2,256	3,958	1.75

Source: Data from the 1996 National Hospital Discharge
Survey, as reported in Centers for Disease Control and
Prevention, "Surveillance Injuries and Violence among
Older Adults," *MMWR, CDC Surveillance Summaries* 48, no.
SS-8 (December 17, 1999): Table 2.

than their youngest cohorts (aged 65 to 74) to be hospitalized for a hip fracture (see Table 8.18).

■ Hip fractures are costly

Seniors account for about 88 percent of all health care expenditures for osteoporosis-related fractures. Hip fractures are the most frequent, devastating, and costly type of fracture for seniors. A 1997 study finds that hip fractures cost the patient between $16,300 and $18,700 in direct medical care, formal nonmedical care, and informally provided family care during the first year following a hip fracture.[66]

■ Hip replacement procedures among the elderly are on the rise

Hip replacement procedures among seniors increased threefold to tenfold from 1987 to 1995. Hip replacements are most common among women aged 85+ (1,444 replacements per 100,000 in 1995) followed by women aged 80 to 84 (965 per 100,000).[67]

■ Seniors experience loss of bone density—women more so than men

Hip bone density is a strong predictor of future fractures, especially of the hip.[68] Osteopenia, the less severe form of reduced bone density, is quite prevalent among

TABLE 8.19
Detailed Data for Chart 8.9: Percent of Adults with Reduced Hip Bone Density, by Age and Sex, 1988–1994

	Men	Women	Ratio of Women to Men
Osteopenia			
65+ years	22%	46%	2.11
65–74	18	47	2.62
75–84	28	46	1.64
85+	40	40	0.99
Osteoporosis			
65+ years	3.8	26	6.87
65–74	2.0	19	9.50
75–84	6.4	33	5.08
85+	14	51	3.69
Osteopenia or osteoporosis			
65+ years	26	72	2.79
65–74	20	66	3.30
75–84	34	79	2.32
85+	54	91	1.69

Source: National Center for Health Statistics, *Health, United States, 1999 with Health and Aging Chartbook* (Hyattsville, MD, 1999), Figure 14.

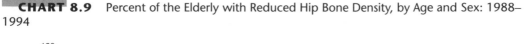

CHART 8.9   Percent of the Elderly with Reduced Hip Bone Density, by Age and Sex: 1988–1994

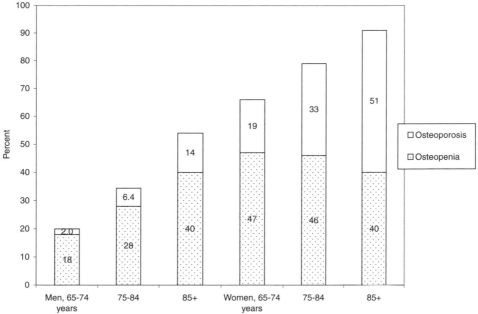

Source: National Center for Health Statistics, *Health, United States, 1999 with Health and Aging Chartbook* (Hyattsville, MD, 1999), Figure 14.

elderly women, with 40 percent or more of them suffering osteopenia in the hip bone (see Table 8.19 and Chart 8.9). The likelihood of osteopenia is relatively stable by age among elderly women, but for elderly men, the likelihood is higher among the older aged cohort. Among the oldest-old, men are as likely as women to suffer from this less severe form of reduced bone density.

However, osteoporosis (the more severe form of reduced bone density) of the hip bone is substantially more prevalent among elderly women than elderly men. Although the gender gap narrows with age, the oldest-old women are still more than three times more likely than their male counterparts to have osteoporosis in the hip bone (see Table 8.19). Osteoporosis is more prevalent than osteopenia among the oldest-old women. In fact, one-half of the oldest-old women have osteoporosis in the hip bone.

Overall, one-quarter of elderly men and nearly three-quarters of elderly women suffer from either osteopenia of the hip bone or the more severe osteoporosis. Among the oldest-old, these figures increase to more than one-half of men and 91 percent of women.

■ The risk factors for reduced bone density are numerous

Women's higher risk of reduced bone density is in part due to their lower body mass index. However, their higher risk of hypertension may also be a contributing

What role might osteoporosis play in height?

As is commonly known, men are taller than women, on average. Interestingly, the height differential between men and women widens across increasing age groups. Among the youngest adults, aged 20 to 29, men are 5.2 inches taller than women, on average; among those aged 80+, the differential widens to 5.7 inches (see Table 8.20). On a proportional basis, the youngest adult men are 8.1 percent taller than their female counterparts, on average. At the oldest ages, the gap widens such that men are 9.3 percent taller than women. Some of this widening differential might be attributable to the stature-shortening effects of osteoporosis, which affect women (especially older women) more than men.

TABLE 8.20
Average Height in Inches, by Age and Sex: 1988–1994

	Men	Women	Ratio of Men to Women	Height Differential in Inches		
				Men versus Women	Men versus Prior Age Group	Women versus Prior Age Group
20–29 years	69.3	64.1	1.081	5.2	NA	NA
30–39	69.5	64.3	1.081	5.2	0.2	0.2
40–49	69.4	64.1	1.083	5.3	–0.1	–0.2
50–59	69.2	63.7	1.086	5.5	–0.2	–0.4
60–69	68.5	63.1	1.086	5.4	–0.7	–0.6
70–79	67.7	62.2	1.088	5.5	–0.8	–0.9
80+	66.7	61.0	1.093	5.7	–1.0	–1.2

Note: NA = Not Available.
Source: National Health and Nutrition Examination Survey (unpublished), Table 1. Available online at www.cdc.gov/nchs/about/major/nhanes/datatblelink.htm.

In this snapshot data, older people are shorter, on average, than younger people. Men aged 80+ are 2.6 inches shorter, on average, than men aged 20 to 29. For women, the differential is 3.1 inches. Given womens' shorter stature to begin with, the proportionate differential is even greater (4.8 percent for women versus 3.8 percent for men) and may be attributable, at least in part, to osteoporosis.

factor. A three-and-a-half year study of 3,700 older women finds that those with the highest blood pressure experienced the greatest bone loss in the hip.[69]

Another study of postmenopausal women finds that osteoporosis risk is most affected by increasing age. Specifically, women aged 65 to 69 are six times more likely than women aged 50 to 54 to have osteoporosis, and those aged 80+ are 23 times more likely than the youngest postmenopausal women.[70] Osteoporosis is also more likely among those with a personal or family history of fractures, those of Asian or

Hispanic heritage, or those who smoke. Lower risk is associated with higher body mass index, African American heritage, estrogen or diuretic use, exercise, and alcohol consumption. Among elderly women, non-Hispanic whites are twice as likely as non-Hispanic blacks to have osteoporosis.

About one-half of senior women are very familiar with osteoporosis.[71] Based on survey results of 400 American women, one-half (53 percent) of women aged 60 to 69 have had a bone density test to test for the presence of osteoporosis.[72]

Cholesterol Levels

■ Senior women are twice as likely as senior men to have high cholesterol

Elevated serum cholesterol levels are a major risk factor for coronary heart disease but are not clearly linked to mortality among older adults.[73] About 40 percent of senior women have high serum cholesterol levels, compared with about 20 percent of senior men.[74] On average, elderly women have serum cholesterol levels of about 230, compared with men's levels of about 210.

DEFINITION: High serum cholesterol is defined as greater than or equal to 240 mg/dl.

Over a more than 30-year period, cholesterol levels among all adults have decreased (see Table 8.21), with dramatic declines in the percent of people with high serum cholesterol levels. In 1988–1994, men and women aged 65 to 74 were 40 percent less likely to have high cholesterol than similarly aged people were in the early 1960s. Average serum cholesterol levels have also declined, although not as dramatically (see Table 8.22).

TABLE 8.21
Percent of Population with High Serum Cholesterol (240 mg/dl), by Age and Sex: 1960–1962 and 1988–1994

	Men			Women		
	1960–1962	1988–1994	Percent Change	1960–1962	1988–1994	Percent Change
20–34 years	15%	8%	−46%	12%	7%	−41%
35–44	34	19	−43	23	12	−47
45–54	39	27	−32	47	27	−43
55–64	42	28	−33	70	41	−42
65–74	38	22	−42	69	41	−40
75+	NA	20	NA	NA	38	NA

Note: NA = Not Available.
Source: National Center for Health Statistics, *Health, United States, 2001 with Urban and Rural Health Chartbook* (Hyattsville, MD, 2001), Table 68. Data from the National Health and Examination Survey.

TABLE 8.22
Mean Serum Cholesterol Level (mg/dl), by Age and Sex: 1960–1962 and 1988–1994

	Men			Women		
	1960–1962	1988–1994	Percent Change	1960–1962	1988–1994	Percent Change
20–34 years	198	186	–6%	194	184	–5%
35–44	227	206	–9	214	195	–9
45–54	231	216	–6	237	217	–8
55–64	233	216	–7	262	235	–10
65–74	230	212	–8	266	233	–12
75+	NA	205	NA	NA	229	NA

Note: NA = Not Available.

Source: National Center for Health Statistics, *Health, United States, 2001 with Urban and Rural Health Chartbook.* (Hyattsville, MD, 2001), Table 68. Data from the National Health and Examination Survey.

Treatment-caused Injuries

The elderly can get caught in a cascading series of medical interventions. One intervention can unleash a series of other complications and further interventions, all of which amplify the overall risk and the consequences can be severe.[75]

■ The elderly have an increased risk of hospital-related injury

Because of their more intense exposure to medical services, the elderly have an increased risk of medical-related injury.[76] One study of more than 30,000 patient records found that 5.9 percent of the hospitalized elderly had experienced an adverse event, compared with 4.7 percent of those aged 45 to 64 and 2.6 percent of those aged 16 to 44. More than two-thirds of these injuries were due to medical errors.

DEFINITION: In medical parlance, an "adverse event" is defined as an unintended injury caused by medical management that results in measurable disability.

■ Functional capabilities affect hospitalization and vice versa

Functional decline (such as confusion, incontinence, loss of appetite, and tendency to fall) is particularly likely to occur in elderly patients when they are hospitalized.[77] Such declines lead to more medical intervention and subsequent adverse medical events.

■ The elderly pose challenges to physicians

Physiological differences in the elderly make them less tolerant of some physician errors (such as those related to excessive fluid administration, inappropriate drug usage, or dehydration).[78] Additionally, illnesses in the elderly are more commonly underdiagnosed or delayed, and many diseases are presented atypically. Older patients are more likely to be underdiagnosed if they are under the care of a nongeriatric physician.

Exacerbating these challenges is the tendency of many elderly patients to dismiss symptoms as part of their normal "aches and pains" or to believe that a symptom is another manifestation of a chronic condition they already have.[79] The elderly also tend to be less assertive with doctors and often accept explanations without voicing their concerns. On the other side of the equation are physician-related biases against older patients and conflicting attitudes about death and dying, which can also complicate matters.[80]

■ There are six common types of medical injuries

Six common types of medical injuries involve seniors: adverse drug events, falls, infections, pressure sores, delirium, and surgical complications.

Adverse Drug Events.   Adverse drug events (ADEs) are the most common type of treatment-caused injury in hospitalized elderly as well as younger patients, with about one-third due to preventable errors.[81] However, the elderly are more susceptible to such events due to normal age-related changes in their bodies' abilities to metabolize and respond to certain drugs, multiple drug reactions, the challenge of complying with complex medication routines, and inappropriate drug prescribing. One study among more than 9,000 patients found that the ADE incidence rose from 3.3 percent for patients under age 50, to 6.3 percent for those aged 50 to 69 and 6.5 percent for those aged 70 to 79.

ADEs are also a problem in nursing homes. A year-long cohort study of 2,916 residents in 18 nursing homes in Massachusetts found that ADEs commonly occur in nursing homes.[82] An average of 1.9 ADEs per 100 resident-months occurred, one-half of which were deemed preventable. If this rate is generalized to all U.S. nursing homes, 24 adverse drug events would be identified over a 1-year period in an average facility of 106 beds, for an annual total of 350,000 ADEs in all nursing homes. Psychoactive medications and anticoagulants are the most common medications associated with preventable ADEs.[83] Errors in ordering and monitoring are the most common sources of preventable ADEs.

Other studies report that in a 4-year period, two-thirds of 332 nursing home residents had an ADE.[84] In 1 day, medication errors occurred in 8 percent of ordered or administered doses in 56 long-term care facilities.

ADEs also occur, of course, among the noninstitutionalized elderly.[85] In a study of 167 older veterans who each took an average of eight drugs, 35 percent reported a drug reaction in the prior year. Twenty-eight percent of them required hospitalization or an emergency room visit. National Ambulatory Medical Care Survey data of 8,700 patient records for visits when prescriptions were written found that 7.5 percent of elderly patients were prescribed at least one of 20 drugs deemed inappropriate for older patients.

A 1997 study reported that among the nearly 1 in 5 adults aged 60+ who regularly takes medication for chronic pain, 1 in 4 suffered from drug-related side effects.[86]

Additionally, nearly 40 percent said that doctors do not discuss possible side effects, and one-half said that doctors do not warn them about potential drug interactions.

Nonsteroidal anti-inflammatory drugs (NSAIDs), such as ibuprofen, are the most common type of prescription medication taken for pain by the elderly.[87] However, 1 in 4 elderly who take NSAIDs experiences side effects such as ulcers.

The majority of the elderly who take prescription NSAIDs, do so for 6 months or longer despite warnings about gastrointestinal complications associated with long-term NSAID use.[88] On average, those who take nonprescription NSAIDs have taken them daily for 5 years, despite product label cautions against more than 10 days of consecutive use.

A recent study found that the combination of alcohol and over-the-counter pain medications is the most common source of adverse drug reactions among older patients.[89]

Falls. Falls account for 31 percent of all accident-related causes of death among the elderly. Among the elderly aged 85+, this percentage increases to 39 percent.[90] Falls are most common among nursing home patients. Each year, falls occur in about one-half of elderly nursing home patients, one-third of those living at home, and 2 percent of those in the hospital.[91] About 1 percent of falls result in a hip fracture. Among elderly nursing home patients who fall, about 9 percent incur serious injury.

More than one-half of falls are due to medically diagnosed conditions, and 37 percent are due to environmental hazards such as stairs or obstacles.[92] Depressed older women have a 40 percent higher chance of falling.

Infections. The elderly are particularly susceptible to infections, such as pneumonia and urinary tract infections, acquired as a result of medical intervention.[93] Hospital-acquired infection rates range from 4 percent to 19 percent of elderly patients. Among nursing home patients, one study of more than 4,000 patients found a 4.4 percent 1-day infection rate of newly acquired infections.

Pneumonia and urinary tract infections together account for about one-half of the infections acquired in long-term care facilities.[94] Nursing home patients are most commonly hospitalized due to pneumonia. Twenty-nine percent of those who acquire pneumonia in nursing homes are admitted to a hospital.

Pressure sores. Immobilization increases the chances of developing pressure sores. A survey of more than 31,000 hospital patients found that at any one time, 11 percent have pressure sores and 80 percent of these patients are aged 60+.[95] The incidence of pressure sores among hospitalized older patients who are bed or chair bound ranges up to 30 percent.

A study among nearly 20,000 nursing home residents found that 11 percent had pressure sores on admission, and the 1-year incidence for remaining residents was 13 percent.[96] In another study, pressure sores were found in 7.7 percent of residents in Department of Veterans Affairs long-term care facilities in 1993.[97] Among those still institutionalized 6 months later, ulcers had healed in 54 percent of the cases. The more severe the ulcer, the less likely it was to have healed: 31 percent of stage 4 ulcers, 45 percent of stage 3 ulcers, and 72 percent of stage 2 ulcers were healed. Older age and rehabilitation therapy increase the odds of healing, whereas incontinence and immobility decrease the odds.

Delirium.   Surgery and drug therapy are frequent causes of delirium in the elderly and can often mistakenly be attributed to dementia or aging-related mental changes. The prevalence of delirium at the time of hospitalization ranges from 14 to 24 percent for older patients and is a predictor of poor hospital outcome.[98] Anywhere from 9 to 31 percent of older patients develop delirium during hospitalization, and as many as 25 percent of older patients experience delirium following surgery.

Surgical complications.   Studies suggest that age alone is not an important risk factor for surgical complications.[99] However, older patients often have functional impairments and other diseases that increase the risks. The result is that the elderly are twice as likely as younger patients to incur surgical complications. Additionally, the elderly account for one-half of all surgical emergencies and three-fourths of operative deaths.

An additional factor is that physicians may delay surgery in the elderly for fear of such complications.[100] Such delays themselves can increase surgical risks substantially by allowing the disease to advance further, thereby further sapping the patients' physical reserves. A study of 613 surgical patients aged 70+ found that mortality rates were more than 10 times greater in those who had emergency operations (21 percent) compared to elective procedures (2 percent).

Recent studies indicate that the elderly who undergo surgery are at risk of cognitive decline as a result of the surgery: the older the patient and the more severe the surgery, the greater the likelihood of cognitive decline.[101] Anywhere from 10 to 30 percent of elderly patients may suffer from decline, such as impaired concentration or memory skills after major surgery. The decline is usually short-term but can persist for years. Major surgeries, such as vascular, abdominal, and orthopedic surgeries, appear to increase the risk, whereas less invasive surgeries are less risky.

NOTES

1. Thomas R. Cole and Mary G. Winkler, *The Oxford Book of Aging* (New York: Oxford University Press, 1999), 33.
2. Jennifer L. Wolff, Barbara Starfield, and Gerard Anderson, "Prevalence, Expenditures, and Complications of Multiple Chronic Conditions in the Elderly," *Archives of Internal Medicine* 162, no. 20 (2002): 2269–2276.
3. Debra L. Blackwell, John Gary Collins, and Richard Coles, "Summary Health Statistics for U.S. Adults: National Health Interview Survey," series 10, no. 205 (National Center for Health Statistics, Vital and Health Statistics, May 2002). Additional calculations made by authors.
4. National Center for Health Statistics. *Health, United States, 2001 with Urban and Rural Health Chartbook* (Hyattsville, MD, 2001): Table 57. 1999 data from the National Health Interview Survey.

5. Patricia F. Adams, Gerry E. Hendershot, and Marie A. Marano, "Current Estimates from the National Health Interview Survey, 1996," series 10, no. 200 (National Center for Health Statistics, Vital and Health Statistics, October 1999), Table 67.

6. Blackwell, Collins, and Coles, "Summary Health Statistics for U.S. Adults." Additional calculations made by authors.

7. Centers for Disease Control and Prevention, "Surveillance for Use of Preventative Health-Care Services by Older Adults, 1995–1997," *MMWR, CDC Surveillance Summaries* 48, no. SS-8 (December 17, 1999).

8. Karen Davis, "Health and Aging in the 21st Century," *The Commonwealth Fund: 1999 Annual Report, President's Message.* Available online at www.cmwf.org/annreprt/1999/president99.asp.

9. Blackwell, Collins, and Coles, "Summary Health Statistics for U.S. Adults." Additional calculations made by authors.

10. National Council on the Aging, "What Older Americans Know about High Blood Pressure," *National Hypertension Survey* (March 9, 2000). Available online at www.ncoa.org/news/hypertension.

11. Blackwell, Collins, and Coles, "Summary Health Statistics for U.S. Adults." Additional calculations made by authors.

12. Centers for Disease Control and Prevention, "Surveillance for Sensory Impairment, Activity Limitation, and Health Related Quality of Life among Older Adults—United States, 1993–1997," *MMWR, CDC Surveillance Summaries* 48, no. SS-8 (December 17, 1999): Table 2. Data from the 1994 National Health Interview Second Supplement on Aging among adults 70+.

13. National Center for Health Statistics, *1999 National Nursing Home Survey*, CD-ROM series 13, no. 28 (Hyattsville, MD, November 2001).

14. Centers for Disease Control and Prevention, "Surveillance for Sensory Impairment," Table 2. Data from the 1994 National Health Interview Second Supplement on Aging.

15. National Center for Health Statistics, *1999 National Nursing Home Survey.*

16. National Council on the Aging, "The Consequences of Untreated Hearing Loss in Older Persons" (May 1999). Available online at www.ncoa.org.

17. Ibid.

18. Blackwell, Collins, and Coles, "Summary Health Statistics for U.S. Adults." Additional calculations made by authors.

19. Ibid.

20. RoperASW, 1999.

21. Blackwell, Collins, and Coles, "Summary Health Statistics for U.S. Adults." Additional calculations made by authors.

22. Robin Leonard, "Statistics on Vision Impairment: A Resource Manual," *Lighthouse International,* February 1999.

23. Centers for Disease Control and Prevention, "Surveillance for Sensory Impairment," Table 2. Data from the 1994 National Health Interview Second Supplement on Aging.

24. National Center for Health Statistics, *1999 National Nursing Home Survey.*

25. Robin Leonard, "Statistics on Vision Impairment."

26. Ibid.

27. Centers for Disease Control and Prevention, "Surveillance for Sensory Impairment," Table 2. Data from the 1994 National Health Interview Second Supplement on Aging.

28. Ibid.

29. Ibid., Table 3.

30. Mediamark Research Inc. Spring 2000.

31. Ibid.

32. Centers for Disease Control and Prevention, "Surveillance for Sensory Impairment," Table 1. Data from the 1994 National Health Interview Second Supplement on Aging.

33. Blackwell, Collins, and Coles, "Summary Health Statistics for U.S. Adults." Additional calculations made by authors.
34. Ali H. Mokdad et al., "Diabetes Trends in the U.S.: 1990–1998," *Diabetes Care* 23, no. 9 (September 2000): 1278–1283, Table 3.
35. National Cancer Institute, *SEER Cancer Statistics Review 1973–1998* (Bethesda, MD, 2001) or *SEER Cancer Statistics Review 1973–1996* (Bethesda, MD, 1999).
36. Mediamark Research Inc. Spring 2000.
37. National Center for Health Statistics, *1999 National Nursing Home Survey.*
38. Centers for Disease Control and Prevention, "Surveillance for Morbidity and Mortality among Older Adults—United States, 1995–1996," *MMWR, CDC Surveillance Summaries* 48, no. SS-8 (December 17, 1999).
39. Centers for Disease Control and Prevention, "Surveillance for Use of Preventative Health-Care Services."
40. National Center for Health Statistics, *Health, United States, 1999.* Data for 1988–1994 from the National Health and Nutrition Examination Survey.
41. Clemencia M. Vargas, Ellen A. Kramarow, and Janet A. Yellowitz, "The Oral Health of Older Americans," *Aging Trends,* no. 3 (National Center for Health Statistics, March, 2001).
42. Sarah Greene Burger, Jeanie Kayser-Jones, and Julie Prince Bell, "Malnutrition and De-hydration in Nursing Homes: Key Issues in Prevention and Treatment" (National Citi-zen's Coalition for Nursing Home Reform, June 2000). Available online at www.cmwf.org/programs/elders.
43. U.S. Department of Health and Human Services, *Oral Health in America: A Report of the Surgeon General* (Rockville, MD: U.S. Department of Health and Human Services, Na-tional Institutes of Health, National Institute of Dental and Craniofacial Research, 2000).
44. Blackwell, Collins, and Coles, "Summary Health Statistics for U.S. Adults." Additional calculations made by authors.
45. National Center for Health Statistics, *1997 National Nursing Home Survey.*
46. Burger, Kayser-Jones, and Bell, "Malnutrition and Dehydration."
47. Blackwell, Collins, and Coles, "Summary Health Statistics for U.S. Adults." Additional calculations made by authors.
48. U.S. Department of Health and Human Services, *Oral Health in America.*
49. National Center for Health Statistics, *Health, United States, 1999 with Health and Aging Chartbook* (Hyattsville, MD, 1999), Figure 19. Data from the National Health Interview Survey.
50. Mediamark Research Inc. Spring 2000.
51. National Center for Health Statistics, *1999 National Nursing Home Survey.*
52. Burger, Kayser-Jones, and Bell, "Malnutrition and Dehydration."
53. Mediamark Research Inc. Spring 2000.
54. Centers for Disease Control and Prevention, "Surveillance for Injuries and Violence among Older Adults," *MMWR, CDC Surveillance Summaries* 48, no. SS-8 (December 17, 1999).
55. Centers for Disease Control and Prevention, "The Costs of Fall Injuries among Older Adults," National Center for Injury Prevention and Control Fact Sheet (January 27, 2000).
56. Debra L. Blackwell and Luong Tonthat, "Summary Health Statistics for the U.S. Popula-tion: National Health Interview Survey, 1997," *Vital and Health Statistics,* series 10, no. 204 (Centers for Disease Control and Prevention, March 2002). Additional calculations made by authors.
57. Centers for Disease Control and Prevention, "Surveillance for Injuries and Violence."

58. Centers for Disease Control and Prevention, "CDC Recommendations Regarding Selected Conditions Affecting Women's Health; Reducing Falls and Hip Fractures among Older Women," *MMWR, CDC Recommendations and Reports* 49, no. RR-2 (March 31, 2000).
59. Centers for Disease Control and Prevention, "Surveillance for Injuries and Violence."
60. National Council on the Aging, "Osteoporosis: A Behind-the-Scenes Look." Available online at www.ncoa.org/press/what60/facts.html.
61. Centers for Disease Control and Prevention, "Surveillance for Injuries and Violence."
62. National Center for Health Statistics, *Health, United States, 1999.* Data from the 1996 National Hospital Discharge Survey.
63. Centers for Disease Control and Prevention, "Surveillance for Injuries and Violence."
64. Centers for Disease Control and Prevention, "CDC Recommendations."
65. Ibid.
66. Davis, "Health and Aging."
67. Victor R. Fuchs, "Health Care for the Elderly: How Much? Who Will Pay for It?" *Health Affairs* (January/February, 1999): 11–21, Exhibit 2.
68. National Center for Health Statistics, *Health, United States, 1999.* Data from the 1988–1994 National Health and Nutrition Examination Survey.
69. "High Blood Pressure, Thin Bones?" *Consumer Reports on Health* (December 2000).
70. Ethel S. Siris et al., "Identification and Fracture Outcomes of Undiagnosed Low Bone Mineral Density in Postmenopausal Women; Results from the National Osteoporosis Risk Assessment," *Journal of the American Medical Association* 286, no. 22 (December 12, 2001): 2815–2822.
71. Davis, "Health and Aging."
72. National Council on the Aging, "Ann-Margaret Personifies."
73. Centers for Disease Control and Prevention, "Surveillance for Use of Preventative Health-Care Services."
74. National Center for Health Statistics, *Health, United States, 2001,* Table 68. Data from the 1988–1994 National Health and Nutrition Examination Survey.
75. Jeffrey M. Rothschild and Lucian L. Leape, "The Nature and Extent of Medical Injury in Older Patients," Public Policy Institute, AARP (September 2000).
76. Ibid.
77. Rothschild and Leape, "Nature and Extent of Medical Injury in Older Patients."
78. Ibid.
79. Ibid.
80. Ibid.
81. Ibid.
82. Jerry Gurwitz et al. "Incidence and Preventability of Adverse Drug Events in the Nursing Home Setting," *American Journal of Medicine* 109, no. 2 (August 1, 2000): 87–94.
83. Ibid.
84. Rothschild and Leape, "Nature and Extent of Medical Injury in Older Patients."
85. Ibid.
86. National Council on the Aging, "Nearly One in Five Seniors Takes Medication for Chronic Pain." Available online at www.ncoa.org/news/archives/pain_results061097 .htm.
87. Ibid.
88. Ibid.
89. National Council on the Aging, "Substance Abuse among Older Americans." Available online at www.ncoa.org/news/subabuse.
90. Donna L. Hoyert et al., "Deaths: Final Data for 1999," *National Vital Statistics Reports* 49, no. 8 (National Center for Health Statistics, National Vital Statistics System, September 21, 2001): Table 9.

91. Rothschild and Leape, "Nature and Extent of Medical Injury in Older Patients."
92. Ibid.
93. Ibid.
94. Ibid.
95. Ibid.
96. Ibid.
97. Dan R. Berlowitz, Gary H. Brandeis, Jennifer Anderson, and Harriet K. Brand, "Predictors of Pressure Ulcer Healing among Long-Term Care Residents," *Journal of the American Geriatrics Society* 45, no. 1 (January 1997).
98. Rothschild and Leape, "Nature and Extent of Medical Injury in Older Patients."
99. Ibid.
100. Ibid.
101. Vicki Haddock, "Going under the Knife," *WebMDHealth* (August 2000). Available online at http://my.webmd.com/content/article/1674.50802.

CHAPTER 9

Mental Health and Illness

Older individuals are sometimes thought to be "normally" depressed. "After all," people sometimes ask, "wouldn't you be depressed about being old?" The fact is that most older people evidence a significant ability to confront the problems that often accompany aging and still maintain emotional equilibrium.

—Gregory Hinrichsen, Mental
Health and Older Adults

The problems of alcoholism and drug addiction have strong links to depression. The search for highs may often begin as a flight from lows.

—Nathan S. Kline, M.D.,
The Nathan S. Kline Institute
for Psychiatric Research

Alzheimer's disease doesn't make special arrangements for presidents or first ladies or anyone else for that matter. When it takes hold, it follows its own course of destruction, frequently ravaging not only its direct victim but also the caregivers and loved ones along with it. This disease is a thief that sneaks into the brain and robs its victims of so much of what is precious about life—our memories and our experiences, ultimately life itself.

—Maureen Reagan, testimony
presented to the Senate
Appropriations Committee,
March 21, 2000

The aging process has you firmly in its grasp if you never get the urge to throw a snowball.

—Doug Larson

Most elderly maintain emotional equilibrium as they adapt to the challenges of aging, but an estimated 15 to 25 percent of seniors have significant symptoms of such mental health problems as depression.[1] Tragically, severe memory impairment is a widespread problem of aging and is more likely in the oldest age groups.

This chapter provides information about issues relating to the elderly's mental health. It covers such topics as depression in the elderly, memory problems, Alzheimer's disease, and mental health care.

Highlights of this chapter include:

- As many as 1 in 4 seniors suffers from mental problems, and as many as 1 in 4 seniors aged 85+ has symptoms of severe depression.
- Two of every three seniors who need mental health care do not get it.
- Memory complaints among older people are very common; one report stating that 50 to 80 percent of older people report memory complaints.
- New research finds that memory problems in the elderly may be declining.
- Nearly one-half of the oldest-old are afflicted with Alzheimer's disease.

MENTAL HEALTH CARE

■ Two of every three seniors who need mental health care do not get it

Researchers estimate that up to 63 percent of seniors with a mental health problem may not be treated,[2] and an estimated one-half of all older adults who acknowledge a mental health problem are actually treated.[3] Although the elderly make up 12 percent of the population, they account for only 6 percent of community-based mental health services clients and 9 percent of private psychiatric patients.

■ Mental health problems in the elderly may go unrecognized

More than one-half of older people who receive mental health care receive it from their primary health care physician.[4] However, many of these primary-care physicians lack adequate geriatric or mental health training, and this can contribute to inadequate treatment and diagnosis of mental disorders in the elderly.

Mental health problems in older people can be more difficult to diagnose because the symptoms can manifest differently than in young people. Depression, in particular, is often underdiagnosed in the elderly due to many reasons:[5]

- Depression is expected to be a normal part of aging.
- Older people tend to underreport psychological symptoms and emphasize physical symptoms.
- Cognitive impairment is common in depressed older people and can limit their ability to accurately report depressive symptoms.
- Depression in older people often occurs along with other illnesses with symptoms that can be very similar to, or masked by, depression.

- Some medical conditions (e.g., stroke or hypothyroidism) can predispose or trigger depression.
- Older people are more likely to take medications, some of which can cause or contribute to depression (e.g., beta blockers and anti-Parkinson's drugs).

Thus, it is not surprising to find that only 55 percent of internists feel confident in diagnosing depression and only 35 percent feel confident in prescribing antidepressants to older persons.[6] A study of elderly health maintenance organization (HMO) patients indicated an apparent failure to recognize depression in older adults and to enter them into treatment.[7] Even when these depressed patients were treated, the treatments lacked intensity and continuity. In particular, the majority of depressed patients who were treated received antidepressant prescriptions that usually did not meet recommended guidelines for dose and duration. Another study found that only about 11 percent of depressed patients in primary care received adequate antidepressant treatment; 34 percent received inadequate treatment; and 55 percent received no treatment.[8]

Additionally, psychiatric symptoms can be incorrectly attributed to other physical disorders or to normal age-related changes, or the condition can be left unnoticed. One longitudinal study of elderly HMO patients found relatively high rates of minor tranquilizer use among depressed elderly patients, raising the concern that primary-care physicians may have been treating insomnia rather than depression.[9] Studies among older adults who have committed suicide reveal that despite having seen their physician within a short period before the suicide, few were receiving mental health treatment.[10] One study found that 20 percent of older adults who committed suicide had visited their primary-care physician on the same day, 40 percent within one week, and 70 percent within one month of the suicide.[11]

■ Age bias can affect support

Age bias is another factor that can contribute to the lack of mental health support afforded the elderly. A study of 215 primary-care physicians revealed that physicians exhibited less willingness to treat older suicidal patients than younger ones.[12] The study randomly assigned one group of physicians a vignette of a retired, geriatric patient who was depressed and suicidal. Another group received the identical vignette, but the patient was younger and employed. Both groups of physicians recognized depression and suicidal risk. However, the physicians presented with the older patient were more likely to feel that the suicidal ideation was rational and normal. In addition, they were less willing to use therapeutic intervention and were not optimistic that psychiatric or psychological assistance would help.

■ Barriers prevent nursing home residents from receiving adequate treatment

According to the Administration on Aging of the Department of Health and Human Services, despite the higher prevalence of mental illness in nursing homes (most commonly depression and dementia), numerous barriers prevent most residents from receiving adequate treatment. Such barriers include:

- a shortage of specialized geriatric mental health professionals,
- nursing home staff who lack the knowledge and adequate training in mental health issues,
- inadequate Medicare/Medicaid reimbursement for behavioral mental health problems, and
- inadequate reimbursement policies that make it difficult to obtain professional mental health services.[13]

MENTAL ILLNESS

■ As many as 1 in 4 seniors suffers from mental illness

An estimated 15 to 25 percent of seniors suffer from significant symptoms of mental illness.[14] Mental health and physical problems commonly coexist with seniors. According to a sweeping report by the Surgeon General's office, some physical disorders can cause mental health problems due to the disorder itself or medication for the treatment. Likewise, some mental disorders can cause or exacerbate physical conditions by diminishing the ability of older adults to care for themselves or by impairing physiological functions.[15]

Depression

■ As many as 1 in 4 seniors aged 85+ has severe depressive symptoms

Eight to twenty percent of older adults in the community and 17 to 35 percent of those in primary care settings have depressive symptoms and syndromes.[16] A recent national survey indicated that 15 to 23 percent of seniors have severe depressive symptoms, with women aged 65 to 84 more likely than men of the same age to be afflicted (see Chart 9.1).[17]

Major depression has been found among 11 percent of older patients hospitalized for medical illnesses, 12 percent of those in long-term care settings, 15 percent of Alzheimer's patients, and 17 to 31 percent of dementia patients.[18] The less severe, but still clinically significant, depressive symptoms are more prevalent (see Table 9.1).

Depression has been found in about 25 percent of patients with cerebrovascular disease, 30 to 60 percent of stroke victims (within 24 months of having a stroke), and up to 40 percent of Parkinson's patients.[19]

■ Depression is more chronic in older adults

Depression tends to be more chronic in older people than in younger adults, with longer duration and shorter remission intervals. The cycles of recurrence and remission are more persistent as well.[20] As a result, although treatment has been success-

CHART 9.1   Percent of Elderly with Severe Depressive Symptoms, by Age and Sex: 1998

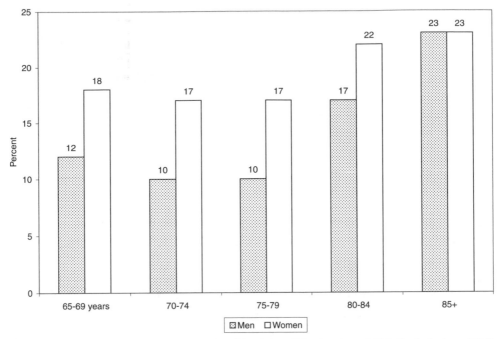

Source: Federal Interagency Forum on Aging Related Statistics, *Older Americans 2000: Key Indicators of Well-Being* (Hyattsville, MD, 2000), Table 16. Data from the Health and Retirement Study.

TABLE 9.1
Approximate Percent of Older Adults Afflicted with Major Depression or Depressive Symptoms

	Major Depression	Depressive Symptoms
Patients hospitalized for medical illnesses	11%	25%
Long-term settings	12	30
Dementia patients	17–31	50
Alzheimer's patients	15	30–40

Source: Data extracted and summarized from studies in George S. Alexopoulos, Ira R. Katz, Charles F. Reynolds III, Daniel Carpenter, and John P. Docherty, *Expert Consensus Pocket Guide to the Pharmacotherapy of Depressive Disorders in Older Patients* (White Plains, NY: Expert Knowledge Systems, 2001).

ful, with 60 to 80 percent response rates, the response generally takes longer than it does with younger adults.

■ Chronic illnesses and loss of a spouse increase the likelihood of depression

Significant lifestyle changes that result from health-related events or the loss of loved ones are often stressful as people try to adapt to new situations. Fewer than 5 percent of the older population are estimated to be severely depressed, but about 25 percent of those with chronic illnesses are estimated to have clinically significant depression. Furthermore, an estimated 10 to 20 percent of widowers and widows suffer from clinically significant depression during the first year of bereavement.[21]

■ Other stresses contribute to depression

A study of the health effects of caregiving found that caregivers experiencing strain had significantly higher levels of depressive symptoms and anxiety and lower levels of perceived health, compared to a control group of age-and-sex-matched noncaregivers.[22] Caregivers also tended to get less rest and have less time to exercise.

Heavy alcohol consumption, a less than high school education, and persistent insomnia are also factors associated with late-onset depression.[23] An estimated 5 to 10 percent of older adults suffer from chronic, primary insomnia, which is one of the symptoms of depression.[24]

DEFINITION: Late-onset depression is defined as depression first diagnosed later than age 60.

■ Late-life depression is costly

Late-life depression is costly because it increases disability and may have detrimental effects on physical health. Primary-care patients with depression have more doctor and emergency room visits, longer hospital stays, and higher outpatient charges, and they use more medication.[25]

■ Depression is associated with physical decline

A study of 1,300 Iowa residents over the age of 70 found that those who showed signs of depression were about 50 percent more likely than those who were not depressed to exhibit substantial physical decline over a 4-year period.[26] The researchers speculated that depression and physical decline reinforce each other, resulting in a downward spiral. In particular, psychological stress may increase susceptibility to disease, thereby further compromising health. Sleeping problems that are common with depression can result in declining physical health, and a depressed mood may keep patients from seeking out medical intervention or following recommended treatment.

Another study followed 4,500 elderly people, who were initially free of heart disease, for a 6-year period.[27] It found that those who most often reported symptoms of depression were 40 percent more likely to develop heart disease than those who least often reported these symptoms. In addition, these more-depressed people were 60 percent more likely to die. The study's researchers suggested that the results may be explained by the fact that depression is associated with less physical activity and more smoking. Depression also increases mental stress, which may increase plaque formation and vessel blockage. Depression is also thought to increase free radical and fatty acid production, which can damage the lining of blood vessels.

◼ Depression and stress increase the likelihood of death

Depression among seniors is associated with increased mortality from suicide or physical illness. Among nursing home patients, major depression increases the likelihood of mortality by 59 percent, regardless of physical condition.[28] A recent epidemiological study found that chronic depression (lasting an average of about 4 years) increased the risk of cancer in older adults by about 88 percent.[29]

A longitudinal study found that elderly caregivers providing support for their spouses and indicating they are experiencing caregiver strain were 63 percent more likely to die within 4 years than were those whose spouses were not disabled.[30] Caregivers who experienced no strain and those who had disabled spouses but provided no help had mortality rates similar to those for the elderly whose spouses were not disabled.

◼ Suicidal thoughts are more prevalent among depressed seniors

If older people are not depressed, they generally do not fear or dread death, even in the face of a recent diagnosis of a terminal illness or a recent serious loss.[31] However, suicidal thoughts are more prevalent among the depressed elderly, with elderly men of all ages having the highest suicide rate of any age group.[32] Depression is the most common diagnosis in elderly suicides.[33]

Memory Problems and Alzheimer's Disease

Each man's memory is his private literature.

—Aldous Huxley

◼ More than one-half of seniors complain about their memory

Memory complaints among older people are very common; one report stated that 50 to 80 percent of older people communicate subjective memory complaints.[34] However, these complaints do not necessarily correspond to actual performance and may be perceptual in nature. Several studies indicate that memory complaints in older people may be more a result of depression than of actual memory decline.

A national study indicated that moderate to severe memory impairment ranges from an incidence of 4.4 percent among those aged 65–69 to 36 percent among those aged 85+ (see Chart 9.2).[35] The ratio of moderate to severe impairment

CHART 9.2 Percent of Noninstitutionalized Elderly with Moderate or Severe Memory Impairment, by Age: 1998

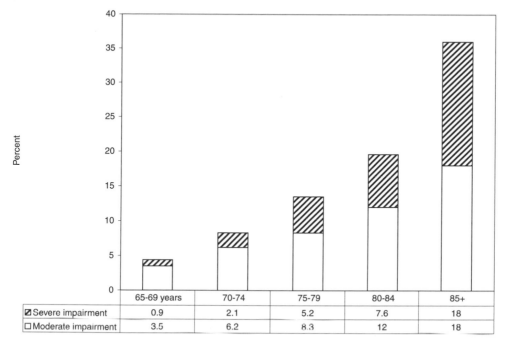

	65-69 years	70-74	75-79	80-84	85+
☑ Severe impairment	0.9	2.1	5.2	7.6	18
☐ Moderate impairment	3.5	6.2	8.3	12	18

Source: Federal Interagency Forum on Aging Related Statistics, *Older Americans 2000: Key Indicators of Well-Being* (Hyattsville, MD, 2000), Table 15. Data from the Health and Retirement Study.

changes across age groups. Among the youngest seniors, aged 65 to 69, severe memory impairments are less than one-third the level of moderate impairments. However, among the oldest seniors, aged 85+, severe memory impairment is just as likely as moderate impairment. Memory impairments are more likely among elderly men than elderly women (see Table 9.2).

■ Seniors' memories may be improving

An encouraging study showed that the typical senior in 1998 performed much better on memory tests than the typical senior in 1993.[36] The study, based on interviews with more than 10,000 seniors, found that only 3.6 percent of community-dwelling adults aged 70 had memory problems in 1998, down from 6.1 percent in 1993. The study's authors cautioned that these results are preliminary and need to be replicated by other scientists before understanding their full implications.

■ Cognitive impairments are most likely among the oldest-old

Very little research has examined the prevalence of cognitive impairment that is short of dementia. A recent two-phase longitudinal study, the first reported in the United States, was conducted on 351 elderly African American residents in Indian-

TABLE 9.2
Percent of Noninstitutionalized Elderly with Moderate or Severe Memory Impairment, by Age and Sex: 1998

| | Moderate Memory Impairment | | | Severe Memory Impairment | | |
	Men	Women	Ratio of Men to Women	Men	Women	Ratio of Men to Women
65–69 years	4.5%	2.9%	1.55	0.8%	0.9%	0.89
70–74	7.5	5.1	1.47	2.6	1.8	1.44
75–79	9.8	7.3	1.34	6.4	4.4	1.45
80–84	14	12	1.15	9.2	6.7	1.37
85+	18	17	1.02	20	18	1.11

Source: Federal Interagency Forum on Aging Related Statistics, *Older Americans 2000: Key Indicators of Well-Being* (Hyattsville, MD, 2000), Table 15. Data from the Health and Retirement Study.

apolis, Indiana, to generate age-specific estimates.[37] The group received a full clinical assessment and diagnosis; subsets of this group were again assessed and diagnosed at 18 and 48 months. The results indicated that 23 percent of noninstitutionalized elderly had cognitive impairments, with 26 percent of them becoming demented after 18 months. Cognitive impairments increased with age: 19 percent for those aged 65 to 74, 28 percent for those aged 75 to 84, and 38 percent for those aged 85+.

■ Nearly one-half of seniors aged 85+ are afflicted with Alzheimer's disease

Alzheimer's disease is a progressive, degenerative brain disorder that causes memory loss, a decline in cognitive abilities, and behavioral changes. Presently, about 12 million people worldwide are afflicted with Alzheimer's disease, including 4 million in the United States.[38] By 2025, an expected 22 million people worldwide will be afflicted. Among those with Alzheimer's disease, 30 to 50 percent experience delusions, 10 to 25 percent have hallucinations, and 40 to 50 percent have depression symptoms.[39]

Alzheimer's disease primarily afflicts an estimated 10 percent of the elderly.[40] In fact, age is the greatest risk factor for developing Alzheimer's disease: 3 percent of the youngest-old, 19 percent of the middle-old, and 47 percent of the oldest-old are afflicted. The rates of Alzheimer's disease among women are higher than among men, an apparent function of women living longer.[41] One-half of all nursing home residents suffer from Alzheimer's disease or a related disorder.[42]

As many as 12 to 15 percent of seniors with mild cognitive impairment (persistent memory loss but not dementia) develop Alzheimer's disease yearly, but only 1 percent of healthy seniors do.[43] People with Alzheimer's disease live an average of 8 to 10 years from the onset of the symptoms.[44]

■ Genetics, vascular health, and diet may affect likelihood of Alzheimer's disease

A longitudinal study found significantly higher age-standardized annual incidence rates for both dementia and Alzheimer's disease among elderly African Americans compared to Nigerians.[45] The study was conducted between 1992 and 1998 among 2,459 community-dwelling Nigerians and 2,149 community-dwelling African Americans, all of whom were aged 65+ and without dementia. Annually, the Nigerians developed dementia or Alzheimer's disease at less than one-half the rate of the African Americans (1.4 percent versus 3.2 percent for dementia and 1.2 percent versus 2.5 percent for Alzheimer's disease). Genetic, dietary, and vascular health differences are suspected contributors to the variations.

Greater cognitive reserve (which can manifest itself with more education and a greater love of reading) and a diet high in antioxidants may offer protection against Alzheimer's disease and other forms of dementia.[46] Conversely, a high-fat diet in early and mid-adulthood, high blood pressure, and head injury may increase the chances of Alzheimer's disease.[47]

■ Head trauma is a possible risk factor for Alzheimer's disease

Several studies have found that Alzheimer's disease is more common among individuals who have sustained a severe head injury (accompanied by a loss of consciousness) during the course of their lives. One study of more than 1,700 World War II veterans found that the risk of Alzheimer's disease was four times greater for those with severe head injury compared with those with no head injury.[48] According to the Alzheimer's Association, what remains unclear is whether head trauma is a result of falls during the early stages of Alzheimer's or whether Alzheimer's results from an earlier head trauma. Additional research is necessary to understand the association between Alzheimer's disease and head injury.

■ Inactivity in younger adulthood is implicated in Alzheimer's disease

Recent research has shown a relationship between activity levels and the likelihood of developing Alzheimer's disease.[49] Specifically, a survey of people in their seventies showed that those who were relatively inactive (intellectually or physically) in early and middle adulthood were about 3.5 times more likely to develop Alzheimer's than those who were more active. These results held even after controlling for age, gender, income, and education. The researchers suggest that inactivity may be a risk factor for the disease and/or that inactivity is an early manifestation of the disease.

■ Alzheimer's disease is costly

Alzheimer's disease–related costs are an estimated $100 billion each year for medical and long-term care, home care, and loss of caregiver productivity.[50] Even though Medicare pays for almost no long-term care, average Medicare expenditures for Alzheimer's patients are almost 70 percent more than for other Medicare beneficiaries.[51] In fact, in 2000 Medicare spending for people with Alzheimer's disease made up about 14 percent of total Medicare spending, even though Alzheimer's patients comprised less than 10 percent of Medicare beneficiaries.[52] Medicare and Medicaid spending in 2000 was an estimated $50 billion ($32 for Medicare and $18.2 for Medicaid).

NOTES

1. Unless otherwise noted, information in this chapter is sourced from U.S. Department of Health and Human Services, "Chapter 5, Older Adults and Mental Health," in *Mental Health: A Report of the Surgeon General* (Rockville, MD, 1999).
2. Ibid.
3. Administration on Aging, "Older Adults and Mental Health: Issues and Opportunities" (January 2001). Available online at www.aoa.dhhs.gov/mh/report2001.
4. Ibid.
5. George S. Alexopoulos, Ira R. Katz, Charles F. Reynolds III, Daniel Carpenter, and John P. Docherty, *Expert Consensus Pocket Guide to the Pharmacotherapy of Depressive Disorders in Older Patients* (White Plains, NY: Expert Knowledge Systems, 2001).
6. U.S. Department of Health and Human Services, "Chapter 5."
7. Jurgen Unutzer et al., "Care for Depression in HMO Patients Aged 65 and Older," *Journal of the American Geriatrics Society* 48, no. 8 (August 2000): 871–878.
8. U.S. Department of Health and Human Services, "Chapter 5."
9. Jurgen Unutzer et al., "Care for Depression."
10. U.S. Department of Health and Human Services, "Chapter 5."
11. National Institute of Mental Health, "Older Adults: Depression and Suicide Facts," NIH publication no. 99-4593 (1999). Available online at www.nimh.nih.gov/publicat/elderlydepsuicide.cfm.
12. Heather Uncapher and Patricai A. Arean, "Physicians Are Less Willing to Treat Suicidal Ideation in Older Patients," *Journal of the American Geriatrics Society* 48, no. 2 (February 2000): 188–192.
13. Administration on Aging, "Older Adults and Mental Health."
14. U.S. Department of Health and Human Services, "Chapter 5."
15. Ibid.
16. Federal Interagency Forum on Aging Related Statistics, *Older Americans 2000: Key Indicators of Well-Being* (Hyattsville, MD, 2000), Table 16. Data from the Health and Retirement Study.
17. Alexopoulos et al., *Expert Consensus Pocket Guide.*
18. Ibid.
19. U.S. Department of Health and Human Services, "Chapter 5."
20. Ibid.
21. Richard Schulz and Scott R. Beach, "Caregiving as a Risk Factor for Mortality—The Caregiver Health Effects Study," *Journal of the American Medical Association* 282, no. 23 (December 15, 1999): 2215–2219.
22. U.S. Department of Health and Human Services, "Chapter 5."
23. Ibid.
24. Ibid.
25. "Depression Leads to Physical Decline," *Consumer Reports on Health* (December 2000).
26. Abraham A. Ariyo et al., "Depressive Symptoms and Risks of Coronary Heart Disease and Mortality in Elderly Americans," *Circulation* 102, no. 15 (2000): 1773.

27. U.S. Department of Health and Human Services, "Chapter 5."
28. Ibid.
29. Schulz and Beach, "Caregiving as a Risk Factor."
30. U.S. Department of Health and Human Services, "Chapter 5."
31. Ibid.
32. Alexopoulos et al., *Expert Consensus Pocket Guide.*
33. U.S. Department of Health and Human Services, "Chapter 5."
34. Federal Interagency Forum on Aging Related Statistics, *Older Americans 2000.* Data from the Health and Retirement Survey.
35. Vicki A. Freedman, Hakan Aykan, and Linda G. Martin, "Aggregate Changes in Severe Cognitive Impairment among Older Americans," *The Journals of Gerontology Series B: Psychological Sciences and Social Sciences* 56 (March 2001): S100–S111.
36. National Institutes of Health, "Cognitive Impairment High among Older People, Study Suggests," National Institutes of Health News Release (November 12, 2001). Available online at www.nia.nih.gov/news. F. W. Unverzagt et al., "Prevalence of Cognitive Impairment: Data from the Indianapolis Study of Health and Aging," *Neurology* 57 (November 13, 2001): 1655–1662.
37. Alzheimer's Disease and Related Disorders Association, "Alzheimer's Disease Statistics," World Alzheimer's Congress 2000, Newsroom Fact Sheet (2000). Available online at www.alzheimers2000.org/news/alxstats.htm.
38. U.S. Department of Health and Human Services, "Chapter 5."
39. Denis A. Evans et al., "Prevalence of Alzheimer's Disease in a Community Population of Older Persons," *Journal of the American Medical Association* 262, no. 18 (November 10, 1989): 2551–2556.
40. U.S. Department of Health and Human Services, "Chapter 5."
41. Ibid.
42. Alzheimer's Disease and Related Disorders Association, "Alzheimer's Disease Statistics," World Alzheimer's Congress 2000, Newsroom Fact Sheet (2000). Available online at www.alzheimer2000.org/news/alzstats.htm.
43. Alzheimer's Disease and Related Disorders Association, "Recent Research Advances," World Alzheimer's Congress 2000, Newsroom Fact Sheet (2000). Available online at www.alzheimer2000.org/news/advance.htm.
44. U.S. Department of Health and Human Services, "Chapter 5."
45. Hugh C. Hendrie et al., "Incidence of Dementia and Alzheimer Disease in 2 Communities," *Journal of the American Medical Association* 285, no. 6 (February 14, 2001): 739–747.
46. Alzheimer's Association, "Vegetables Rich in Anti-oxidants May Help Protect against Alzheimer's and Other Forms of Dementia," Alzheimer's Association Current News Releases (July 11, 2000). Available online at www.alz.org/media/news/current. Alzheimer's Association, "Education May Protect against Alzheimer's Disease and Other Forms of Dementia," Alzheimer's Association Current News Releases (July 9, 2000). Available online at www.alz.org/media/news/current.
47. Alzheimer's Association, "High-Fat Diet in Early Adulthood May Be Associated with Increased Risk of Alzheimer's," Alzheimer's Association Current News Releases (July 12, 2000). Available online at www.alz.org/media/news/current.
48. B. L. Plassman et al., "Documented Head Injury in Early Adulthood and Risk of Alzheimer's Disease and Other Dementias," *Neurology* 55 (2000): 1158–1166.
49. Robert P. Friedland et al., "Patients with Alzheimer's Disease Have Reduced Activities in Midlife Compared with Healthy Control-Group Members," *Proceedings of National Academy of Sciences* 98, no. 6 (March 13, 2001): 3440–3445.

50. U.S. Department of Health and Human Services, "Chapter 5."
51. Alzheimer's Association, "Race against Time: Alzheimer's Epidemic Hits as America Ages," Alzheimer's Association Current News Releases (March 21, 2000). Available online at www.alz.org/media/news/current.
52. Alzheimer's Association, "Medicare and Medicaid Costs for People with Alzheimer's Disease" (April 3, 2001). Available online at www.alz.org/media/news/current/040301alzreport.htm.

CHAPTER 10

Prescription and Over-the-Counter Drugs

Prescription drugs are central to the appropriate medical care of people of all ages. They are particularly important to the elderly, who often need several or more medications to manage and treat multiple conditions. As this book was going to press, the debate on Capitol Hill over how to guarantee the elderly access to prescription drugs was intense, and the outlook for passage of a Medicare prescription drug benefit was still up in the air.

This chapter covers seniors' use of, and expenditures for, prescription, generic, and over-the-counter drugs; information on the types of medications commonly used by the elderly; drug purchasing behavior and attitudes of the elderly; and drug advertising.

Highlights of this chapter include:

- The elderly disproportionately account for 34 percent of all prescriptions dispensed and 42 percent of all prescription drug expenditures.

- About one-third of the elderly do not have prescription drug coverage and must pay full retail price for their prescriptions.

- Hypertension drugs are the most common prescription medications used by the elderly.

- Pain relievers, such as aspirin, ibuprofen, and acetaminophen, are the most common over-the-counter drugs used by the elderly.

- The elderly are more likely than people under age 65 to use mail-order prescriptions.

- The elderly generally have lower opinions of pharmaceutical companies and HMOs than they do of other health care providers.

MEDICATION USAGE BY THE ELDERLY

■ The elderly are heavy users of prescription drugs

People aged 65+ accounted for only 12 percent of the population in 1998; however, 34 percent of all prescriptions dispensed and 42 percent of all prescription drug

CHART 10.1   Average Number of Drugs Prescribed at Outpatient Physician Offices, by Age and Sex: 1997

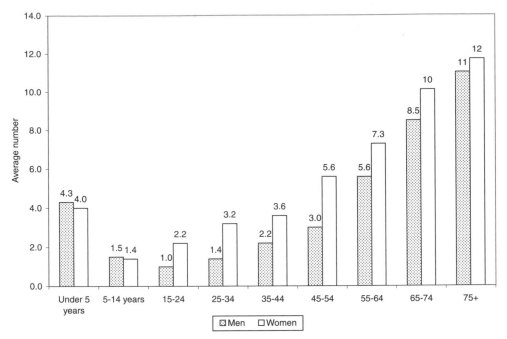

Source: David H. Kreling et al., "Prescription Drug Trends—A Chartbook," The Kaiser Family Foundation (July 2000). Available online at www.kff.org.

expenditures involved this age group.[1] The older the group, the more likely they are to use prescription drugs. According to the 1996 Medical Expenditure Panel Survey, the elderly averaged about 20 prescriptions a year; 1.7 times more than those aged 45 to 64 (12 per year) and four times that of adults aged 19 to 44 (5 per year).[2]

A greater disparity is evident when assessing outpatient physician-generated prescriptions. The 1997 National Ambulatory Medical Care Survey indicated that 75-year-olds used nearly three times more prescriptions annually than 45-year-olds did (see Chart 10.1).[3] Adult women of all ages are prescribed more drugs, on average, than men are, although the gender gap narrows at older ages.

■ Most seniors use prescription drugs

Most noninstitutionalized Medicare beneficiaries (86 percent) used at least one prescription drug in 1995; the average beneficiary used 18 prescriptions during 1995, increasing to 22 in 1998.[4, 5] Medicare beneficiaries in fair or poor health fill at least twice as many prescriptions as those with good to excellent health.[6]

One study of nearly 90,000 drug-insured elderly found that 15 percent incurred at least $3,000 in prescription drug spending in 2000.[7] These "higher-cost" drug users

CHART 10.2   Percent of Household Spending on Prescription and Nonprescription Drugs, by Age of Householder: 1999

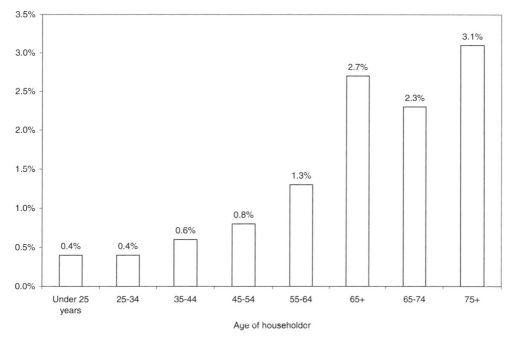

Age of householder

Source: Bureau of Labor Statistics, *1999 Consumer Expenditure Survey,* Table 47. Available online at www.bls.gov.

are similar in average age and sex than lower-cost users but average more chronic conditions and subsequently use more medications, which are expensive and less often generic. Specifically, higher-cost drug users average 65 prescriptions per year at an average price of $70, compared with an average of 24 annual prescriptions at an average cost of $42 for lower-cost drug users.

A 1995 AARP study found that 69 percent of the elderly were at the time of the study taking any prescription drug, with an average of 2.4 prescription drugs. This was higher than the 59 percent of people aged 50–64, who were taking an average of 1.7 drugs.[8]

■ The elderly spend more on drugs

The average elderly household spends 2.5 times more than younger households on prescription and nonprescription drugs ($706 versus $284, respectively, in 1999).[9] These elderly households also devote a higher percentage of their annual household expenses to drugs (see Chart 10.2).[10] Between 1990 and 1999, average annual household inflation-adjusted spending on drugs increased 17 percent among elderly households and 15 percent among younger households.[11]

■ Medicare beneficiaries' drug expenses are increasing

Total drug spending for the Medicare population (which includes the disabled as well as the elderly) was estimated to be $71 billion in 2001, according to the Congressional Budget Office.[12] Average annual drug spending per Medicare beneficiary approximately doubled over a 5-year period to an estimated $1,756 in 2001. Average annual out-of-pocket spending was estimated at $858 in 2001, with 17 percent of beneficiaries expected to have no out-of-pocket drug expenses and an additional 56 percent expected to have expenses under $1,000.[13] Thirteen percent had expenses of $2,000 or more and accounted for 52 percent of the $34 billion out-of-pocket expenditures expected for Medicare beneficiaries in 2001.

■ Price increases are a minor reason for increased prescription drug expenditures

Drug expenditures in the United States increased 79 percent from 1993 to 1998. Forty-three percent of this growth is due to the increased number of prescriptions dispensed, and 39 percent is due to changes from older to newer medications. Manufacturer price increases accounted for only 18 percent of the increased expenditures.[14]

These dynamics have resulted in the elderly spending relatively more on prescription drugs than in the past. In fact, on a constant dollar basis, today's seniors spend, on average, about six times more on prescription drugs than their counterparts did 30 years ago.[15]

Between 1992 and 1996, prescription drug expenditures per senior (on a constant dollar basis) increased at a faster rate than overall health care spending per senior. Prescription drug expenditures accounted for nearly 8 percent of the elderly's total health care expenditures in 1996,[16] and an estimated 10 percent in 2000. By the time the first baby boomers enter the elderly ranks in 2010, that figure could be more than 13 percent.

The increasing influence of prescription drugs on the elderly's pocketbook is being noticed. The elderly are in nearly universal agreement (80 percent have this opinion) that the price of prescription drugs has risen faster than most other expenditures in the past 5 years.[17] However, the elderly are less strongly committed about governmental regulation to limit prescription drug prices, with 54 percent stating there is not as much regulation as there should be. When the elderly are apprised that such regulation might lead to less research and development of new drugs, their support for governmental regulation declines to 43 percent.

Younger adults, on the other hand, are less likely to feel that prescription drug prices have risen faster than other prices (58 percent). They are, however, somewhat more likely to feel that regulation is not as strict as it should be to limit drug prices (62 percent). Their support for governmental regulation also declines (to 41 percent) when told of the potential for less research and development.

▪ Most elderly have prescription drug insurance

About one-third of the elderly overall do not have prescription drug coverage and must pay full retail price for their prescriptions.[18] One breakdown indicates that 53 percent of Medicare beneficiaries had consistent prescription drug coverage throughout 1996, whereas 28 percent had no coverage and 19 percent had coverage for only part of the year.[19]

Geographic residence, income, and chronic conditions are the strongest predictors of prescription drug coverage.[20] Independent of other factors, state of residence can increase the probability of drug coverage by up to 300 percent, with coverage highest for Medicare beneficiaries in the western United States and lowest in the Midwest. Residing in a state with a pharmaceutical assistance program increases continuous coverage by almost 60 percent and partial coverage by nearly 20 percent. Living in an urban area increases coverage by almost 90 percent, compared with rural residency. Those with higher incomes also are more likely to have coverage. Furthermore, for each additional reported chronic condition, the likelihood of continuous coverage increases about 20 percent. Race, age, and ethnicity have little, if any, affect on coverage.

Employer-sponsored drug programs are the single largest source of drug coverage for Medicare beneficiaries; 46 percent of those with drug coverage obtain it from employers or former employers.[21] This figure may decline in the future, given the current trend toward declining retiree health coverage. One recent study reported that 24 percent of employers offered supplemental health coverage to Medicare-eligible retirees in 2000, down from 40 percent in 1994.[22] Another survey of large employers found that 30 percent of employers would seriously consider terminating retiree drug coverage over the next 3 to 5 years.[23]

Among Medicare beneficiaries with prescription drug coverage, individually purchased private policies cover 13 percent, Medicare+Choice HMOs cover 20 percent, and state Medicaid programs cover 18 percent.[24]

As of January 2001, 26 states had enacted state-based pharmacy assistance programs to assist low-income seniors.[25] These programs, along with other public programs such as the Department of Veterans' Affairs, provide drug coverage to about 3 percent of Medicare beneficiaries.[26]

Among the elderly who have drug coverage, more than half are worried that their plan will not cover a drug that they or a family member might need (30 percent are very worried; 23 percent are somewhat worried).[27] More than half are also worried that their plan will raise the share they pay for drugs (25 percent are very worried; 30 percent are somewhat worried). The elderly are less concerned about being required to use generic drugs rather than brand name drugs (28 percent are worried).

Most elderly prescription drug spending is for chronic diseases that tend to require near life-long treatment and subsequently is rather predictable and continuous.[28] Heavy, chronic prescription drug users tend to be the purchasers of prescription drug policies, resulting in high premiums and low enrollment for individual drug coverage policies.

TABLE 10.1

Elderly Medicare Beneficiary Prescription Drug Use and Spending: 1998

	Without Drug Coverage	With Drug Coverage	Ratio of without to with Drug Coverage
Average number of prescriptions per person	16.7	24.4	0.68
Annual out-of-pocket prescription drug expense	$546	$325	1.68

Source: John Poisal and Lauren Murray, "Growing Differences between Medicare Beneficiaries with and without Drug Coverage," *Health Affairs* 20, no. 2 (March/April 2001): 74–86.

■ Lack of drug coverage reduces drug use

Having a higher income and having more comprehensive insurance coverage increase the likelihood that the elderly will use prescription drugs, regardless of whether the drug is for a minor illness or for a serious, chronic condition.[29]

Among Medicare beneficiaries in 1995, 89 percent of those with drug coverage used prescription drugs versus 81 percent of those without drug coverage.[30] Those without drug coverage used one-third fewer prescriptions than those with coverage; however, their out-of-pocket expenditures were 68 percent higher (see Table 10.1).[31]

A study of noninstitutionalized elderly Medicare beneficiaries who had hypertension found that those with no drug insurance coverage were 40 percent more likely than those with coverage to *not* purchase antihypertensive drugs.[32] Even when they purchased the drugs, they purchased fewer tablets and paid more than twice as much per pill, on average, than did their counterparts with drug coverage. Additionally, drug coverage among this group was lowest for those elderly at or just above the poverty level, putting them at greatest risk.

■ Not having prescription drug coverage causes deprivations

An AARP poll among Medicare beneficiaries found that at least one-half of those without prescription drug coverage said that prescription drug expenses caused them to not fill a prescription, use it less often than prescribed, or spend less on food.[33] These deprivations were about twice the rate of those for beneficiaries with drug coverage. Specifically, those without coverage were more likely than those with coverage to:

- use a medication less often than prescribed (57 percent versus 30 percent),
- not fill a prescription (52 percent versus 24 percent),
- spend less on food (50 percent versus 23 percent), or
- incur all three deprivations (27 percent versus 11 percent).

MEDICATIONS USED BY THE ELDERLY

Prescription Drug Use

■ Hypertension drugs are the most common prescription drugs used by seniors

Mediamark Research data on prescription drug use finds that in a 12-month period, two-thirds of the elderly use prescription drugs for at least one of 30 ailments (see Chart 10.3).[34] Hypertension drugs are the most commonly used: 33 percent of all elderly (and one-half of those taking any prescription drug) use a prescription drug for hypertension, compared with 10 percent of younger adults. About one-half as many elderly are treating high cholesterol or rheumatism with prescription drugs (17 percent and 15 percent, respectively). About 1 in 10 elderly (11 percent) is being treated for diabetes with prescription drugs.

Thirteen percent of elderly women are taking estrogen replacement therapy, a lower rate than the 23 percent of women aged 55–64 using this drug.[35] One in ten elderly women is treating osteoporosis with prescription drugs—twice the usage level of the next younger group of women, aged 55–64.

CHART 10.3 Prescription Drug Use by Age: 2000

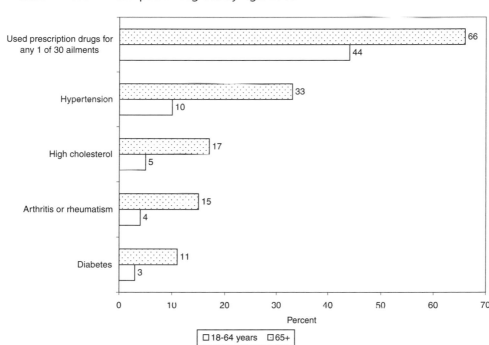

Source: Mediamark Research Inc. Spring 2000.

Among other ailments, urinary tract infections appear to have afflicted 7 percent of elderly women and 4 percent of elderly men over the past year, judging from prescriptions.[36] Seven percent of elderly men were treated with prostate drugs over the past year.[37]

A 1997 study found that nearly 1 in 5 adults aged 60+ regularly takes medication for chronic pain but 2 in 3 said pain still prevents them from doing routine tasks and hobbies.[38] Nonsteroidal antiinflammatory drugs (NSAIDs), such as ibuprofen, are the most common type of prescription medication taken for pain by the elderly.

■ Seniors favor generic drugs

The vast majority of all multisourced drugs dispensed for the elderly are generic products (87 percent).[39] Brand name drug use is highest for drugs that treat diabetes, hyperlipidemia, cardiac rhythm disorders, and osteoporosis and is lowest for drugs that treat acid-peptic disease and depression.

The elderly and younger adults favor generic drugs equally, with 8 in 10 stating that brand name prescription drugs are about the same quality as generic prescription drugs with the same active ingredients.[40]

Over-the-Counter Drug Use

Three in ten elderly state (29 percent) they regularly take over-the-counter drugs (excluding seasonal products).[41] An equal amount (30 percent) say they sometimes use such drugs. Unlike prescription drugs, brand name over-the-counter drugs have the edge, with more than half (54 percent) of the elderly who take any type of over-the-counter drug usually getting a brand name product and one-third (33 percent) usually getting a generic drug.

Oral headache remedies and pain relievers. Oral headache remedies and pain relievers (e.g., aspirin, ibuprofen, and acetaminophen) are the most commonly used over-the-counter drugs; 82 percent of the elderly use such products in a 6-month period, somewhat lower than the 88 percent of younger adults (see Chart 10.4). However, the elderly are more frequent users of these products. In a 30-day period, seniors report having used over-the-counter oral headache remedies and pain relievers an average of 17 times, compared with an average of 12 times by younger adults.[42]

Among users of these products, 71 percent of younger adults use these pain relievers for headaches, whereas only 40 percent of the elderly use them for headaches and 33 percent use them for arthritis or rheumatism. About 1 in 5 elderly uses such products for muscle aches and pains, backaches, or heart attack prevention.[43]

Whereas 86 percent of elderly women use over-the-counter oral pain relievers compared with 77 percent of elderly men, there are no significant differences in how frequently they use the products.[44]

Pain-relieving rubs and liquids. In a 6-month period, pain-relieving rubs and liquids are used by 36 percent of the elderly, compared with one-quarter of younger adults. Elderly users of the products use them 10 times on average over a 30-day period versus 6 times for younger users. As with oral pain relievers, elderly women are

CHART 10.4   Over-the-Counter Drug Usage (Percent Using in Past 6 Months), by Age: 2000

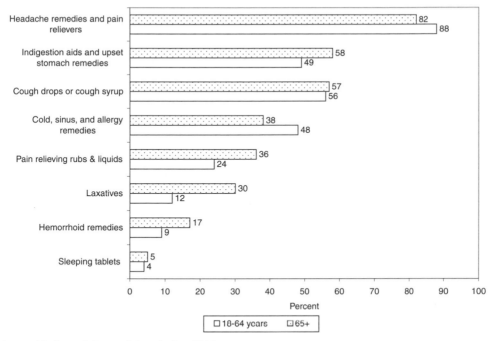

Source: Mediamark Research Inc. Spring 2000.

somewhat more likely than elderly men to use topical pain relievers (39 percent versus 32 percent), but both use the product just as frequently.[45]

Cold, sinus, and allergy remedies.   Only 38 percent of the elderly use cold, sinus, and allergy remedies in a 6-month period compared with 48 percent of younger adults (see Chart 10.4).[46] It is unclear whether this means that the elderly have fewer colds and allergies or that they use fewer of these medications.

Cough medication.   The elderly and younger adults are equally likely to use cough drops or cough syrup, with nearly 6 in 10 of both groups having done so in a 6-month period (see Chart 10.4).[47]

Nonprescription sleeping tablets.   One in twenty elderly has used nonprescription sleeping tablets in a 6-month period, comparable to the rate for younger adults. However, seniors use the product more intensively than younger adults (12 times over a 30-day period versus 8 times for younger adults).[48]

Indigestion aids and upset stomach remedies.   Nearly 6 in 10 elderly people use indigestion aids and upset stomach remedies in a 6-month period, compared with 49 percent of younger adults (see Chart 10.4). The elderly also use the product more intensively, averaging 14 times over a 30-day period versus 10 times among younger users.[49]

Laxatives. Laxative usage increases dramatically with age, rising from 6 percent of adults aged 18 to 24 years, to 18 percent among those aged 55 to 64, and jumping to 30 percent of the elderly. The elderly are also heavier users of laxatives, using them an average of 10 times in a 30-day period compared with 7 times in the same period for younger adults.[50]

Hemorrhoid remedies. The elderly are about half as likely to use hemorrhoid remedies as they are to use laxatives. However, seniors are twice as likely as younger adults to be using hemorrhoid remedies (17 percent versus 9 percent in a 6-month period).[51]

DRUG PURCHASING BEHAVIOR AND ATTITUDES

■ Drug stores are the major source of prescription drugs

The elderly most commonly purchase their prescription drugs at large drug stores or other large chain stores; independent neighborhood drug stores are the next most common source (see Table 10.2).[52] The elderly are more likely to use mail-order prescriptions than the group under age 65, perhaps due to their more regular use of prescription drugs as well as participation in drug plans that might require such purchasing.

■ The elderly are confident of the amount of information received about a new prescription

The last time the elderly got a prescription drug they had never taken before, most of them (84 percent) were confident that they had enough information about the drug (63 percent were very confident; 21 percent somewhat confident).[53] Younger adults are equally confident (87 percent) but are somewhat less strong in their conviction (53 percent were very confident).

TABLE 10.2
Percent of Adults Using Various Prescription Drug Sources, by Age: 2000

Prescription Drug Source	Under 65 Years	65+ Years	Ratio of 65+ to Under 65 Years
At large drug store or other large chain store	77%	65%	0.84
At independent neighborhood drug store	53	54	1.02
By mail-order	10	20	2.00
Directly through health plan	29	19	0.66

Source: "National Survey on Prescription Drugs," *The News Hour with Jim Lehrer*/Kaiser Family Foundation/Harvard School of Public Health (September 2000).

TABLE 10.3
Percent Who Trust Various Sources "a Lot" to Provide Accurate Information about Prescription Medicines, by Age: 2000

Source Trusted "a Lot"	Under 65 Years	65+ Years	Ratio of 65+ to Under 65 Years
Doctor	72%	80%	1.11
Pharmacist	63	77	1.22
Product information inserts in prescription medicines	47	47	1.00
Government agencies	36	27	0.75
Family and friends	23	23	1.00
Advertisements for prescription medicines	7	8	1.14

Source: "National Survey on Prescription Drugs," *The News Hour with Jim Lehrer*/Kaiser Family Foundation/Harvard School of Public Health (September 2000).

■ Doctors and pharmacists are the most trusted sources for drug information

For the elderly, doctors and pharmacists are the most trusted sources of information about prescription medicines, even more so than prescription drug product information inserts (see Table 10.3).[54] The elderly trust doctors and pharmacists more than younger adults do. Advertisements for prescription medicines are the least trusted sources of information.

Friends or family are among the least trusted sources of information on prescription drugs, so they are not consulted very often.[55] Eighty-nine percent of the elderly and 78 percent of younger adults almost never or not very often use these sources for advice about which drugs to take.

■ Direct-to-consumer advertising is a growing influence

Even though prescription drug advertisements are not among the most trusted sources of information, direct-to-consumer advertising has increased dramatically as pharmaceutical companies seek to influence consumers in making prescription drug decisions. In 1998, $1.3 billion was spent on direct-to-consumer advertising—nearly five times more than in 1994.[56] The television portion alone increased nearly 20-fold during the same time period.

According to the September 2000 National Survey on Prescription Drugs, awareness of prescription drug advertising is high: 86 percent of the elderly and 92 percent of younger adults had seen or heard such an advertisement in the past year.[57] Among those aware of such an ad, more than two-thirds of adults had seen or heard such an ad via the major media sources (TV, radio, newspapers, or magazines). How-

TABLE 10.4

Source of Awareness of Prescription Medicine Advertisements in Past Year (among Those Having Seen or Heard Such Advertisements), by Age: 2000

Source of Ads for Prescription Drugs	Under 65 Years	65+ Years	Ratio of 65+ to Under 65 Years
TV or radio	88%	75%	0.85
Newspaper or magazine	74	65	0.88
Mailing	32	37	1.16
Billboard	34	19	0.56
Internet	17	4	0.24

Source: "National Survey on Prescription Drugs," *The News Hour with Jim Lehrer*/Kaiser Family Foundation/Harvard School of Public Health (September 2000).

ever, the elderly were less likely than younger adults to have been exposed to such ads via all sources other than mailings (see Table 10.4).

Prescription drug advertising has not been very effective, however, in communicating benefits, side effects, or what the drug is designed to treat (see Table 10.5).[58] Less than half of the elderly rate the ads as excellent or good at such communication aspects and only about 1 in 10 rates them as excellent. Additionally, the elderly are less likely than younger adults to view the ads as effective at communicating potential benefits or what a drug is designed to treat.

Older Americans are potentially vulnerable to such advertising, given their disproportionate use of prescription drugs. AARP conducted a study to determine how well informed consumers are about such advertisements.[59] As with the National Survey of Prescription Drugs, the AARP study found adults aged 60+ are just as likely as other consumers to notice direct-to-consumer advertisements. However, older adults

TABLE 10.5

Percent Rating the Effectiveness of Prescription Drug Advertising as Excellent or Good (among Those Having Seen or Heard Such Advertisements), by Age: 2000

How Well Drug Advertising Explains:	Under 65 Years	65+ Years	Ratio of 65+ to Under 65 Years
Potential benefits	59%	45%	0.76
Potential side effects	45	46	1.02
What conditions or disease the drug is designed to treat	52	46	0.88

Source: "National Survey on Prescription Drugs," *The News Hour with Jim Lehrer*/Kaiser Family Foundation/Harvard School of Public Health (September 2000).

appeared to obtain less information from the ads because the ads less clearly communicate what the advertised products are for, or even that they are prescription drugs. Fifty percent of the older group versus more than 60 percent of younger adults said it is clear that the advertised drug is available only by prescription. Older consumers also were less likely than adults aged 18 to 39 to feel that the ads had enough information about risks and side effects.

These same older consumers also indicated that their physicians are less communicative about medications.[60] Specifically, 17 percent said their doctors rarely talk to them about the risks and potential side effects of prescribed medications (versus 10 percent of adults aged 18 to 39). More than 4 in 10 older consumers (42 percent) said their doctors rarely or never talk to them about nonprescription options when prescribing (versus about 30 percent of younger adults).

This lack of communication is evident among the nearly 1 in 5 older adults (aged 60+) who regularly take medication for chronic pain.[61] Nearly 40 percent of these people indicate that doctors do not discuss possible side effects of the medications, and one-half say that doctors do not warn them about potential drug interactions.

According to the National Survey on Prescription Drugs, slightly more than one-third of all adults who had seen or heard drug advertisements had subsequently talked with a doctor about the particular medication.[62] Among these adults, only 10 percent of the elderly and 22 percent of the nonelderly asked the doctor to prescribe the medicine they saw or heard advertised. This translates to about 4 percent of all elderly and 8 percent of all the nonelderly who asked their doctor to prescribe a medicine they saw or heard advertised.

■ The elderly hold drug companies in low regard

The elderly generally have lower opinions of drug and pharmaceutical companies and HMOs than they do of other health care providers.[63] Barely 4 in 10 elderly have favorable opinions of drug companies, and less than one-third are favorable toward HMOs; more than one-half have unfavorable opinions of both groups (see Table 10.6). Only tobacco companies are held in significantly less regard than drug companies or HMOs. In contrast, the vast majority of the elderly (more than 7 in 10) have favorable opinions of hospitals and doctors, and they even hold health insurance companies in higher regard than they do drug companies.[64]

The elderly exhibit some differences of opinion with the younger generations (those under age 65) regarding health care providers (see Table 10.6). Interestingly, the elderly have more favorable opinions than younger adults of health insurance companies: nearly 6 in 10 elderly have favorable opinions, whereas 6 in 10 younger adults have unfavorable opinions. Not surprisingly, the elderly favor drug companies less, with only 4 in 10 having favorable opinions, compared with one-half of younger adults.

At least one-half of the elderly feel that various health care providers make too much profit (see Table 10.7).[65] On the lower end of this spectrum are HMOs and hospitals followed by health insurance companies. At the high end are the pharmaceu-

TABLE 10.6
Percent Having a Favorable Opinion of Various Entities, by Age: 2000

Entity Viewed Favorably	Under 65 Years	65+ Years	Ratio of 65+ to Under 65 Years
Banks	69%	82%	1.19
Doctors	81	80	0.99
Hospitals	71	72	1.01
Health insurance companies	39	57	1.46
Airlines	58	46	0.79
Pharmaceutical and drug companies	50	39	0.78
Oil companies	31	33	1.06
HMOs and other managed care plans	36	30	0.83
Tobacco companies	24	16	0.67

Source: "National Survey on Prescription Drugs," *The News Hour with Jim Lehrer*/Kaiser Family Foundation/Harvard School of Public Health (September 2000).

tical and drug companies—a large majority of the elderly (85 percent) feel that the profits made are excessive, even more so than oil and tobacco companies. Older adults have an even stronger opinion regarding drug company profits than younger adults do.[66]

All adults are fairly evenly divided on whether health plans should pay for a brand name prescription drug when a patient requests it, even if a cheaper generic drug is available (see Table 10.8).[67] When a doctor requests a brand name prescrip-

TABLE 10.7
Percent Who Believe Various Industries Make Too Much Profit, by Age: 2000

Industry	Under 65 Years	65+ Years	Ratio of 65+ to Under 65 Years
Airlines	33%	33%	1.00
Banks	51	48	0.94
HMOs and other managed care plans	57	49	0.86
Hospitals	45	55	1.22
Health insurance companies	69	62	0.90
Tobacco companies	78	67	0.86
Oil companies	75	77	1.03
Pharmaceutical and drug companies	70	85	1.21

Source: "National Survey on Prescription Drugs," *The News Hour with Jim Lehrer*/Kaiser Family Foundation/Harvard School of Public Health (September 2000).

TABLE 10.8
Percent of Those Opposed to Having Health Plans Pay for Brand Name Prescription Drugs When Requested (Even If a Cheaper Generic Drug Is Available), by Age: 2000

	If Patient Requests It			If Doctor Requests It		
	Under 65 Years	65+ Years	Ratio of 65+ to Under 65 Years	Under 65 Years	65+ Years	Ratio of 65+ to Under 65 Years
Opposed	47%	50%	1.06	32%	36%	1.13
Additional opposed if it means higher premiums	19	26	1.37	23	22	0.96
Total opposed	65	76	1.17	55	58	1.05

Source: "National Survey on Prescription Drugs," *The News Hour with Jim Lehrer*/Kaiser Family Foundation/Harvard School of Public Health (September 2000).

tion, they are less opposed to having the health plan pay for it. Opposition increases substantially, though, when they are presented with the possibility of having to pay higher premiums.

NOTES

1. Families USA Foundation, "Cost Overdose: Growth in Drug Spending for the Elderly, 1992–2010," Families USA publication no. 00-107 (2000). Available online at www.familiesusa.org.
2. Patricia Neuman, "Improving Prescription Drug Coverage: Opportunities and Challenges for Reform," Henry J. Kaiser Family Foundation (March 22, 2001). Available online at www.kff.org.
3. David H. Kreling et al., "Prescription Drug Trends—A Chartbook," The Kaiser Family Foundation (July 2000). Available online at www.kff.org.
4. Margaret Davis et al., "Prescription Drug Coverage, Utilization, and Spending among Medicare Beneficiaries," *Health Affairs* 18, no. 1 (January/February 1999): 231–243.
5. John Poisal and Lauren Murray, "Growing Differences between Medicare Beneficiaries with and without Drug Coverage," *Health Affairs* 20, no. 2 (March/April 2001): 74–86.
6. Bruce Stuart, Dennis Shea, and Becky Briesacher, "Prescription Drug Costs for Medicare Beneficiaries: Coverage and Health Status Matter," The Commonwealth Fund (January 2000).
7. Cindy Parks Thomas, Grant Ritter, and Stanley S. Wallack, "Growth in Prescription Drug Spending among Insured Elders," *Health Affairs* 20, no. 5 (September/October 2001): 264–277.
8. American Association of Retired Persons, "Survey on Prescription Drug Issues and Usage among Americans Aged 50 and Older" (September 1995). Available online at http://research.aarp.org.
9. Bureau of Labor Statistics, *1999 Consumer Expenditure Survey*, Table 4500. Available online at www.bls.gov.

10. Ibid., Table 47.
11. Sharon Ynetman, ed., *Americans 55 and Older: A Changing Market*, 3rd ed. (Ithaca, NY: New Strategist Publications, 2001), 343. Additional calculations made by authors.
12. The Kaiser Family Foundation, "Medicare and Prescription Drugs," *The Medicare Program* (May 2001). Available online at www.kff.org.
13. Michael E. Gluck and Kristina W. Hanson, *Medicare Chart Book*, 2nd ed. The Kaiser Family Foundation (Fall 2001). Available online at www.kff.org.
14. David H. Kreling et al., "Prescription Drug Trends."
15. David Brown, "For Medicare Patients, Drug Costs Are a Bitter Pill," *The Washington Post National Weekly Edition* (July 3, 2000): 29.
16. Families USA Foundation, "Cost Overdose."
17. "National Survey on Prescription Drugs," *The News Hour with Jim Lehrer*/Kaiser Family Foundation/Harvard School of Public Health (September 2000). Available online at www.kff.org/content/2000/3065/summaryandchartpack.pdf.
18. Mark McClellan, Ian D. Spatz, and Stacie Carney, "Designing a Medicare Prescription Drug Benefit: Issues, Obstacles, and Opportunities," *Health Affairs* 19, no. 2 (March/April 2000): 26–41. Davis et al., "Prescription Drug Coverage."
19. The Commonwealth Fund, "Prescription Drug Coverage Is Fragile for Medicare Beneficiaries" (February 2, 2000). Available online at www.cmwf.org/media/releases.
20. Bruce Stuart, Dennis Shea, and Becky Briesacher, "Dynamics in Drug Coverage of Medicare Beneficiaries: Finders, Losers, Switchers," *Health Affairs* 20, no. 2 (March/April 2001): 86–99.
21. David Gross and Normandy Brangan, "Medicare Beneficiaries and Prescription Drug Coverage: Gaps and Barriers," AARP Research, Public Policy Institute (June 1999). Available online at www.research.aarp.org/health.
22. Families USA Foundation, "Cost Overdose." David Gross, "Trends in the Costs, Coverage, and Use of Prescription Drugs by Medicare Beneficiaries," AARP Research Center, Public Policy Institute (July 2001). Available online at http://research.aarp.org/health/dd63_trends.html.
23. Neuman "Improving Prescription Drug Coverage."
24. Gross and Brangan, "Medicare Beneficiaries and Prescription Drug Coverage."
25. Neuman "Improving Prescription Drug Coverage."
26. Gross and Brangan, "Medicare Beneficiaries and Prescription Drug Coverage."
27. "National Survey on Prescription Drugs," *The News Hour with Jim Lehrer*/Kaiser Family Foundation/Harvard School of Public Health.
28. McClellan, Spatz, and Carney, "Designing a Medicare Prescription Drug Benefit."
29. Davis et al., "Prescription Drug Coverage."
30. Ibid.
31. Poisal and Murray, "Growing Differences."
32. Jan Bluestein, "Drug Coverage and Drug Purchases by Medicare Beneficiaries with Hypertension," *Health Affairs* 19, no. 2 (March/April 2000): 219–230.
33. "Drug Poll Reveals Array of Problems," *AARP Bulletin* (November 2000).
34. Mediamark Research Inc. Spring 2000.
35. Ibid.
36. Ibid.
37. Ibid.
38. National Council on the Aging, "Nearly One in Five Seniors Takes Medication for Chronic Pain." Available online at www.ncoa.org/news/archives.
39. Earl P. Steinberg et al., "Beyond Survey Data: A Claims-based Analysis of Drug Use and Spending by the Elderly," *Health Affairs* 19, no. 2 (March/April 2000): 198–211.
40. "National Survey on Prescription Drugs," *The News Hour with Jim Lehrer*/Kaiser Family Foundation/Harvard School of Public Health.

41. Ibid.
42. Mediamark Research Inc. Spring 2000.
43. Ibid.
44. Ibid.
45. Ibid.
46. Ibid.
47. Ibid.
48. Ibid.
49. Ibid.
50. Ibid.
51. Ibid.
52. "National Survey on Prescription Drugs," *The News Hour with Jim Lehrer*/Kaiser Family Foundation/Harvard School of Public Health.
53. Ibid.
54. Ibid.
55. Ibid.
56. Kreling et al., "Prescription Drug Trends."
57. "National Survey on Prescription Drugs," *The News Hour with Jim Lehrer*/Kaiser Family Foundation/Harvard School of Public Health.
58. Ibid.
59. Lisa Foley and David Gross, "Are Consumers Well Informed about Prescription Drugs?" AARP Public Policy Institute (April 2000). Available online at http://research.aarp.org.
60. Ibid.
61. National Council on the Aging, "Nearly One in Five Seniors Takes Medication for Chronic Pain." Available online at www.ncoa.org/news/archives.
62. "National Survey on Prescription Drugs," *The News Hour with Jim Lehrer*/Kaiser Family Foundation/Harvard School of Public Health.
63. Ibid.
64. National Council on the Aging, "Nearly One in Five Seniors."
65. "National Survey on Prescription Drugs," *The News Hour with Jim Lehrer*/Kaiser Family Foundation/Harvard School of Public Health.
66. National Council on the Aging, "Nearly One in Five Seniors."
67. "National Survey on Prescription Drugs," *The News Hour with Jim Lehrer*/Kaiser Family Foundation/Harvard School of Public Health.

CHAPTER 11

Long-Term Care: An Overview

American families are being stressed to the breaking point because of the emotional and financial strains of providing long-term care.

—The Long-Term Care Campaign

Generally, older people pay more for long-term care than for anything else they buy.

—AARP consumer information

In our society, informal caregivers often go unnoticed except by those who depend on their care.

—Jeannette Takamura and Bob Williams, Informal Caregiving: Compassion in Action

---

DEFINITION: Long-term care (LTC) is a comprehensive range of services that meet the physical, social, and emotional needs of persons of all ages with disabilities. LTC differs from other types of health care in that the goal is not to cure illness, but to help reach and maintain the best level of functioning possible.

Long-term care (LTC) services range from skilled medical treatment to help with such basic activities and routines of daily living as bathing, dressing, eating, and housekeeping. The elderly, particularly the oldest-old, are the primary users of LTC.

The need for LTC is often determined by how much help individuals need to perform activities of daily living (ADLs) or instrumental activities of daily living (IADLs). ADLS include such actions as bathing and getting dressed. IADLs include such actions as preparing meals and managing money. (See Chapter 5 for more complete definitions.) Some of the conditions that can cause limitations on these activities are heart disease, stroke, Parkinson's disease, and Alzheimer's disease.

This chapter presents an overview of long-term care covering: the LTC population, who provides LTC, the types of professional services, who pays for LTC, LTC insurance, and LTC for veterans.

Highlights of this chapter include:

- Sixty-seven percent of elderly LTC recipients rely totally on informal caregiving.
- If informal caregivers to the elderly were reimbursed for their services, the cost would run from $45 billion to $94 billion a year.
- Paraprofessional workers provide 80 percent of nursing home care and more than 90 percent of in-home services.[1]
- Almost 40 percent of the elderly with LTC needs do not get help.
- The federal government is the largest purchaser of long-term care. In 1995, Medicare and Medicaid together accounted for about 56 percent of LTC expenditures for the elderly.
- Medicaid is the biggest purchaser of nursing home care. Medicare is the biggest purchaser of home health care.
- LTC expenses are expected to grow at 2.6 percent a year for the next 40 years.

THE LONG-TERM CARE POPULATION

The most recent estimates of the entire LTC population that are available are based on 1994–1995 surveys. According to this analysis, 17 percent of the elderly need some level of LTC. Of the estimated 12.8 million Americans reporting LTC needs in 1995, measured by the need for assistance with ADLs or IADLs, 57 percent were aged 65+.

In 1999, about 4 percent of all elderly adults—1.5 million individuals—were in nursing homes, down from 5 percent in 1994.[2] An estimated 1,293,000 elderly people were current home health care patients in 1998, a decrease of 26 percent from 1996.[3]

WHO PROVIDES LONG-TERM CARE FOR THE ELDERLY?

The majority of long-term care is provided by informal caregivers.[4] According to the U.S. Department of Health and Human Services, almost 1 in 3 Americans (31 percent), totaling 52 million persons, voluntarily provides informal care to ill or disabled people of all ages.[5]

DEFINITION: Informal caregivers are family members, friends, and other helpers who provide long-term care and are not paid for their services.

■ Two-thirds of elderly LTC recipients rely on unpaid help

Informal caregiving is the foundation of LTC for the elderly. Almost 67 percent of elderly LTC recipients rely solely on informal caregiving.[6] More than seven million Americans—mostly family members—provide 120 million hours of unpaid care to elders with functional disabilities living in the community.[7] If these caregivers were reimbursed for their services, the cost would run from $45 billion to $94 billion a year. Fifty percent of elderly people with LTC needs who lack family members to care for them live in nursing homes, compared with only 7 percent of those who do have family caregivers.[8]

■ The majority of caregivers of the disabled elderly are helping family members

Informal caregivers to the elderly include a range of family members and friends.[9] Statistical facts about family caregivers include the following:

- The majority of caregivers of the disabled elderly are helping out family members.
- The average number of caregivers per disabled elder is 1.7, and each caregiver provides an average of almost 20 hours of unpaid help each week.
- Almost three-quarters of primary informal caregivers to the elderly are women.
- The average age of primary caregivers to the elderly is 60+. Half are age 65+; and slightly over one-third are between the ages of 45 and 64.
- More than two-thirds (68 percent) of primary caregivers to the elderly live in the same household with the disabled person for whom they provide care.
- The majority of primary caregivers are spouses (40 percent) or adult children (36 percent).

■ Most primary informal caregivers do not hold paying jobs

The following facts describe the employment characteristics of unpaid caregivers.

- Most primary informal caregivers do not hold paying jobs. Among the 31 percent who are in the labor force,[10] 67 percent work full time.
- Employed caregivers donate 18 hours of unpaid help per week.
- Employed primary caregivers of the elderly with severe disabilities—those with three or more ADL limitations—provide between 32 and 39 hours of care per week.
- Two-thirds of caregivers with paying jobs report conflicts between jobs and caregiving obligations that have caused them to rearrange their work schedules, to work fewer paid hours than they otherwise would have, or to take unpaid leaves of absence from work. Nearly one-half of female caregivers with part-time paid jobs report working less because of elder care responsibilities. Sixteen percent of caregivers with full-time jobs say that caregiving has caused them to work fewer paid hours than they otherwise would.

■ More than one-third of disabled seniors with LTC needs use paid care

Slightly over one-third (35.1 percent) of disabled seniors with LTC needs use formal (paid) home care.[11] Only 5.4 percent rely entirely on paid helpers. Other facts about paid caregiving for the elderly include:

- The use of paid home care is much greater among seniors with moderate to severe disabilities. About half of the most severely disabled seniors (having three or more ADL limitations) use paid home care.

- Disabled seniors who live with their spouses are least likely to rely on formal help. They receive an average of 5 hours of help per week from paid caregivers, compared to 36 hours of help they receive from informal caregivers.

- Disabled elderly men cared for by their wives use the least amount of paid care, averaging about 4 hours of formal care and about 40 hours of informal help per week.

- Disabled elderly women who live with their husbands receive about 6.5 hours of paid help and 32 hours of informal help from their spouses per week.

DEFINITION: Moderate to severe disability is defined by individuals requiring help with one or more ADL tasks.

■ Paraprofessionals are the backbone of the paid LTC workforce

Second to informal caregivers, paraprofessionals are the most frequent providers of care for the elderly. In 1998, nursing assistants held about 750,000 jobs in nursing homes, and home health and personal care aides held about 746,000 jobs.[12]

DEFINITION: Paraprofessional caregivers are home health aides, certified nursing assistants (CNAs), personal attendants, and related nonprofessional workers employed in nursing homes, assisted living facilities, adult care homes, group homes, and individual clients' residences.

According to the Paraprofessional Healthcare Institute:[13]

Nationwide, paraprofessionals in all formal health care sectors total more than 2.1 million, 86 percent of whom are women, and 30 percent of whom are women of color. More than 28 percent return from work to a family living in poverty. In addition, beneath the formal sector lies a "gray-market" workforce of paid caregivers who are hired directly by consumers but whose income is not reported. The size of this unreported workforce is significant but unquantifiable.

The paraprofessional workforce is projected to grow in the future, increasing by 31 percent between 2000 and 2010 (see Table 11.1). Experts predict a shortage of workers due to high turnover and related problems.[14] Estimated turnover rates range from about 45 percent to 100 percent for nursing home paraprofessionals.[15]

Other health professionals who are key to LTC delivery are physicians, registered nurses (RNs), licensed practical nurses (LPNs), and physical therapists (PTs). All of

TABLE 11.1
Number of Employees in Paraprofessional Occupations: 2000 and 2010 Projections

	2000	2010	Percent Change from 2000 to 2010
Home health aides	615,000	907,000	47%
Other health care aides*	1,660,000	2,068,000	25
Total	2,275,000	2,975,000	31

*Includes nursing aides, orderlies, attendants, occupational therapist aides and assistants, physical therapist aides and assistants, and other health care support workers.
Source: Bureau of Labor Statistics, "Employment and Occupation 2000 and Projected 2010," Monthly Labor Review 124, no. 11 (November 2001).

these specialties are facing personnel shortages that will worsen with the aging of the baby boomers.

In 1996, Alliance for Aging research estimated that at least 20,000 physicians with geriatric training were needed to provide appropriate care for the current population of more than 30 million Americans.[16] According to the Alliance: "Meanwhile, the United States has less than one-third the needed number of primary care physicians with geriatric training and less than one-fourth the number of academic physician-scientists necessary to train present and future doctors in the principles of geriatrics." This shortage in health care expertise will become more severe as the older population continues to grow in size. By the year 2030, the United States will need more than 36,000 physicians with geriatric training to care for more than 65 million older Americans.

The nursing supply also faces shortages. According to a preliminary survey by the Health Resources and Services Administration (U.S. Department of Health and Human Services), the nation's RNs continue to grow older, and the rate of students entering the profession has slowed over the past 4 years.[17] Comparisons of data from 1980 and 2000 surveys show a significant shift in the age of the RN population. In 1980, 53 percent of RNs were under age 40, but by 2000, only 32 percent were under age 40. In addition, the rate of nurses entering the workforce was just 4.1 percent between 1996 and 2000, down from 14.2 percent growth between 1992 and 1996.

■ Almost 40 percent of the elderly with LTC needs do not get help

Thirty-seven percent of elderly people living in the community who need LTC report that they do not receive it or receive less help than necessary.[18] Most of the unmet needs are in the area of IADLs, such as meal preparation and outdoor mobility. Only 1.4 percent report unmet ADL needs; another 13.1 percent report undermet ADL needs.

Additional analyses indicate that the proportion of the elderly who report not receiving help with ADLs declined from 5 percent in 1984 to a little over 1 percent in

1994.[19] Robyn Stone pointed out the implications of these findings in her 2000 paper, *Long-Term Care for the Elderly with Disabilities*: "These findings are interesting because they suggest that most elderly people with long-term care needs believe their needs are being met. It is important to remember, however, that most of the care is being provided 'free' by family and friends; as the availability of such caregivers declines in the future, unmet needs may grow."

TYPES OF PROFESSIONAL LONG-TERM CARE SERVICES

Long-term care is a fragmented system of programs from institutional care for extremely frail patients to community-based agencies providing Meals-on-Wheels and transportation to homebound seniors. LTC usually consists of low-tech services, although more high-tech equipment is being developed, such as emergency alert systems and robots to perform daily tasks.

The major types of long-term care services include the following:

Home care. Home care encompasses a variety of services in the patient's home, including rehabilitative therapy, personal assistance, personal care, and homemaker or chore services. Patients requiring home care do not necessarily require medical care, but they almost always require assistance in essential everyday tasks. An older person who receives just three home health visits per week could pay about $12,000 for home care each year.[20] Those with severe impairments will pay more.

According to the National Association for Home Care, in 2001 there were more than 20,000 home care agencies in the United States. Of those agencies, 7,152 were Medicare-certified home health agencies. In 2000 there were 2,273 Medicare-certified hospices. For recent statistics on home health care, see the analysis of the 1998 National Home and Hospice Care Survey in Chapter 12.

Nursing homes. The most extensive and costly long-term care services are provided by nursing homes. Nursing home residents are typically frail and require nursing care and round-the-clock supervision or they are technology dependent. Nursing homes can have special units to manage certain illnesses such as Alzheimer's-type dementia. The proportion of elderly people spending one or more nights in a nursing home has dropped over the past decade, and current residents are more cognitively impaired.[21] The cost of nursing home care ranges from $35,000 to $60,000 a year.

In 1998 there were 17,458 nursing homes,[22] 1.81 million skilled nursing and nursing facility beds, and an average of 53 beds per 1,000 elderly people in the United States. For recent statistics on nursing homes, see the analysis of the National Nursing Home Survey in Chapter 13.

Adult day care. As a community-based group program, adult day care provides a variety of health, social, and related support services in a protective setting during any part of a day, but it provides less than 24-hour care. Individuals who participate in adult day care attend on a planned basis during specified hours. Adult day care enables participants to remain in the community and provides relief for caregivers. Twenty-seven states reported 3,590 licensed day care centers in 1998.[23]

Respite care. Respite care is intermittent care for a disabled person to provide relief to the regular caregiver. Care can be provided in the patient's home or at an outside setting for anywhere from a few hours to a few days. Unlike other forms of long-term care that are aimed at benefiting the frail individual, respite care also is a service to the caregiver, who is usually a family member.

Assisted living and other types of supportive housing. Services such as meals and housekeeping can be provided to frail residents on an as-needed basis. Such residents normally live in separate quarters. The most common monthly rate for assisted living facilities offering either high service or high privacy was approximately $1,800 in 1998.[24]

Continuing care retirement communities. Continuing care retirement communities (CCRCs) involve special housing that covers the entire spectrum of long-term care. Older people enter a CCRC by paying an entrance fee, and they also pay a monthly fee. There are approximately 2,100 CCRCs in the United States, with an estimated 625,000 residents, or about 2 percent of the elderly population. CCRCs often are seen as a form of LTC insurance because they protect residents against the future cost of specified health and nursing home care.

Community services. A host of other programs are part of the LTC continuum because they offer access to other services or they provide specialized services such as Meals-on-Wheels. Examples of these services are transportation, information and referral, case management, and nutrition services. Many of these programs are provided through the Older Americans Act (OAA) and the Social Services Block Grant (SSBG), which are discussed next.

Government-funded LTC programs. Three major government programs provide community-based care for elderly LTC patients: the Older Americans Act (OAA), Social Services Block Grants (SSBG), and Community Service Block Grants (CSBGs).

The Older Americans Act, enacted in 1965, is the most important vehicle for the organization and delivery of supportive and nutrition services to older persons. Title III of the OAA specifically authorizes funding for many community-based LTC services, including homemaker/home health aide services, adult day care, respite care, and chore services. Title III also funds a variety of other supportive services and nutrition services. Home care services have been a priority for Title III funding since 1975.

Title III supports 57 state agencies on aging, 660 area agencies on aging, and more than 27,000 service providers, and it currently funds six separate service programs. States receive separate allotments of funds for supportive services and centers, congregate and home-delivered nutrition services, USDA commodities or cash in lieu of commodities, disease prevention and health promotion services, and in-home services for the frail elderly.

Social Services Block Grants are designed to protect individuals from abuse and neglect, help them become self-sufficient, and reduce the need for institutional care.

Community Service Block Grants fund services to fulfill unmet local needs and complement those services provided by other agencies, including temporary housing, transportation, and services for the elderly.

WHO PAYS FOR LONG-TERM CARE?

■ Most people are not informed about how to pay for long-term care

According to a survey by the American Association of Retired Persons (AARP), 60 percent of Americans aged 45+ say they are at least "somewhat familiar" with LTC services currently available.[25] But most are uninformed about the costs of, and funding sources for, LTC services. The AARP survey asked 1,800 Americans aged 45+ a range of questions designed to measure their level of understanding of the costs and funding sources associated with LTC. The results showed that Americans aged 45+ generally do not know how much LTC services cost. For example, only 15 percent could identify the cost of nursing home care within 20 percent of the national average cost. Another quarter (24 percent) said they did not know the cost. And more than half (51 percent) were too low in estimating the cost. (According to AARP's estimates, the national average monthly cost of nursing home care is $4,654.)

About 3 in 10 (31 percent) Americans aged 45+ say they have insurance that covers the costs of long-term care, but they probably do not. Another survey commissioned by the Kaiser Family Foundation and Harvard School of Public Health found that 69 percent of Americans favor expanding Medicare to cover LTC, "even if it means higher premiums or taxes."[26] Interestingly, 70 percent of those under age 65 supported covering LTC, compared to 64 percent of those aged 65+. The survey also found that a majority of Americans mistakenly believe that Medicare covers long-term care. Only 36 percent said they were aware that the program does not cover such costs. Among respondents aged 65+, 44 percent said they knew Medicare doesn't cover long-term care.

Government and Consumer Spending for Long-Term Care

■ The federal government is the largest payer for LTC

The federal government is the largest purchaser of LTC services. Family members and other informal caregivers provide many hours of unpaid care. As mentioned earlier, the value of such donated care ranges from $45 billion to $94 billion per year.[27] The elderly face significant uncovered liability for LTC care, including $30 billion for nursing home care. In recent years, the private long-term care insurance market has grown, but only a small percentage of the elderly are covered.

■ Government spending for LTC is close to $100 billion

At least 80 federal programs assist persons with LTC, either directly or indirectly, through cash assistance, in-kind transfers, or the provision of goods and services. The two largest programs covering LTC costs are Medicare and Medicaid.

TABLE 11.2

Elderly Long-Term Care Expenditures (in billions of dollars), by Source of Payment: 2000

Source of Payment	Nursing Home Care	Home Care
Medicaid	$31.0	$4.9
Medicare	11.2	8.1
Other public funds (e.g., OAA, SSBG, states)	>1 million	2.8
Out-of-pocket and other payments	28.2	11.3
Long-term care insurance	0.3	0.2
Total	70.7	27.3
Total long-term care: $98 billion		

Source: S. Lutzsky et al., "Preliminary Data from a Survey of Employers Offering Group Long-Term Care Insurance to Their Employees" (Washington, DC: Lewin Group, June 1999).

Table 11.2 indicates that significant public and private funds are spent on LTC for the elderly, estimated at $98 billion in 2000. Medicaid and Medicare account for $55 billion of this spending, or 56 percent of the total.

■ Approximately 72 percent of LTC spending on the elderly is for institutional care

The elderly face significant uncovered liability for long-term care. Approximately 72 percent of LTC spending on the elderly is for institutional care. An estimated 40 percent of institutional care is paid by the elderly themselves. Medicaid accounts for another 43 percent of institutional care.

Table 11.2 also indicates that nearly all private spending for nursing home care is paid directly by consumers out-of-pocket. Private insurance coverage for long-term nursing home care is very limited, with private insurance payments estimated to be only about 0.3 percent of total spending for nursing home care in 2000. Even though most persons needing LTC live in the community, and not in institutions, comparatively little LTC spending is for the home and community-based services that the elderly and their families prefer. In 2000, expenditures for home and community-based care for the elderly was estimated to be about $27 billion, or 27 percent of total LTC spending for the elderly. This spending does not take into account the substantial support provided to the elderly by family and friends.

Medicare plays a relatively small role in financing LTC services. Medicare covers acute health care costs. It was never envisioned to provide protection for long-term care. Coverage of nursing home care is limited to short-term stays in skilled nursing facilities, and only for those people who demonstrate a need for daily skilled nursing care or other skills and rehabilitation services following a hospitalization. Many people who require long-term nursing home care do not need daily skilled care, and therefore they do not qualify for Medicare's benefit. As a result of this restriction,

Medicare paid for only an estimated 15 percent of the elderly's nursing home spending in 2000. For similar reasons, Medicare pays for only limited amounts of community-based LTC services, through the program's home health benefit. Medicare's spending for home health care for the elderly is estimated to be about 27 percent of home and community-based LTC in 2000.

Other federal programs such as the Social Services Block Grant, the Older Americans Act, and the Supplemental Security Income (SSI) program, provide support for community-based LTC services for impaired elderly people. In addition to these federal programs, states devote significant state funds to home and community-based LTC services.

■ Expenditures for LTC for the elderly are expected to grow 2.6 percent per year

The Congressional Budget Office (CBO) estimates that inflation-adjusted expenditures for long-term care for the elderly will grow annually by 2.6 percent between 2000 and 2040.[28] The CBO estimates that LTC expenditures will reach $207 billion in 2020 and $346 billion in 2040.*

Long-Term Care Insurance

■ Long-term care insurance is a growing market

Long-term care insurance is a relatively new product. LTC policies have been sold for about 30 years, compared with 200 years for life insurance. The number of people purchasing LTC insurance is growing rapidly. In seven years, the number of policies sold doubled, from about 3.4 million in 1993 to more than 6.8 million by the end of 1999.[29] In 1999, more than 750,000 policies were sold. By December 31, 1999, 124 companies had sold more than 6.8 million LTC policies. The LTC insurance market grew an average of 18 percent a year between 1987 and 1999.

In 2000, 77 percent of LTC policies covered both nursing home and home health care, up from 37 percent in 1990.[30] Over the past five years, the average nursing home benefit has increased by 28 percent.

■ In 1999, 5 percent of older adults purchased, or considered purchasing, LTC insurance

Most people age 60+ (74 percent) have at least a fairly good understanding of LTC insurance.[31] Five percent of older adults purchased, or thought about purchasing,

---

* The CBO assumptions are based on a rising proportion of home health care and assumes that Medicaid will pick up a growing share of those expenditures. They also assume that private insurance spending for long-term care will rise during the 2000–2020 period. Without that assumption, CBO would have projected expenditures to be lower in 2020 and the proportion of expenditures paid by Medicare, Medicaid, and out of pocket to be higher. Expenditures are projected to be higher when private insurance is included because insurance lowers the price faced by long-term care users, which encourages greater utilization.

LTC insurance during 1999.[32] One-third of all LTC policies are sold to people be-tween the ages of 55 and 64. The median income of purchasers is $42,500.

■ LTC premiums are too costly for most elderly

Most elderly cannot afford LTC insurance. Average annual LTC insurance premi-ums have increased 11 percent between 1995 and 2000, from $1,505 to $1,677.[33] In 1999, average premiums were $300 a year at age 40, $409 a year at age 50, and $1,002 at age 65.[34] However, premiums for LTC policies vary widely, based on the age of the policyholder and policy options. For example, LTC insurance premiums may be $5,880 or more per year at age 75.[35]

■ One-quarter of the elderly have preexisting conditions that prevent them from purchasing LTC insurance

About 1 in 4 elderly people has preexisting conditions that prevent them from purchasing LTC insurance, even if they can afford it.[36] However, according to the Health Insurance Association of America (HIAA), 9 of the top 10 LTC insurance sell-ers no longer have a preexisting condition limitation as long as pertinent medical conditions are disclosed at the time of application.[37]

Age limits for purchasing LTC policies are expanding. Companies now offer indi-vidual policies to people as young as 18 and as old as 99.

■ Forty-two states comply with HIPAA long-term care regulations

The National Association of Insurance Commissioners (NAIC) has established a model act and regulations for LTC insurance products sold within their jurisdic-tions. Among other things, this act includes an inflation protection requirement of benefits increasing at an annual 5 percent compounded rate. The Health Insurance Portability and Accountability Act (HIPAA) of 1996 required LTC policies to meet many of the standards specified in the NAIC model act and regulations to receive fa-vorable tax treatment. The HIAA reports that 42 states are at least 60 percent compli-ant with HIPAA.

■ Employer-based policies are increasing

LTC insurance policies include individual, group association, and employer-sponsored, as well as riders to life insurance policies.[38] According to HIAA, employer-based policy sales have increased steadily over the years. By the end of 1999, more than 3,200 employers offering LTC insurance had sold 1 million policies to employ-ees and retirees.[39] Most of these plans require employees to pay all the costs of the premiums.

■ Long-term care insurance sales are concentrated in nine states

Only nine states accounted for one-half of all individual and group LTC policies sold by the end of 1999:[40] Florida, California, Pennsylvania, Illinois, Texas, Ohio, Washington, Iowa, and Missouri. Florida accounted for nearly 10 percent of all LTC insurance policies sold in the United States. Based on 1999 statistics, 124 companies sell LTC insurance.

LONG-TERM CARE FOR VETERANS

■ The Veterans Administration provides an array of LTC services

Although the Veterans Administration (VA) provides a comprehensive array of services, not all programs are available in all VA locations.[41] In March 1990, 139,000 male veterans were in nursing homes. Nearly 75 percent were aged 65+. Through 1996, the average daily census of patients in VA nursing homes continued historic annual increases, reaching a peak of 13,642. However, this trend has slowed. The average daily census of patients in VA nursing homes decreased to 12,742 in fiscal year (FY) 1999. Some key VA programs for elderly veterans with long-term care needs include the following.

State veterans' homes. Through the State Home Grant program, the VA provides grants to states for the construction and support of state veterans' homes to provide LTC for frail, elderly veterans. In fiscal year 1998, more than 22,400 veterans were provided nursing home care in state veterans' homes.

The Geriatric Evaluation and Management program. Currently, 110 VA medical centers have Geriatric Evaluation and Management (GEM) programs that include inpatient units or outpatient clinics, as well as consultation services. The GEM programs provide both primary and specialized care services to a targeted group of elderly patients.

Nursing home care units. VA nursing homes provide skilled nursing and related medical services. Many also provide subacute and postacute care. In fiscal year 1998, more than 46,000 veterans received care in VA's 132 nursing home care units (NHCUs).

Alzheimer's and other dementia care programs. Approximately 56 VA medical centers have developed specialized programs for the care of veterans with dementia.

Homemaker/Home Health Aide program. The Homemaker/Home Health Aide (H/HHA) program enables selected patients who meet the criteria for nursing home placement to remain at home through the provision of personal care services. During fiscal year 1998, 118 VA facilities purchased these services for approximately 2,400 veterans on any given day.

NOTES

1. R. C. Atchley, *Frontline Workers in Long-Term Care: Recruitment, Retention, and Turnover Issues in an Era of Rapid Growth* (Oxford, OH: Scripps Gerontology Center at Miami University, 1996).

2. Authors' analysis of 1999 National Nursing Home Survey.
3. Authors' analysis of 1998 National Home and Hospice Care Survey.
4. U.S. Department of Health and Human Services, *Informal Caregiving: Compassion in Action* (Washington, DC, June 1998).
5. Ibid.
6. Robyn I. Stone, *Long-Term Care for the Elderly with Disabilities: Current Policy, Emerging Trends, and Implications for the Twenty-First Century* (New York: Milbank Memorial Fund, 2000). Available online at www.milbank.org.
7. U.S. Department of Health and Human Services, *Informal Caregiving.*
8. National Academy of Aging, reported in Stone, *Long-Term Care.*
9. U.S. Department of Health and Human Services, *Informal Caregiving.*
10. Ibid.
11. Ibid.
12. Robyn Stone and Joshua Wiener, "Who Will Care for Us?" (Washington, DC: Urban Institute, U.S. Department of Health and Human Services, American Association of Homes and Services for the Aged, and Robert Wood Johnson Foundation, October 2001), 3. Available online at www.urban.org.
13. Paraprofessional Healthcare Institute, *Direct Care Health Workers: The Unnecessary Crisis in Long-Term Care* (Aspen, CO: Aspen Institute, January 2001), 12. Available online at www.paraprofessional.org.
14. Stone and Wiener, "Who Will Care for Us?"
15. Ibid.
16. Alliance for Aging Research, "Will You Still Treat Me When I'm 65?" (May 1996). Available at www.agingresearch.org/features.html.
17. U.S. Health Resources and Services Administration, "Health Workforce Analysis: National Sample Survey of Registered Nurses" (not dated). Available online at www.hrsa.gov.
18. B. Jackson and P. Doty. "Unmet and Undermet Need for Functional Assistance among the U.S. Disabled Elderly." Paper presented at the 1997 annual meeting of the Gerontological Society of America, Cincinnati. Reported in Stone, *Long-Term Care.*
19. National Long Term Care Survey. Reported in Stone, *Long-Term Care.*
20. AARP consumer information. Available online at http://aarp.gov.
21. Stone, *Long-Term Care.*
22. C. Harrington et al., "1998 State Data Book on Long-Term Care Program and Market Statistics" (University of California–San Francisco and Wichita State University, November 1999).
23. Ibid.
24. C. Hawes et al., "A National Study of Assisted Living for the Frail Elderly: Results of a National Telephone Survey of Facilities" (Beachwood, OH: Menorah Park Center for the Aging, 1999).
25. American Association of Retired Persons, *Most Americans Unprepared for Long-Term Care Costs* (December 2001). Available online at www.aarp.org.
26. Kaiser Family Foundation, *National Survey on Medicare* (October 20, 1998). Available online at www.kff.org.
27. Department of Health and Human Services, *Informal Caregiving.*
28. Congressional Budget Office (not dated). Available online at www.cbo.gov.
29. Health Insurance Association of America, "Long-Term Care Insurance in 1998–1999" (Washington, DC, not dated). Available online at www.hiaa.org.
30. Health Insurance Association of America, "Buyers and Non-Buyers of Long-Term Care Insurance: A Decade of Experience," *Older Americans Reports* (October 20, 2000): 352.
31. RoperASW, 1999.
32. RoperASW, 2000.

33. Health Insurance Association of America, "Who Buys Long-Term Care Insurance in 2000?" (not dated). Available online at www.hiaa.org.

34. Health Insurance Association of America, "Number of Americans with Long-Term Care Insurance Triples over 10 Years" (February 22, 2002). Available online at www.hiaa.org.

35. American Association of Retired Persons, "Private Long-Term Care Insurance" (not dated).

36. Long Term Care Campaign, "All About Long-Term Care" (Washington, DC, 2000).

37. Health Insurance Association of America, "Number of Americans."

38. Health Insurance Association of America, "Long-Term Care Insurance."

39. Ibid.

40. Ibid.

41. Statement of Kenneth W. Kizer, M.D., M.P.H, Undersecretary for Health, Department of Veterans Affairs, on long-term care within the Veterans Health Administration, before the House Veterans' Affairs Committee, Subcommittee on Health (April 22, 1999). Available online at www.va.gov.

CHAPTER 12

Long-Term Care: Home Health Care

The future is more and more about management of chronic disease and less about acute care. By definition, this means that home care will become the heart of health care.

—Val J. Halamandaris, President, National Association for Home Care

This chapter incorporates a special analysis performed by Kris Hodges of newly available statistics from the 1998 National Home and Hospice Care Survey along with other key statistics.[1] An overview of home health care and its role in long-term care appears in Chapter 11.

Highlights of this chapter include:

- Nearly 3 percent of elderly people were current home health care patients in 2000, a decrease of 49 percent from 1996.

- At least some of the decline is due to decreases in Medicare reimbursements. In fact, Medicare spending for home health care was $9.5 billion in 1999, a nearly 50 percent decline from 1997.

- At age 65, the elderly have a 72 percent chance that they will use home health care in their lifetime compared to a 49 percent likelihood of entering a nursing home.

- The oldest-old women are most likely to be home health care patients.

- The lightest users of home health care are those who live with their primary caregiver.

- Most elderly home health care discharges meet their goals.

CURRENT HOME HEALTH CARE PATIENTS

■ Home health care use is decreasing

According to the National Home and Hospice Care Survey, the elderly accounted for 71 percent of all home health care patients, or an estimated 955,000 elderly people in 2000.[2] On an age-adjusted basis, this represents 2.8 percent of all elderly adults and is a decrease of 49 percent from 1996 (see Table 12.1). This decline reflects the closing of many home health agencies resulting from changes in the reimbursement system enacted by Congress as part of the Balanced Budget Act in 1997.

These changes are also evident in Medicare spending for home health care, which rose from $3.7 billion in 1990 to $17.8 billion in 1997 but then declined to $9.5 billion in 1999.[3]

■ The elderly are more likely to use home health care than nursing home care

According to one estimate, at age 65 the elderly have a 72 percent chance of using home health care in their lifetime versus a 49 percent likelihood of entering a nursing home.[4] Nearly 3 percent of all elderly are current home health care patients (see Table 12.1).

More than one-half (56 percent) of elderly home health care patients live with family members and more than one-third (38 percent) live alone.[5]

Almost all elderly home health care patients (87 percent) receive care from an agency that has been certified by Medicare or Medicaid as a home health agency.[6] Less than one-half of elderly home health care recipients (45 percent) receive serv-

TABLE 12.1
Rate of Home Health Care Use (per 100 Persons), by Age and Sex: 1996, 1998, and 2000

	Rate per 100 Persons			Percent Change		
	1996	1998	2000	1998 versus 1996	2000 versus 1998	2000 versus 1996
65+ years*	5.47	3.81	2.77	−30%	−27%	−49%
65–74	2.40	2.02	1.30	−16	−36	−46
75–84	7.54	4.70	3.48	−38	−26	−54
85+	12.5	8.85	6.94	−29	−22	−44
Men, 65+ years*	4.38	2.78	2.16	−37	−22	−51
65–74	1.87	1.60	1.01	−14	−37	−46
75–84	5.99	3.21	2.70	−46	−16	−55
85+	10.4	6.53	5.54	−37	−15	−47
Women, 65+ years*	6.15	4.46	3.16	−27	−29	−49
65–74	2.83	2.36	1.55	−17	−34	−45
75–84	8.54	5.69	4.00	−33	−30	−53
85+	13.4	9.82	7.55	−27	−23	−44

*Age-adjusted to the year 2000 population standard using the following three age groups: 65–74 years, 75–84 years, and 85+ years.
Source: National Center for Health Statistics, *Health, United States, 2002 with Chartbook on Trends in the Health of Americans* (Hyattsville, MD, 2002): Table 88.

CHART 12.1 Rate of Current Home Health Care Use, by Age and Sex: 2000

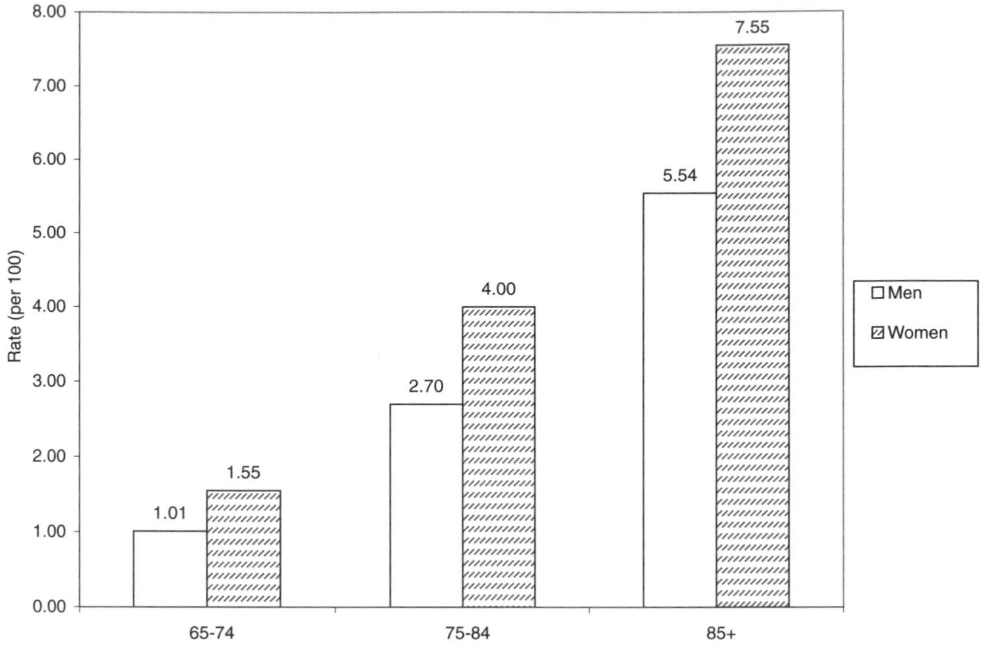

Source: National Center for Health Statistics, *Health, United States, 2002 with Chartbook on Trends in the Health of Americans* (Hyattsville, MD, 2002), Table 88.

ices from proprietary organizations, with nonprofit or other types of organizations providing care for the remaining 55 percent.[7]

■ Oldest-old women are the most likely to be home health care patients

The likelihood of being a current home health care patient is higher among older age groups. With each successive 10-year age increment, the likelihood of the elderly being a home health care patient increases at least twofold (see Chart 12.1). Elderly women of every age group are more likely than elderly men to receive home health care. The oldest-old women are the most likely to be home health care patients, with about 7.6 percent currently using such services.

■ Home health care patients are predominantly women

Elderly women, the predominant users of home health care services, outnumber elderly male patients 2.6 to 1 (see Table 12.2). Seventy-two percent of elderly home health care patients are women, and more than one-half are women aged 75+.

Although men are in the minority, those aged 85+ are 1.7 times more likely than the average elderly person to be home health care patients (see ratios in Table 12.2). Elderly women aged 75+ have a greater than average likelihood of being a home

TABLE 12.2
Percent Distribution of Elderly Home Health Care Patients and Total
U.S. Elderly, by Age, Sex, Race, Marital Status, and Region: 1998

	Current Home Health Care Patients	Total U.S. Elderly	Ratio of Patients to Total U.S. Elderly
Total 65+ years	100%	100%	1.00
65–74	29	53	0.54
75–84	43	35	1.25
85+	28	12	2.36
Men 65+	28	41	0.68
65–74	10	24	0.43
75–84	12	14	0.86
85+	6.0	3.5	1.74
Women 65+	72	59	1.23
65–74	19	29	0.63
75–84	32	21	1.51
85+	22	8.3	2.61
Race*			
White	84	89	0.94
Men	27	37	0.73
Women	57	52	1.09
Black	15	8.3	1.86
Men	3.6	3.2	1.11
Women	12	5.0	2.34
Marital status*			
Men, married	20	32	0.64
Women, married	17	25	0.69
Census region			
Northeast	34	21	1.58
Midwest	21	24	0.90
South	36	35	1.03
West	9.1	20	0.46

*Current patient demographics based on those of known status.

Source: Special analysis conducted by Kris Hodges based on data from Home health care data from National Center for Health Statistics, *1998 National Home and Hospice Care Survey*, CD-ROM series 13, no. 27 (Hyattsville, MD, October 2000); U.S. population data from Bureau of the Census, *Statistical Abstract of the United States: 1999*, 119th ed. (Washington, DC, 1999), Tables 21 and 63.

health care patient. In fact, the oldest-old women are 2.6 times more likely than the average elderly person to use the services. Black elderly women and the elderly from the Northeast also are more likely to be home health care patients.

CHART 12.2   Distribution of Elderly Home Health Care Patients by Length of Service since Admission: 1996 and 1998

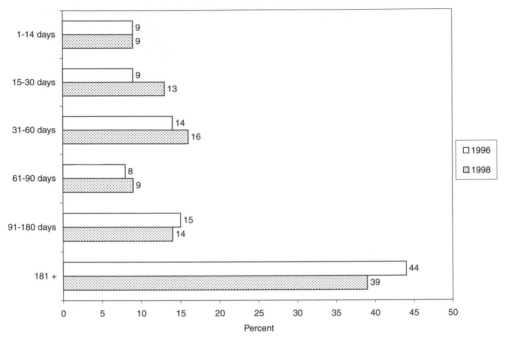

Sources: For 1996 data: Martha Little Munson, "Characteristics of Elderly Home Health Care Users: Data from the 1996 National Home and Hospice Care Survey," no. 309 (Hyattsville, MD: National Center for Health Statistics, December 22, 1999). For 1988 data: National Center for Health Statistics, *1998 National Home and Hospice Care Survey*, CD-ROM series 13, no. 27 (Hyattsville, MD, October 2000).

■ **Married elderly are much less likely than unmarried elderly to be home health care patients**

Conversely, married elderly are much less likely to be home health care users: 37 percent of home health care patients are married, compared to 57 percent of all elderly. This reflects, at least in part, the availability of a spouse to provide care in lieu of professional care.

■ **The average elderly home health care patient has been using the service for almost a year**

Elderly home health care patients in 1988 had received service for just less than a year (337 days, on average), with one-half using the service for 107 days or longer.[8] This length of service distribution skews lower than in 1996, again reflecting the decline in Medicare reimbursement that may be shortening the length of service available to the elderly (see Chart 12.2).[9]

CHART 12.3   Average Length of Home Health Care Services (in Days) among Elderly Patients, by Caregiver Status: 1998

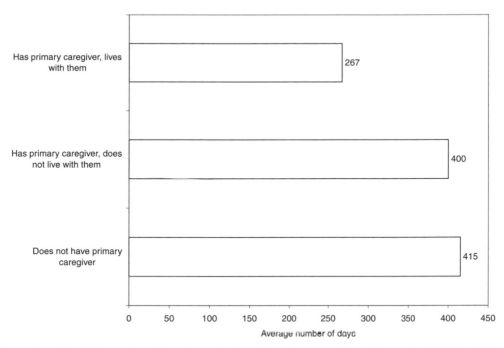

Source: Special analysis conducted by Kris Hodges based on data from National Center for Health Statistics, *1998 National Home and Hospice Care Survey*, CD-ROM series 13, no. 27 (Hyattsville, MD, October 2000).

■ Elderly patients living with primary caregivers are lighter users of home health care

Most elderly home health care patients (80 percent) have a primary caregiver, and 72 percent of them live with that caregiver.[10] Interestingly, those who live with a primary caregiver have been using home health care for the least amount of time, whereas those who have no primary caregiver have been using it for the greatest amount of time (see Chart 12.3). Those who have a primary caregiver but do not live with them have been using home health care for about as long as those who have no primary caregiver. One possible explanation for this differential is that those without immediate caregiver access are more dependent upon outside services for their care.

Elderly men who use home health care have a greater likelihood than do their female counterparts of having a primary caregiver (89 percent versus 78 percent) as well as living with that caregiver (82 percent versus 67 percent).[11] In part, this may account for men's shorter use of home health care (see Table 12.3). Elderly women use home health care services anywhere from 10 to more than 50 percent longer than their male counterparts do.

TABLE 12.3

Average Length of Home-Health Care Services among Elderly Patients
(in Days), by Age and Sex: 1998

	Total	Men	Women	Ratio of Women to Men
65+ years	337	262	366	1.40
65–74	280	261	290	1.11
75–84	372	264	412	1.56
85+	341	261	363	1.39

Source: Special analysis conducted by Kris Hodges based on data from National
Center for Health Statistics, *1998 National Home and Hospice Care Survey*, CD-
ROM series 13, no. 27 (Hyattsville, MD, October 2000).

■ **Circulatory problems are the most common reason for receiving home
health care**

The most frequently listed primary admission diagnosis for elderly home health
care patients is diseases of the circulatory system (mostly heart disease), accounting
for 30 percent of all primary diagnoses (see Table 12.4). Heart disease alone accounts
for nearly 1 in 5 primary diagnoses. Diseases of the musculoskeletal system and con-
nective tissue, injuries and poisonings, diabetes, chronic obstructive pulmonary disease, and blood-related diseases round out the most common primary diagnoses.

TABLE 12.4

Percent of Current Elderly Home Health Care Patients by Primary
Admission Diagnosis: 1998

	Percent
Diseases of circulatory system	30%
Heart disease	17
Cerebrovascular disease	5.6
Essential hypertension	4.3
Other circulatory diseases	3.1
Diseases of musculoskeletal system and connective tissue	9.3
Injuries and poisonings	8.9
Diabetes mellitus	7.1
Chronic obstructive pulmonary disease	5.3
Diseases of the blood and blood forming organs	4.9

Source: National Center for Health Statistics, *1998 National Home and
Hospice Care Survey*, CD-ROM series 13, no. 27 (Hyattsville, MD, October
2000).

■ Most elderly home health care patients are not incontinent

One in four elderly home health care patients has difficulty controlling either bowels or bladder, and about 1 in 8 has a catheter and/or ostomy (see Table 12.5). Incontinence increases with age.

Elderly home health care patients most commonly receive skilled nursing services; 79 percent received these services in the past 30 days.[12] Homemaker-household services are a distant second (24 percent), followed by physical therapy (22 percent). These patients also receive more ADL assistance than IADL assistance (see Table 12.5). ADL assistance increases with age, whereas IADL assistance remains relatively stable. (See Chapter 5 for complete definitions of ADLs and IADLs.)

More than 90 percent of elderly home health care patients use some type of aid, most commonly eyeglasses and walkers (see Table 12.6). As might be expected, younger patients are less likely than older patients to use aids. The greatest age dif-

TABLE 12.5
Percent of Elderly Home Health Care Patients with Stated Functional Status: 1998

	All Elderly Patients	65–74 Years	75–84 Years	85+ Years
Has a catheter and/or ostomy*	12%	12%	12%	13%
Has difficulty controlling:				
Bladder and/or bowels*	25	18	26	31
Bladder*	24	18	24	29
Bowels*	8.9	5.0	8.5	13
Receives help with ADLs**				
Bathing	52	41	53	60
Dressing	45	36	47	50
Transferring	29	24	28	33
Walking	28	21	28	33
Using toilet room	23	19	21	27
Eating	9.4	9.0	7.2	13
Receives help with IADLs**				
Doing light housework	38	34	39	40
Preparing meals	21	22	20	22
Taking medications	19	20	16	22
Shopping	14	15	14	13
Using the telephone	3.9	3.8	2.7	5.8
Managing money	2.1	1.7	1.9	2.9

*Among those with known catheter, ostomy, bladder and bowel status.

**Based on those of known status.

Source: Special analysis conducted by Kris Hodges based on data from National Center for Health Statistics, *1998 National Home and Hospice Care Survey,* CD-ROM series 13, no. 27 (Hyattsville, MD, October 2000).

TABLE 12.6

Percent of Elderly Home Health Care Patients Using a Particular Aid: 1998

	All Elderly Patients	65–74 Years	75–84 Years	85+ Years
Eyeglasses	54%	50%	54%	58%
Walker	45	35	46	53
Dentures	27	25	28	27
Cane	26	21	26	32
Wheelchair	24	23	30	22
Commode	19	15	17	24
Hospital bed	15	12	16	19
Oxygen	9.4	8.7	11	7.2
Grab bar	9.0	11	7.7	9.2
Hearing aid	8.0	3.4	7.5	14
Blood glucose monitor	6.2	6.6	8.0	3.1
Transfer equipment	3.6	3.8	4.0	2.9
No aids used	7.4	13	6.2	3.6

Source: National Center for Health Statistics, *1998 National Home and Hospice Care Survey,* CD-ROM series 13, no. 27 (Hyattsville, MD, October 2000).

ferential exists for ambulatory aids, such as walkers and canes, as well as hearing aids and hospital beds.

HOME HEALTH CARE DISCHARGES

According to the 1988 National Home and Hospice Care Survey, an estimated 5,301,000 elderly discharges from home health care services occurred during 1998. The elderly accounted for 70 percent of all discharges.[13]

Most elderly discharges met their goals, such as recovering or stabilizing, with women more likely than men to have done so because they are more likely to have stabilized (see Table 12.7). Men are more likely to have died or been discharged to the hospital.

A recent study focusing on Medicare patients who were discharged from a hospital to home health care found that during a 2-month period in 1999, nearly 4 in 10 Medicare patients (38 percent) were readmitted to the hospital.[14] This is a 3 percentage point drop from a similar time period in 1997. One in five of these Medicare patients (19 percent) had an emergency room visit, which also represents a 3 percentage point drop from the same period 2 years earlier.

■ Elderly home health care discharge status varies by age, sex, and race

Middle-old men are the most likely to have been discharged due to death; in 1998, for instance, 11 percent died, which is more than three times the likelihood of their older and younger counterparts (see Chart 12.4). More specifically, death be-

TABLE 12.7
Percent of Elderly Home Health Care Discharges with Given Disposition Status,
by Sex: 1998

	Men	Women	Ratio of Men to Women	Ratio of Women to Men
Goals met	61%	71%	0.86	1.16
Recovered	20	19	1.04	0.96
Stabilized	30	39	0.78	1.29
Family or friends resumed care	5.9	7.7	0.77	1.30
Other	5.2	5.2	1.01	0.99
Transferred to:	23	21	1.08	0.93
Hospital	14	11	1.31	0.76
Nursing home	3.3	5.1	0.65	1.55
Other	5.4	5.3	1.01	0.99
Moved out of area	3.6	1.7	2.06	0.48
Deceased	7.1	2.9	2.40	0.42
Other	5.3	3.1	1.68	0.59

Source: Special analysis conducted by Kris Hodges based on data from National Center for Health Statistics, *1998 National Home and Hospice Care Survey*, CD-ROM series 13, no. 27 (Hyattsville, MD, October 2000).

falls elderly black men at a disproportionate rate; they are almost three times more likely to have died than their white counterparts (see Chart 12.5). In contrast, elderly white men are more than four times as likely to be discharged to a hospital than their black counterparts.

The likelihood of family or friends resuming care or of stabilization declines with age for both elderly men and women (see Chart 12.4).

The oldest-old are about twice as likely as their youngest counterparts to be discharged to a hospital (see Chart 12.4). Nursing home discharges are most likely among the oldest-old men and women and middle-old women as well as elderly black men and women. In fact, elderly black men are four times more likely, and elderly black women are 1.7 times more likely, than their white counterparts to be admitted to a nursing home (see Chart 12.5).

■ Elderly home health care discharges used services for less than 4 months, on average

Elderly home health care discharges had used the services for an average of 104 days, less than one-third the length of current home health care patients. Except among the middle-old discharges, elderly women used the services for a longer time than men (see Table 12.8).

Home health care patients who died had used the services the longest—more than 7 months on average. Those who recovered or stabilized had used it the shortest, less than 2 months on average (see Chart 12.6).

CHART 12.4   Percent of Elderly Home Health Care Discharges with Given Disposition Status, by Age and Sex: 1998

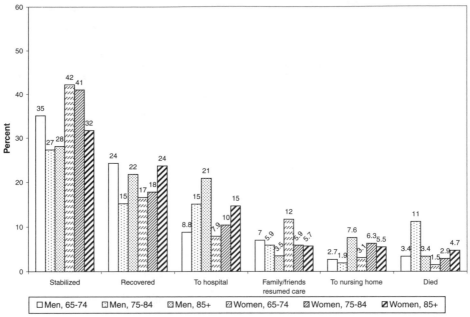

Source: Special analysis conducted by Kris Hodges based on data from National Center for Health Statistics, *1998 National Home and Hospice Care Survey,* CD-ROM series 13, no. 27 (Hyattsville, MD, October 2000).

CHART 12.5   Percent of Elderly Home Health Care Discharges with Given Disposition Status, by Sex and Race: 1998

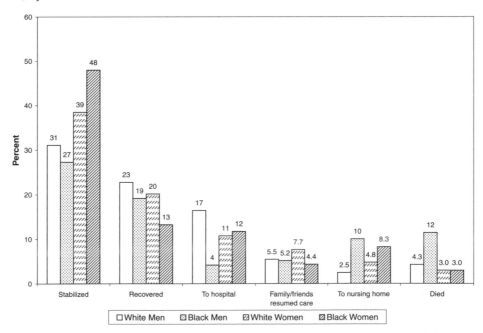

Source: Special analysis conducted by Kris Hodges based on data from National Center for Health Statistics, *1998 National Home and Hospice Care Survey,* CD-ROM series 13, no. 27 (Hyattsville, MD, October 2000).

TABLE 12.8

Average Length of Home Health Care Use (in Days) among Elderly Home Health Care Discharges, by Age and Sex: 1998

	Men	Women	Ratio of Women to Men
65+ years	92	111	1.21
65–74	68	121	1.78
75–84	110	88	0.80
85+	93	135	1.45

Source: National Center for Health Statistics, *1998 National Home and Hospice Care Survey,* CD-ROM series 13, no. 27 (Hyattsville, MD, October 2000).

■ Aids used by discharges who died reflect their more severe health status

Elderly home health care patients who died had the highest use of hospital beds and oxygen, reflecting their more severe health status (see Table 12.9). Those who were discharged to a hospital or nursing home have the highest use of ambulatory aids such as wheelchairs, canes, and walkers.

CHART 12.6   Average Length of Service among Elderly Home Health Care Discharges (in days), by Reason for Discharge: 1998

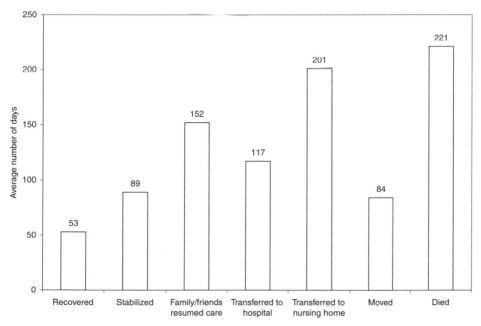

Source: Special analysis conducted by Kris Hodges based on data from National Center for Health Statistics, *1998 National Home and Hospice Care Survey*, CD-ROM series 13, no. 27 (Hyattsville, MD, October 2000).

TABLE 12.9

Percent of Elderly Home Health Care Discharges Using a Particular Aid, by Reason for Discharge: 1998

	All Elderly Discharges	Reason for Discharge		
		Recovered or Stabilized	To Hospital or Nursing Home	Died
Eyeglasses	48%	49%	53%	38%
Walker	42	41	48	23
Cane	28	29	36	22
Dentures	20	20	27	22
Wheelchair	17	15	25	20
Commode	15	12	21	14
Hospital bed	11	6.3	16	29
Oxygen	10	11	11	21
Hearing aid	6.4	5.9	10	8.4
Grab bar	6.3	6.5	6.6	7.6
Blood glucose monitor	4.8	4.5	7.4	4.2
Transfer equipment	1.5	1.0	1.3	0.6
No aids used	13	14	12	6.9

Source: Special analysis conducted by Kris Hodges based on data from National Center for Health Statistics, *1998 National Home and Hospice Care Survey*, CD-ROM series 13, no. 27 (Hyattsville, MD, October 2000).

Not surprisingly, those who have recovered or stabilized have the least need for ADL and IADL assistance and have the least problems with incontinence (see Table 12.10).

NOTES

All percents in data are based on totals that exclude missing values and those of unknown status.

1. National Center for Health Statistics, *1998 National Home and Hospice Care Survey*, CD-ROM series 13, no. 27 (Hyattsville, MD, October 2000).
2. National Center for Health Statistics, *Health, United States, 2002 with Chartbook on Trends in the Health of Americans* (Hyattsville, MD, 2002): Table 88.
3. Department of Health and Human Services, Office of Inspector General, "Adequacy of Home Health Services: Hospital Re-Admissions and Emergency Room Visits," OEI-02-99-00531 (September 2000).
4. Lewin-VHI. Based on the Brookings-ICF Long-Term Care Financing Model. Cited in Robyn I. Stone, *Long-Term Care for the Elderly with Disabilities: Current Policy, Emerging Trends, and Implications for the Twenty-First Century* (New York: Milbank Memorial Fund, 2000); available online at www.milbank.org.
5. National Center for Health Statistics, *1998 National Home and Hospice Care Survey*.
6. Ibid.
7. Ibid.

TABLE 12.10
Percent of Elderly Home Health Care Discharges, by Functional Status: 1998

	All Elderly Discharges	Reason for Discharge		
		Recovered or Stabilized	Transferred to Hospital or Nursing Home	Died
Has a catheter or ostomy*	6.4%	3.5%	14%	12%
Has difficulty controlling:				
Bladder and/or bowels*	17	14	22	34
Bladder*	15	12	21	32
Bowels*	7.6	5.8	11	20
Receives help with ADLs**				
Bathing	41	33	63	56
Dressing	34	27	54	51
Transferring	24	18	38	43
Walking	23	19	31	29
Using toilet room	18	12	30	35
Eating	6.4	1.8	17	20
Receives Help with IADLs**				
Doing light housework	23	18	32	28
Taking medications	13	8.6	20	18
Preparing meals	10	6.8	21	12
Shopping	3.7	1.5	9.0	7.7
Using the telephone	1.4	0.5	4.1	4.9
Managing money	0.6	0.5	0.1	1.7

*Based on those with known catheter, ostomy, bladder and bowel status.

**Based on those of known status.

Source: Special analysis conducted by Kris Hodges based on data from National Center for Health Statistics, *1998 National Home and Hospice Care Survey*, CD ROM series 13, no. 27 (Hyattsville, MD, October 2000).

8. Ibid.
9. Martha Little Munson, "Characteristics of Elderly Home Health Care Users: Data from the 1996 National Home and Hospice Care Survey," no. 309 (Hyattsville, MD: National Center for Health Statistics, December 22, 1999).
10. National Center for Health Statistics, *1998 National Home and Hospice Care Survey*.
11. Ibid.
12. Ibid.
13. Ibid.
14. Department of Health and Human Services, Office of Inspector General, "Adequacy of Home Health Services."

CHAPTER 13

Long-Term Care: Nursing Home Care

Very often nursing home placement is the only solution to a particular set of problems.

—Sarah Green Burger and Martha D'Erasmo, Living in a Nursing Home

This chapter incorporates a special analysis conducted by Kris Hodges of newly available data from the 1999 National Nursing Home Survey,[1] along with other statistics. An overview of nursing home care and its role in long-term care appears in Chapter 11.

Highlights of this chapter include:

- Nursing home usage has declined since the 1970s. Today, only about 4 percent of the elderly are in a nursing home.
- The oldest-old women are the most likely seniors to be nursing home residents, accounting for 40 percent of all elderly residents.
- The average nursing home resident has lived there for more than 2 years.
- Married nursing home residents have resided for substantially less time in a nursing home than have their never-married counterparts.
- Most nursing home residents are incontinent.
- Death accounts for more than 1 in 4 elderly nursing home discharges overall, but 1 in 3 among the oldest-old discharges.
- Elderly discharges had resided in a nursing home for an average of about 10 months. Those who had recovered or stabilized had the shortest residencies, whereas those who died had the longest.
- Regardless of the reason for discharge, elderly discharges who are married had substantially shorter residencies than did their never-married counterparts.

NURSING HOME RESIDENTS

■ Nursing home usage has declined among the elderly

Despite the aging of the population, the demand for nursing home care has been decreasing since the mid-1970s. On an age-adjusted basis, 5.9 percent of the elderly population in 1973–1974 was in a nursing home versus 4.3 percent in 1999, a decline of 26 percent (see Table 13.1).[2] The declines have been most dramatic for older age groups, especially among the oldest-old men. As mentioned in Chapter 5, part of this decline appears to be associated with declining disability among the elderly.

■ About 1 in 25 seniors is in a nursing home

An estimated 1,469,500 elderly adults were nursing home residents in 1999, representing 1 in 25 elderly (4.3 percent; see Table 13.1). Nine in ten nursing home residents are elderly.[3]

Two-thirds of elderly nursing home residents reside in for-profit facilities. A slightly greater percent (69 percent) reside in urban-setting nursing homes.

The elderly usually become nursing home residents at the initiation of a spouse, child, other family member, or a friend. Typically, families make the decision at the point that unpaid, informal caregiving approaches 60 hours per week.[4]

TABLE 13.1
Nursing Home Residency Rate (per 100 Persons), by Age and Sex:
1973–1974 and 1999

	1973–1974	1999	Percent Change, 1999 versus 1973–1974
65+ years*	5.85	4.33	−26%
65–74	1.23	1.08	−12
75–84	5.77	4.30	−25
85+	25.7	18.3	−29
Men, 65+ years*	4.25	3.06	−28
65–74	1.13	1.03	−8.8
75–84	3.99	3.08	−23
85+	18.3	11.7	−36
Women, 65+ years*	6.75	4.98	−26
65–74	1.31	1.12	−15
75–84	6.89	5.12	−26
85+	29.5	21.1	−29

*Age adjusted to the year 2000 population standard using the following three age groups: 65–74 years, 75–84 years, and 85+.
Source: National Center for Health Statistics, *Health, United States, 2002 with Chartbook on Trends in the Health of Americans* (Hyattsville, MD, 2002), Table 97.

The probability for using nursing home care increases with age. Although only 4.3 percent of the U.S. elderly resided in nursing homes in 1999, research has shown that many more are expected to use nursing home care at some time in their lives. Projections of nursing home use during one's lifetime vary from 39 to 49 percent.[5] According to 1995 estimates, 39 percent of the elderly living in the community were expected to use nursing home care for some period in their lives: 20 percent for more than 1 year and 10 percent for more than 5 years. Older age groups have a greater likelihood of needing nursing home care. Of those aged 85+ living in the community in 1995, 49 percent were expected to use nursing home care at some point in their lives.[6]

■ One in five of the oldest-old women lives in a nursing home

The likelihood of being a nursing home resident is higher among older age groups. With each successive 10-year age increment, the likelihood of the elderly being in a nursing home increases about three- to fourfold (see Chart 13.1 and detailed data in Table 13.2). The oldest-old women are the most likely to be nursing home residents, with 1 in 5 residing there in 1999 (see Table 13.2).

Among the youngest-old, women are somewhat more likely than men to be in a nursing home. However, the gender gap widens with age, with the oldest-old

CHART 13.1   Rate of Nursing Home Residency (per 100 Persons), by Age and Sex: 1999

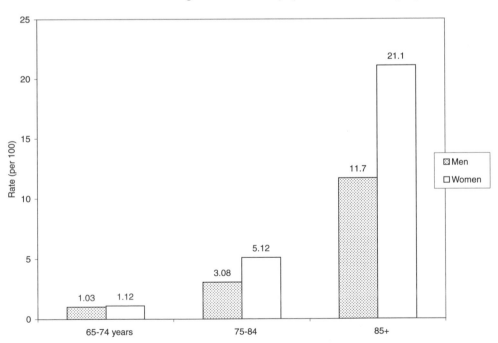

Source: National Center for Health Statistics, *Health, United States, 2002 with Chartbook on Trends in the Health of Americans* (Hyattsville, MD, 2002), Table 97.

TABLE 13.2

Detailed Data for Chart 13.1: Nursing Home Residency (Rate per 100 Persons), by Age and Sex, 1999

	Men		Women		
	Rate	Ratio to Prior 10-Year Age Category	Rate	Ratio to Prior 10-Year Age Category	Ratio of Women to Men
65+ years*	3.06	NA	4.98	NA	1.63
65–74	1.03	NA	1.12	NA	1.09
75–84	3.08	2.99	5.12	4.57	1.66
85+	11.7	3.80	21.1	4.12	1.81

*Age adjusted to the year 2000 population standard using the following three age groups: 65–74 years, 75–84 years, and 85+.

Note: NA = Not Available.

Source: National Center for Health Statistics, *Health, United States, 2002 with Chartbook on Trends in the Health of Americans* (Hyattsville, MD, 2002), Table 97.

women being nearly twice as likely as their male counterparts to be nursing home residents (see Table 13.2).

■ Elderly women greatly outnumber elderly men in nursing homes

In the general population, elderly women outnumber elderly men 3 to 2. However, in nursing homes, women constitute three-quarters of elderly nursing home residents, outnumbering men 3 to 1 (see Table 13.3).

■ Four in ten seniors in nursing homes are women aged 85+

Compared with the average elderly adult, elderly nursing home residents are more likely to be the oldest-old men, older women (aged 75+ and especially aged 85+), black or white women, and from the Midwest (see Table 13.3).

In fact, women aged 85+ are 4.9 times more prevalent in the nursing home population than in the total U.S. elderly population, and account for 42 percent of the elderly people in nursing homes. Two-thirds of elderly nursing home residents are women aged 75+.[7]

■ Elderly nursing home residents have lived there for more than 2 years, on average

About 4 in 10 elderly nursing home residents have lived there for 1 year or less (see Table 13.4). Slightly more than one-quarter have lived there for more than 3 years, and 1 in 10 has resided for more than 6 years. On average, an elderly nursing home resident has lived there for nearly 2.5 years (885 days), and half of all residents have lived there for 1.4 years (496 days) or longer.[8]

TABLE 13.3

Percent of Elderly Nursing Home Residents versus Percent of Total U.S. Elderly, by Age, Sex, Race, Marital Status, and Region: 1999

	Nursing Home Residents	Total U.S. Population	Ratio of Nursing Home Residents to Total U.S. Population
65+ years	100%	100%	1.00
65–74	13	53	0.25
75–84	35	35	1.00
85+	52	12	4.26
Men 65+	26	41	0.62
65–74	5.7	24	0.24
75–84	10	14	0.72
85+	9.8	3.6	2.73
Women 65+	74	59	1.27
65–74	7.5	29	0.26
75–84	25	21	1.19
85+	42	8.5	4.91
Race*			
White	88	89	0.99
Men	22	37	0.59
Women	66	52	1.27
Black	10	8.3	1.20
Men	3.0	3.3	0.91
Women	7.0	5.1	1.38
Marital status*			
Men, married	10	30	0.33
Women, married	7.8	24	0.33
Census region			
Northeast	24	22	1.10
Midwest	31	24	1.29
South	33	35	0.93
West	13	19	0.67

*Resident demographics based on those of known status.

Sources: Special analysis conducted by Kris Hodges based on data from National Center for Health Statistics, *1999 National Nursing Home Survey*, CD-ROM series 13, no. 28 (Hyattsville, MD, November 2001). 1999 U.S. population data from Bureau of the Census, *Statistical Abstract of the United States: 2000*, 120th ed. (Washington, DC, 2000).

Elderly women reside in nursing homes longer than elderly men do (see Table 13.5). This gender difference is most evident at the oldest age group (85+): the oldest-old women have resided in a nursing home 1.3 times longer than comparably aged men. Among the middle-old (75–84 years), men have resided somewhat longer than women have.

TABLE 13.4
Length of Nursing Home Residency among
Elderly Residents: 1998

	Percent	Cumulative Percent
30 days or less	8.3%	8.3%
31–90 days	9.3	18
91–180 days	9.9	28
181–365 days	15.2	43
1–2 years	18.4	61
2–3 years	12.0	73
3–4 years	8.2	81
4–5 years	5.1	86
5–6 years	4.1	91
6–7 years	2.3	93
7 or more years	7.2	100

Source: Special analysis conducted by Kris Hodges based on data from National Center for Health Statistics, *1999 National Nursing Home Survey,* CD-ROM series 13, no. 28 (Hyattsville, MD, November 2001).

■ Married nursing home residents have lived in nursing homes for less time than their nonmarried counterparts

The elderly who are married are substantially less likely to be nursing home residents: 18 percent of the nursing home elderly are married, compared with 54 percent of all elderly (see Table 13.3). This likely reflects the availability of a spouse or offspring to provide informal care in lieu of professional care. This reasoning is supported by the length of time residents have resided in a nursing home. Married resi-

TABLE 13.5
Average Length of Nursing Home Residency (in Days) among Elderly
Residents, by Age and Sex: 1999

	Total	Men	Women	Ratio of Women to Men
65+ years	885	815	909	1.12
65–74	921	896	940	1.05
75–84	766	815	746	0.92
85+	957	768	1,001	1.30

Source: Special analysis conducted by Kris Hodges based on data from National Center for Health Statistics, *1999 National Nursing Home Survey*, CD-ROM series 13, no. 28 (Hyattsville, MD, November 2001).

CHART 13.2   Average Length of Nursing Home Residency among Elderly Residents, by Marital Status: 1999

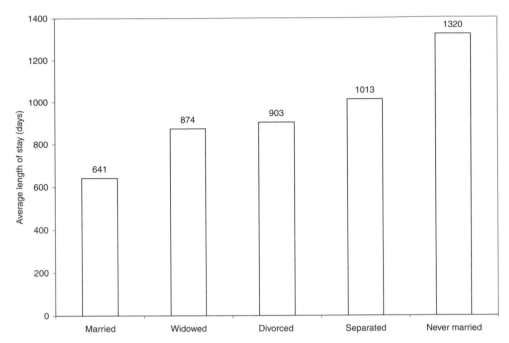

Source: Special analysis conducted by Kris Hodges based on data from National Center for Health Statistics, *1999 National Nursing Home Survey*, CD-ROM series 13, no. 28 (Hyattsville, MD, November 2001).

dents have the shortest length of residence: 641 days (1.75 years) on average, compared with significantly higher figures for those who no longer or never had a spouse (see Chart 13.2). In fact, those who have never been married have been residents for twice as long as those who are married.

■ Nursing home residents are most commonly admitted from a hospital

Nearly one-half (47 percent) of nursing home residents are admitted from a hospital, 31 percent from a private residence, and 11 percent from another nursing home.[9] More than one-quarter (28 percent) of current nursing home residents had resided at the same nursing home at some prior time. Most of these prior residents are admitted from the hospital (60 percent) or from a private residence (23 percent); fewer than 1 in 10 (8 percent) is admitted from other nursing homes.

■ The elderly are as likely to receive skilled care as intermediate care

Forty-eight percent of nursing home residents receive skilled care, and a similar percentage receive intermediate care. The remaining 4 percent receive residential care.[10]

■ Average nursing home costs for the elderly exceed $45,000 per year

The average daily cost for elderly nursing home residents is $124.[11] This ranges from an average of $89 for residential care, to $107 for intermediate care, to $146 for skilled care.

■ Medicaid support for nursing home residents is more than twice as likely among the longest residents

More than one-half of all nursing home residents (57 percent) rely on Medicaid as their primary source of payment.[12] Fewer than 1 in 5 rely primarily on their own income (17 percent) or on Medicare (16 percent). Private insurance is the primary source of payment for fewer than 1 in 10 residents (8 percent).

As might be expected, the primary source of payment varies by the length of residency. Medicaid is least prevalent among those who have recently entered into nursing home care and is highest among those with the longest residencies: 30 percent for those with 100 or fewer days versus 71 percent for those who have resided for 4 or more years.[13] This reflects the asset depletion common among long-term nursing home residents who then become Medicaid patients.

Private insurance declines as a primary source of payment from 11 percent among the newest residents (100 days or less) to just 3.4 percent of those with the longest residency (4 or more years). Interestingly, the proportion who primarily pay from their own personal incomes remains relatively constant across increasing lengths of residency, ranging from 17 percent of the newest residents to 14 percent of the longest residents.[14]

■ Elderly nursing home residents most commonly use eyeglasses and wheelchairs

More than 9 in 10 elderly nursing home residents use some type of aid. Eyeglasses and wheelchairs are the most commonly used aids, each of which are used by more than 6 in 10 elderly residents (see Table 13.6). Nearly one-half have dentures, and 1 in 4 uses a walker. The likelihood of using any particular aid is usually higher among older residents.

Eyeglass use is similar among institutionalized and noninstitutionalized elderly. The National Nursing Home Survey indicated that 65 percent of elderly nursing home patients wear eyeglasses.[15] This compares to 69 percent of noninstitutionalized elderly.[16] Eyeglass use is highest among elderly nursing home residents who have partial sight impairments (70 percent); it declines to 62 percent of those with severe sight impairments and 29 percent of those who are blind.[17]

Eleven percent of elderly residents use a hearing aid, but usage varies considerably by hearing status.[18] Among those who are partially impaired (even with a hearing aid), 26 percent use a hearing aid. Usage increases to 42 percent of those who are severely impaired and drops to 25 percent of those who are deaf.

Elderly nursing home residents are 16 times more likely to use a wheelchair than are their noninstitutionalized counterparts (63 percent versus 3.9 percent; see Chapter 5).[19]

TABLE 13.6
Percent of Nursing Home Residents Using a Particular Aid, by Age: 1999

Aid	65+ Years	65–74 Years	75–84 Years	85+ Years
Eyeglasses	65%	55%	62%	69%
Wheelchair	63	59	61	65
Dentures	45	36	42	50
Walker	26	17	24	30
Transfer equipment	14	15	14	14
Hearing aid	11	3.5	6.9	15
Commode	6.8	5.8	6.7	7.1
Oxygen	6.3	8.2	6.4	5.8
Cane	5.6	6.7	4.5	6.0
No aids used	4.5	9.7	5.0	2.8

Source: National Center for Health Statistics, *1999 National Nursing Home Survey,* CD-ROM series 13, no. 28 (Hyattsville, MD, November 2001).

■ Incontinence is common among elderly nursing home residents

More than one-half of elderly nursing home residents have difficulty controlling either their bowels or bladder; the likelihood of this difficulty is higher among older residents.[20] Fewer than 1 in 10 elderly residents has a catheter or ostomy (see Table 13.7). According to the 1998 Medicare Current Beneficiary Survey, 64 percent of institutionalized elderly have urinary incontinence, compared with 20 percent of their noninstitutionalized counterparts (see Chapter 8 for more details).[21]

■ Many more nursing home residents are chairfast than bedfast

Four in ten elderly nursing home residents are chairfast; but fewer than 10 percent are bedfast (see Table 13.7).

■ ADL and IADL assistance and other personal care activities do not vary greatly by resident age

Not surprisingly, elderly nursing home residents have substantially greater needs for ADL and IADL assistance than their noninstitutionalized counterparts. (See Chapter 5 for complete definitions of ADL and IADL.) According to the Census Bureau's 1999 Survey of Income and Program Participation (SIPP), fewer than 1 in 10 noninstitutionalized elderly has difficulty with ADLs or IADLs.[22] These levels are substantially lower than the 50 percent and higher levels among elderly nursing home residents (see Table 13.7; Chapter 5 presents detailed data on the noninstitutionalized elderly), although these rates do not vary substantially with age in the nursing home setting.

TABLE 13.7

Percent of Elderly Nursing Home Residents with Particular Functional Status, by Age: 1999

Functional Status	All Elderly Residents	65–74 Years	75–84 Years	85+ Years
Has a catheter/ostomy*	8.2%	9.8%	8.6%	7.5%
Has difficulty controlling:				
Bladder and/or bowels*	57	49	55	61
Bladder*	56	46	53	60
Bowels*	44	38	43	46
Is bedfast	6.2	6.8	6.7	5.7
Is chairfast	40	37	39	42
Does not use toilet room	18	17	18	18
Receives help with ADLs**				
Bathing	95	92	95	96
Dressing	88	84	89	89
Using toilet room	58	52	57	60
Eating	47	43	47	49
Transferring	30	26	31	32
Receives help with IADLs**				
Caring for personal possessions	76	68	76	79
Securing personal items	75	70	75	76
Managing money	73	69	74	74
Using the telephone	65	61	64	67

*Among those with known catheter/ostomy, bladder and bowel status.

**Based on those of known status.

Source: Special analysis conducted by Kris Hodges based on data from National Center for Health Statistics, *1999 National Nursing Home Survey*, CD-ROM series 13, no. 28 (Hyattsville, MD, November 2001).

NURSING HOME DISCHARGES

■ Death accounts for more than 1 in 4 elderly nursing home discharges

An estimated 2,229,000 elderly people were discharged from nursing homes in 1999. The elderly account for 88 percent of all nursing home discharges.

Overall, the elderly are about equally likely to have died in a nursing home as to have been discharged to a hospital; more than one-half of all elderly discharges are for these two reasons (see Chart 13.3). One-third of elderly discharges are due to either patient stabilization or recovery. Fewer than 1 in 10 discharges is admitted to another nursing home. Elderly men and women have similar discharge profiles.

Discharges due to hospitalization remain relatively stable with age. The oldest-old women are three times more likely, and the oldest-old men 1.7 times more likely, than their youngest-old counterparts to have died (see Chart 13.4).

CHART 13.3 Percent of Elderly Nursing Home Discharges with Given Disposition Status, by Sex: 1999

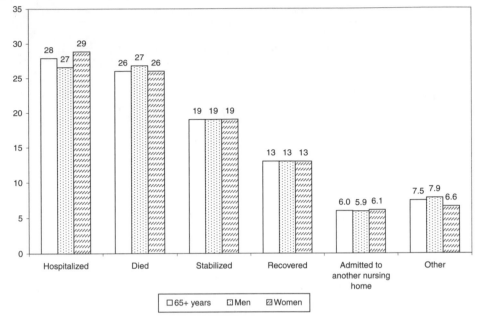

Source: Special analysis conducted by Kris Hodges based on data from National Center for Health Statistics, *1999 National Nursing Home Survey*, CD-ROM series 13, no. 28 (Hyattsville, MD, November 2001).

Elderly white men and women are more likely than their black counterparts to have been discharged due to stabilization, recovery, or death (see Chart 13.5). In contrast, elderly black men and women are substantially more likely than their white counterparts to have been admitted to the hospital.

■ Elderly nursing home discharges resided for less than 10 months, on average

The average length of residency among elderly nursing home discharges was less than 10 months (282 days), less than one-third the average length of stay of current elderly residents. Except among the youngest-old discharges (for which lengths of stays for both genders was about equal), elderly women resided for substantially longer periods of time than did elderly men (see Table 13.8).

■ Elderly nursing home patients who recovered or stabilized had an average stay of less than 2 months

Length of residency is highly related to the reason for discharge. Not surprisingly, those elderly residents who recovered or stabilized had the shortest nursing home stays, an average of 2 months or less (see Chart 13.6). Those who died had the longest residency, 19 months on average.

CHART 13.4   Percent of Elderly Nursing Home Discharges with Given Disposition Status, by Age and Sex: 1999

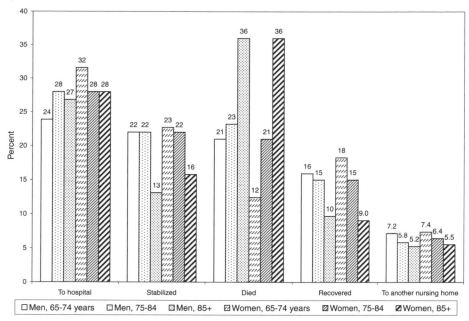

Source: Special analysis conducted by Kris Hodges based on data from National Center for Health Statistics, *1999 National Nursing Home Survey,* CD-ROM series 13, no. 28 (Hyattsville, MD, November 2001).

CHART 13.5   Percent of Elderly Nursing Home Discharges with Given Disposition Status, by Sex and Race: 1999

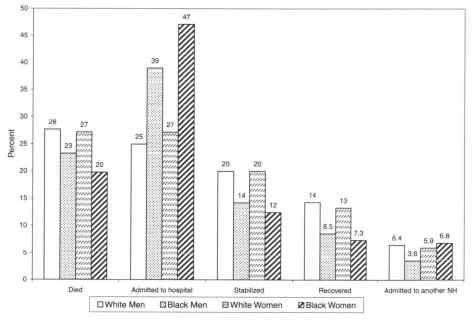

Source: Special analysis conducted by Kris Hodges based on data from: National Center for Health Statistics, *1998 National Nursing Home Survey,* CD-ROM series 13, no. 28 (Hyattsville, MD, November 2001).

TABLE 13.8

Average Length of Nursing Home Residency (in Days) among Elderly
Nursing Home Discharges, by Age and Sex: 1999

	Total	Men	Women	Ratio of Women to Men
65+ years	282	196	332	1.69
65–74	147	149	145	0.97
75–84	216	173	246	1.42
85+	405	262	460	1.76

Source: Special analysis conducted by Kris Hodges based on data from National
Center for Health Statistics, *1999 National Nursing Home Survey*, CD-ROM series
13, no. 28 (Hyattsville, MD, November 2001).

CHART 13.6   Average Length of Nursing Home Residency among Elderly Nursing Home
Discharges, by Reason for Discharge: 1999

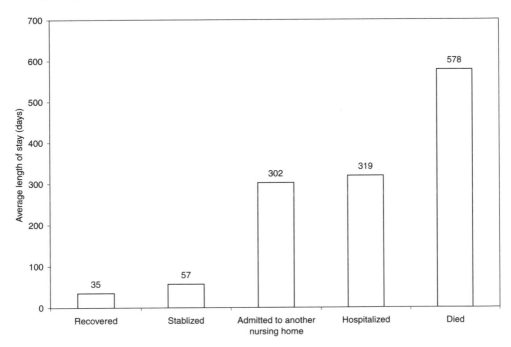

Source: Special analysis conducted by Kris Hodges based on data from National Center for Health Statistics,
1999 National Nursing Home Survey, CD-ROM series 13, no. 28 (Hyattsville, MD, November 2001).

CHART 13.7   Average Length (in Days) of Nursing Home Residency among Elderly Nursing Home Discharges, by Discharge Status and Marital Status: 1999

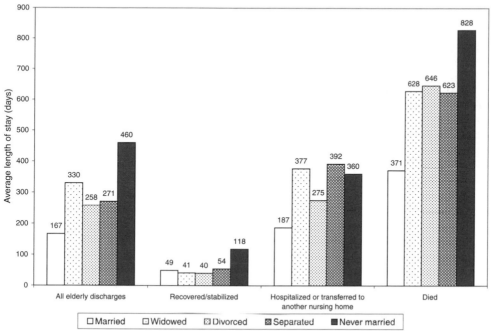

Source: Special analysis conducted by Kris Hodges based on data from National Center for Health Statistics, *1999 National Nursing Home Survey*, CD-ROM series 13, no. 28 (Hyattsville, MD, November 2001).

■ **Never-married discharges reside in a nursing home nearly three times longer than their married counterparts**

Elderly nursing home patients who have never been married spend the longest time in a nursing home prior to discharge, nearly three times longer than their married counterparts (see Chart 13.7). This large differential may reflect the greater lack of available caretakers among those who have no spouse or offspring. A similar pattern exists by the reason for discharge.

■ **Recovered or stabilized discharges are more ambulatory than other discharges**

Recovered or stabilized elderly discharges are more ambulatory than other discharges, as evidenced by the highest use of walkers and canes among the former, but the lowest use of wheelchairs (see Table 13.9). The recovered or stabilized elderly are also the least likely to use oxygen. In fact, those who died were three times more likely to be using oxygen at the time of death (discharge) as those who had recovered or stabilized.

TABLE 13.9
Percent of Nursing Home Discharges Using a Particular Aid, by Reason for Discharge: 1999

Aid	All Elderly Discharges	Recovered or Stabilized	Transferred to Hospital or Other Nursing Home	Died
		Reason for Discharge		
Eyeglasses	68%	74%	64%	63%
Wheelchair	52	38	62	60
Dentures	44	47	43	41
Walker	32	53	23	15
Oxygen	20	11	18	33
Transfer equipment	13	8.1	15	16
Hearing aid	12	14	11	13
Cane	8.4	15	5.4	3.9
Commode	7.6	7.1	6.3	8.0
No aids used	3.6	3.3	3.0	4.3

Source: Special analysis conducted by Kris Hodges based on data from National Center for Health Statistics, *1999 National Nursing Home Survey*, CD-ROM series 13, no. 28 (Hyattsville, MD, November 2001).

A similar disparity among discharges is also evidenced in ADL and IADL assistance and other personal care areas (see Table 13.10). Those who died had the highest needs for ADL and IADL assistance as well as the highest incontinence levels prior to death, whereas those who recovered or stabilized had the least.

MALNUTRITION AND DEHYDRATION IN NURSING HOMES

Recent research indicates that from 8 to 31 percent of nursing home residents suffer from malnutrition.[23] A small-scale study of 100 elderly patients admitted to a nursing home found that 39 percent showed signs of malnutrition.[24] Those who were admitted from acute-care facilities had lower nutritional reserves than those coming from home. (There is little comparable research on the prevalence of either borderline or overt dehydration.)

DEFINITION: Dehydration is defined as a rapid weight loss of greater than 3 percent of body weight.

The average cost of hospitalization for dehydration in the elderly is estimated at $1.36 billion.[25] Hospitalized seniors with malnutrition, dehydration, or both have longer hospital stays and increased mortality. In addition, poorly nourished nursing

TABLE 13.10

Percent of Elderly Nursing Home Discharges with Particular Functional Status, by Reason for Discharge: 1999

Functional Status	All Elderly Discharges	Reason for Discharge		
		Recovered or Stabilized	Transferred to Hospital or Other Nursing Home	Died
Has a catheter or ostomy*	18%	7.3%	22%	28%
Has difficulty controlling:				
Bladder and/or bowels*	39	20	46	56
Bladder*	38	19	44	55
Bowels*	31	10	37	51
Is bedfast	22	2.0	20	55
Is chairfast	26	13	37	27
Does not use toilet room	24	5.3	30	43
Receives help with ADLs**				
Bathing	90	78	96	99
Dressing	85	69	93	96
Using toilet room	53	53	55	49
Among those who use toilet room	68	56	76	83
Eating	51	22	59	78
Transferring	34	45	31	18
Among those who are not bedfast or chairfast	58	51	64	72
Receives help with IADLs**				
Caring for personal possessions	61	33	73	82
Securing personal items	63	42	72	79
Managing money	56	29	68	73
Using the telephone	52	27	64	69

*Among those with known catheter or ostomy, bladder, and bowel status.

**Based on those of known status.

Source: Special analysis conducted by Kris Hodges based on data from National Center for Health Statistics, *1999 National Nursing Home Survey*, CD-ROM series 13, no. 28 (Hyattsville, MD, November 2001).

home patients have greater risks of developing fever, infections, and pressure sores. A 1998 study found that 67 percent of residents with eating problems received liquid supplements.[26]

Many factors can contribute to inadequate food intake among the elderly, including:[27]

- age-related declines in taste, smell, and appetite;
- depression;

- medications that can cause loss of appetite or gastrointestinal irritation;
- functional or cognitive impairments that can limit the ability to feed oneself (about 50 percent of nursing home residents cannot eat independently and are nearly twice as likely to suffer weight loss as those who eat independently);
- poor oral health; and
- dysphagia (swallowing disorders, which affect an estimated 40 to 60 percent of institutionalized seniors) and other neurological disorders.

In nursing homes, lack of individualized care, inadequate staffing, and lack of mealtime supervision by professional staff can contribute to poor nutritional intake.[28] In contrast, residents whose family members assist them with eating are unlikely to lose weight.

A large study in 1995 conducted among nearly 7,000 residents in more than 200 nursing homes found that about 25 percent had a low body-mass index (BMI), and 10 percent suffered a 5 percent loss of body weight in 1 month or 10 percent in 6 months. (All of these symptoms are indicators of poor nutritional status.[29])* Residents with low BMIs have been shown to have increased mortality within 1 year, and 85 percent of those that lived showed no improvement. The worst nursing home facilities have been found to have resident weight loss almost double that of the best facilities.

NURSING HOME STAFFING AND ADMINISTRATION

■ The majority of care received in nursing homes is from certified nursing assistants

On average, nursing home residents at Medicare- or Medicaid-certified facilities receive 3.5 hours of direct and indirect care from all sources in a 24-hour period.[30] The majority of the care is from certified nursing assistants (CNAs). Staffing levels are the highest in Medicare (skilled care)-only facilities, where almost 6 hours of care is provided daily per resident. CNAs again provide the bulk of the care, but the average time spent by registered nurses (RNs) is three times the level for all certified facilities (see Table 13.11). Most states require from 2 to 2.5 hours of direct and indirect care per patient per day, but some have lower standards, and many have no standards.

A recent analysis found that 54 percent of nursing home facilities do not have enough nurses aides to provide the recommended 2 hours of care per resident per day.[31] At least 2.9 hours are considered the minimal level for providing optimal care in delivering five specific daily care services that are linked to good resident outcomes. When the minimum of 2.9 hours is specified, more than 92 percent of nurs-

---

* This study excluded residents with terminal prognoses and tube-fed or parenterally fed residents.

TABLE 13.11

Average Minutes Spent per Day with Each Resident by Various Nursing
Home Staff: 1997

	Type of Certified Facility	
	Medicare/ Medicaid	Medicare (skilled care)-Only
Registered nurses	42	130
Licensed practical nurses or licensed visiting nurses	42	78
Certified nursing assistants	126	150
All staff	210	358

Note: Data are self-reported.

Source: Sarah Greene Burger et al., "Malnutrition and Dehydration in Nursing
Homes: Key Issues in Prevention and Treatment," National Citizen's Coalition
for Nursing Home Reform (June 2000). Available online at www.cmwf.org/
programs/elders.

ing homes do not meet the threshold, and nearly one-half of these facilities would
need to increase nurse aide staffing by 50 percent or more to reach the threshold.

An average of 5.5 health deficiencies were reported in nursing homes in 1999,
with more than one-half of them attributable to nursing deficiencies.[32] Deficiencies
are more common among for-profit nursing homes (6.2 deficiencies) and less common among government and nonprofit facilities (4.5 and 4.1 deficiencies, respectively).[33]

The most common deficiencies cited are food sanitation (25 percent of facilities
cited), highest practicable care (20 percent), hazard-free environment (19 percent),
pressure sore prevention and treatment (17 percent), and accident prevention (16
percent).[34]

NURSING HOME FACILITIES

▬ Nursing homes have an 87 percent occupancy rate

According to the National Nursing Home Survey, an estimated 18,000 nursing
home facilities existed in 1999.[35] Nursing homes average 105 beds, with a current
occupancy rate of 87 percent and an annual discharge rate of 134 per 100 beds.
Nursing homes in the Northeast are the largest (129 beds per nursing home, on average) and have the highest occupancy rates (93 percent). Those in the West are the
smallest (89 beds, on average) and have discharge rates that are twice that of other
regions.

■ Two-thirds of the 18,000 U.S. nursing homes are proprietary

Two-thirds (67 percent) of the nursing home facilities are proprietary, one-quarter (27 percent) are nonprofit, and 7 percent are governmental or other types of facilities.[36] More than one-half (60 percent) are part of a franchise. The Midwest and South each account for one-third of all nursing home facilities.

NOTES

All percents in data are based on totals that exclude missing values and those of unknown status.

1. National Center for Health Statistics, *1999 National Nursing Home Survey*, CD-ROM series 13, no. 28 (Hyattsville, MD, November 2001).
2. National Center for Health Statistics, *Health, United States, 2001 with Urban and Rural Health Chartbook* (Hyattsville, MD, 2001), Table 97.
3. National Center for Health Statistics, *1999 National Nursing Home Survey*.
4. Office of the Assistant Secretary for Planning and Evaluation report on the 1989 Informal Caregiver's Supplement to the National Long-Term Care Survey. Available online at http://aspe.hhs.gov/daltcp/projects.htm#Duke4.
5. Robyn I. Stone, *Long-Term Care for the Elderly with Disabilities: Current Policy, Emerging Trends, and Implications for the Twenty-First Century* (New York: Milbank Memorial Fund, 2000). Available online at www.milbank.org.
6. Harriet L. Komisar et al., *Long-Term Care for the Elderly: A Chart Book* (Institute for Health Care Research and Policy, New York, NY, Georgetown University, 1996).
7. National Center for Health Statistics, *1999 National Nursing Home Survey*, CD-ROM series 13, no. 28 (Hyattsville, MD, November 2001).
8. Ibid.
9. Ibid.
10. Ibid.
11. Ibid.
12. Ibid.
13. Ibid.
14. Ibid.
15. National Center for Health Statistics, *1999 National Nursing Home Survey*.
16. Mediamark Research Inc. Spring 2000.
17. National Center for Health Statistics, *1999 National Nursing Home Survey*.
18. Ibid.
19. Centers for Disease Control, "Prevalence of Disabilities and Associated Health Conditions among Adults—United States, 1999," *MMWR Weekly* 50, no. 7 (March 2, 2001): 120–125. Data from the Survey of Income and Program Participation.
20. National Center for Health Statistics, *1999 National Nursing Home Survey*.
21. Health Care Financing Administration, "The Characteristics and Perceptions of the Medicare Population (1998)," *Medicare Current Beneficiary Survey* (2001): Section 2.
22. Centers for Disease Control, "Prevalence of Disabilities."
23. Sarah Greene Burger et al., "Malnutrition and Dehydration in Nursing Homes: Key Issues in Prevention and Treatment," National Citizen's Coalition for Nursing Home Reform (June 2000). Available online at www.cmwf.org/programs/elders.
24. K. Nelson et al., "Prevalence of Malnutrition in the Elderly Admitted to Long-term Care Facilities," *Journal of the American Dietetic Association* 93, no. 4 (April 1993): 459–461.
25. Burger et al., "Malnutrition and Dehydration in Nursing Homes.
26. Ibid.

27. Ibid.
28. Ibid.
29. Ibid.
30. Ibid.
31. Health Care Financing Administration, "Appropriateness of Minimum Nurse Staffing Ratios in Nursing Homes; Executive Summary," Report to Congress (2000). Available online at www.hcfa.gov/medicaid/reports.
32. C. McKeen Cowles, *Nursing Home Statistical Yearbook, 1999* (Washington, DC: American Association of Homes and Services for the Aging, 2000), Table IV-1.
33. Ibid., Table IV-2.
34. Ibid., Table IV-3.
35. National Center for Health Statistics, "Selected Characteristics of Homes, Beds, and Residents," *1999 National Nursing Home Survey Data Highlights.* Available online at www.cdc.gov/nchs/about/major/nnhsd/nnhsd.htm.
36. Ibid.

CHAPTER 14

Care at the End of Life: Hospice Care

Life is hardly more than a fraction of a second. Such a little time to prepare oneself for eternity!!!

—*Paul Gauguin*

Death, as the psalmist saith, is certain to all, all shall die.

—*William Shakespeare,* Henry IV

Hospices provide palliative care, as opposed to curative care, to dying patients. Hospice services are provided by an interdisciplinary team and include supportive physical, social, emotional, and spiritual services to the terminally ill, as well as support for the patient's family. The National Hospice and Palliative Care Organization estimated that 3,100 hospice programs existed in the United States in 2000. An estimated 700,000 patients were admitted in 2000 and 600,000 died, accounting for one-quarter of all deaths in the United States.[1] This chapter incorporates a special analysis conducted by Kris Hodges of newly available statistics from the 1998 National Home and Hospice Care Survey[2] along with other important statistics.

DEFINITION: Palliative care provides pain and symptom management, physical care, counseling, and related services to patients who are terminally ill. It does not attempt to cure disease or health problems.

Highlights of this chapter include:

- The Medicare program provides coverage for more than 2,287 hospices.
- Hospice care usage rates among the elderly increased 73 percent in 4 years.
- Four in five hospice patients are elderly.
- Three-quarters of elderly hospice patients receive care at home.
- More than 90 percent of elderly hospice patients have a primary caregiver.
- Cancer is the leading cause of the elderly's admission to hospice care.

- Nine in ten elderly hospice patients receive skilled nursing services.
- One-half of elderly hospice patients receive social services, medications, personal and spiritual care, and durable medical equipment and supplies.

Two-thirds of older adults (aged 60+) have at least a fairly good understanding of hospice care.[3]

MEDICARE COVERAGE OF HOSPICE CARE

Since 1982, Medicare has provided coverage for hospice care for terminally ill Medicare beneficiaries with a life expectancy of 6 months or less.[4] However, a National Hospice Foundation survey indicated that 90 percent of respondents do not realize that hospice care is fully covered through Medicare.[5] Medicaid in 42 states covers hospice services.

DEFINITION: Hospice is not a place (although some hospice care services have residential facilities); it is a philosophy of care. Hospice is pain and symptom management, physical care, and counseling provided by a Medicare-approved program for people who are terminally ill. The patient's attending physician and the hospice medical director must certify that the patient is terminally ill and is not expected to live longer than 6 months. Nine in ten elderly hospice discharges are due to death.

CURRENT HOSPICE PATIENTS

■ Four in five hospice patients are elderly

According to the National Home and Hospice Survey, an estimated 85,900 elderly people were hospice patients, accounting for 81 percent of all hospice care patients in 2000. On an age-adjusted basis, this means that fewer than 3 in 1,000 elderly adults were current hospice patients in 2000 (see Table 14.1).

Use of hospice care services among the elderly increased 73 percent in a 4-year period with increases substantially higher among the middle and oldest-old.

The likelihood of being a current hospice care patient is higher among the older age groups. With each successive 10-year age increment, the likelihood of the elderly being a current hospice care patient roughly doubles (see Table 14.2). Elderly men of all ages are more likely than are elderly women to be current patients.

The gender profile of elderly hospice care patients is similar to that of the average elderly person (see Table 14.3). In other words, the ratio of men to women in the general elderly population is the same as in the elderly hospice care patient population. However, the elderly hospice care patient population skews much older than the general elderly population. It also skews more to those in the South and to black men. Elderly married women and the elderly in the Northeast tend to be underrepresented in the elderly hospice care patient population.

TABLE 14.1
Rate of Hospice Care Use (per 10,000 Persons), by Age and Sex: 1996, 1998, and 2000

	1996	1998	2000	Percent Change		
				1998 versus 1996	2000 versus 1998	2000 versus 1996
65+ years*	14.4	18.4	24.9	28%	35%	73%
65–74	7.8	9.9	10.1	27	2.0	29
75–84	16.9	22	31.9	30	45	89
85+	34.7	44.7	67.3	29	51	94
Men, 65+ years*	16.1	20.3	26.9	26	33	67
65–74	10.4	10.2	13.0	–2	27	25
75–84	18.5	25.2	32.6	36	29	76
85+	33.9	49.2	69.9	45	42	106
Women, 65+ years*	12.9	17.3	23.3	34	35	81
65–74	5.8	9.6	7.6	66	–21	31
75–84	15.9	19.9	31.5	25	58	98
85+	35	42.9	66.2	23	54	89

*Age adjusted to the year 2000 population standard using the following three age groups: 65–74 years, 75–84 years, and 85+ years.
Source: National Center for Health Statistics, *Health, United States, 2002 with Chartbook on Trends in the Health of Americans* (Hyattsville, MD, 2002), Table 89.

TABLE 14.2
Rate of Hospice Care Use (per 10,000 Persons), by Age and Sex: 2000

	Men		Women		
	Rate	Ratio to Prior 10-Year Age Category	Rate	Ratio to Prior 10-Year Age Category	Ratio of Men to Women
65+ years*	26.9	NA	23.3	NA	1.15
65–74	13.0	NA	7.6	NA	1.71
75–84	32.6	2.51	31.5	4.14	1.03
85+	69.9	2.14	66.2	2.10	1.06

*Age adjusted to the year 2000 population standard using the following three age groups: 65–74, 75–84 and 85+.
Source: National Center for Health Statistics, *Health, United States, 2002 with Chartbook on Trends in the Health of Americans* (Hyattsville, MD, 2002), Table 89.

TABLE 14.3

Percent of Elderly Hospice Care Patients Compared to Percent of Total U.S. Elderly, by Age, Sex, Race, Marital Status, and Region: 1998

	Current Elderly Hospice Patients	Total Elderly U.S. Population	Ratio of Elderly Hospice Patients to Elderly U.S. Population
Total elderly	100%	100%	1.00
65–74	29	53	0.54
75–84	42	35	1.21
85+	29	12	2.46
Men, 65+	42	41	1.01
65–74	13	24	0.56
75–84	19	14	1.38
85+	9.3	3.5	2.71
Women, 65+	58	59	0.99
65–74	16	29	0.53
75–84	23	21	1.09
85+	20	8.3	2.36
Race*			
White	90	89	1.01
Men	38	37	1.03
Women	52	52	1.00
Black	9.1	8.3	1.10
Men	4.3	3.2	1.32
Women	4.8	5.0	0.95
Marital status*			
Men, married	30	32	0.95
Women, married	14	25	0.54
Census region			
Northeast	12	21	0.55
Midwest	24	24	1.01
South	46	35	1.30
West	19	20	0.93

*Current patient demographics based on those of known status.

Sources: Special analysis conducted by Kris Hodges based on 1998 hospice data from National Center for Health Statistics, *1998 National Home and Hospice Care Survey*, CD-ROM series 13, no. 27 (Hyattsville, MD, October 2000); 1998 U.S. population data from Bureau of the Census, *Statistical Abstract of the United States: 1999*, 199th ed. (Washington, DC, 1999), Tables 21 and 63.

■ Most elderly hospice patients receive care at home

The majority of elderly hospice patients, 78 percent, receive in-home care.[6] Sixty-two percent of elderly hospice patients live with family members, 6 percent live with nonfamily members, 21 percent live in nursing homes, and 10 percent live alone.

One-quarter (24 percent) of elderly patients receive hospice care from a proprietary agency; the remaining three-quarters receive care from a nonprofit or other type of agency. Virtually all elderly hospice patients receive care from an agency certified by Medicare (94 percent) or Medicaid (89 percent) as a hospice. About half receive hospice care from a Medicare- or Medicaid-certified home health agency. Medicare is the primary source of payment for almost all elderly hospice patients (95 percent of those of known status).[7]

■ The average elderly hospice patient has been receiving care for more than 4 months

Current elderly hospice patients in 1998 received services for slightly more than 4 months (130 days), on average, with 55 percent using the service for 90 days or less (see Chart 14.1). About 1 in 5 had been using the service for more than 180 days.

CHART 14.1 Distribution of Elderly Hospice Care Patients by Length of Service since Admission: 1998

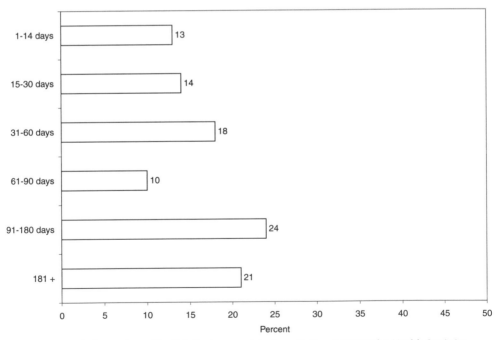

Source: Special analysis conducted by Kris Hodges on data from National Center for Health Statistics, *1998 National Home and Hospice Care Survey*, CD-ROM series 13, no. 27 (Hyattsville, MD, October 2000).

■ Patients living with a caregiver use hospice care less than those living without a primary caregiver at home

Almost all elderly hospice patients (92 percent) have a primary caregiver, and 82 percent of them live with that caregiver.[8] Those who live with their primary caregiver have been using hospice services for the least amount of time, whereas those who have no primary caregiver have been using hospice services for the greatest amount of time (see Chart 14.2)—more than twice as long as those who live with their primary caregiver. This differential reflects the greater dependency on outside services for those who have no caregivers. Even those elderly hospice patients who have a primary caregiver but do not live with them, have been using hospice services for 20 percent longer than those who live with their caregivers.

■ Cancer is leading cause of admission to hospice care

Nearly one-half of elderly hospice patients are admitted with cancer as the primary diagnosis (see Table 14.4). Chronic obstructive pulmonary disease and heart disease are distant runners up for the primary admission diagnoses.

CHART 14.2   Average Length of Hospice Care Services among Elderly Patients, by Caregiver Status: 1998

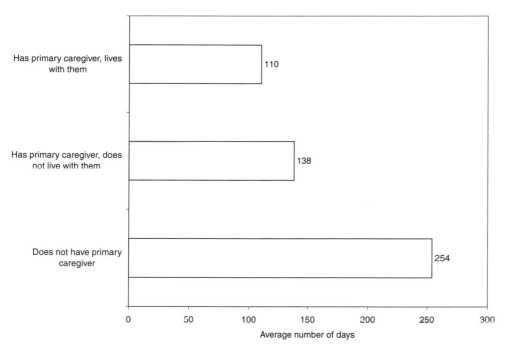

Source: Special analysis conducted by Kris Hodges on data from National Center for Health Statistics, *1998 National Home and Hospice Care Survey*, CD-ROM series 13, no. 27 (Hyattsville, MD, October 2000).

TABLE 14.4

Percent Distribution of Elderly Hospice Care Patients, by Primary Admission Diagnosis: 1998

Diagnosis	Distribution
Cancer	48%
Chronic obstructive pulmonary disease	11
Heart disease	11
Alzheimer's disease	7.3
Cerebrovascular disease	2.1

Source: Special analysis conducted by Kris Hodges on data from National Center for Health Statistics, *1998 National Home and Hospice Care Survey,* CD-ROM series 13, no. 27 (Hyattsville, MD, October 2000).

TABLE 14.5

Percent of Elderly Current Hospice Care Patients, by Functional Status: 1998

Functional Status	Percent
Has a catheter or ostomy*	19%
Has difficulty controlling:	
Bladder and/or bowels*	36
Bladder*	32
Bowels*	22
Receives help with ADLs**	
Bathing	75
Dressing	62
Transferring	55
Using toilet room	45
Walking	41
Eating	29
Receives help with IADLs**	
Taking medications	34
Doing light housework	31
Preparing meals	12
Shopping	4.2
Using the telephone	2.5
Managing money	1.0

*Among those with known catheter, ostomy, bladder and bowel status.

**Based on those of known status.

Source: Special analysis conducted by Kris Hodges on data from National Center for Health Statistics, *1998 National Home and Hospice Care Survey,* CD-ROM series 13, no. 27 (Hyattsville, MD, October 2000).

■ Elderly hospice care patients are quite disabled

One in five elderly hospice care patients has a catheter and/or an ostomy (see Table 14.5). Another one-third are incontinent. ADL assistance is high among elderly patients. Assistance with medications and housework are the most common forms of IADL assistance. (See Chapter 5 for complete definitions of ADL and IADL.)

TABLE 14.6
Percent of Elderly Hospice Care Patients Using a Particular Aid: 1998

Aid	Percent
Hospital bed	59%
Wheelchair	44
Oxygen	40
Eyeglasses	39
Commode	38
Special mattress	32
Walker	31
Shower chair	23
Dentures	18
Cane	10
Hearing aid	7.5
No aids used	4.8

Source: Special analysis conducted by Kris Hodges on data from National Center for Health Statistics, *1998 National Home and Hospice Care Survey,* CD-ROM series 13, no. 27 (Hyattsville, MD, October 2000).

TABLE 14.7
Percent of Elderly Hospice Care Patients Receiving Services in a 30-Day Period: 1998

Service	Percent
Skilled nursing services	90%
Social services	74
Medications	65
Personal care	65
Spiritual care	57
Durable medical equipment and supplies	54
Counseling	45
Physician services	31
Homemaker or household services	20
Dietary or nutritional services	17
Psychological services	15

Source: Special analysis conducted by Kris Hodges on data from National Center for Health Statistics, *1998 National Home and Hospice Care Survey,* CD-ROM series 13, no. 27 (Hyattsville, MD, October 2000).

■ **Six in ten elderly hospice care patients use a hospital bed**

Only 5 percent of all elderly hospice patients do not use an aid (see Table 14.6). Hospital beds, wheelchairs, and oxygen are the most commonly used aids.

■ **Hospice care patients receive many services**

Ninety percent of all elderly hospice patients received skilled nursing services in a 30-day period during 1998 (see Table 14.7). Social services, medications, personal and spiritual care, and durable medical equipment and supplies were provided to more than one-half of all elderly hospice care patients.

HOSPICE CARE DISCHARGES

■ **Most elderly hospice discharges are due to death**

In 1998, an estimated 377,600 elderly were discharged from hospice care, comprising 76 percent of all discharges. Due to the critical condition of patients and the

CHART 14.3   Distribution of Elderly Hospice Care Discharges, by Length of Service since Admission: 1998

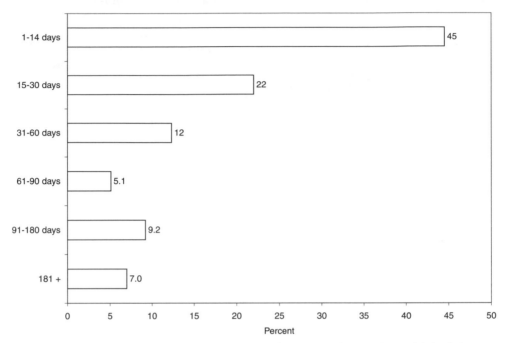

Source: Special analysis conducted by Kris Hodges on data from National Center for Health Statistics, *1998 National Home and Hospice Care Survey,* CD-ROM series 13, no. 27 (Hyattsville, MD, October 2000).

nature of hospice care, most elderly hospice discharges (89 percent) are due to death. The elderly who were discharged received hospice service for 51 days, on average. Forty-five percent received services for 2 weeks or less, and two-thirds received services for no more than 1 month (see Chart 14.3).

Elderly hospice discharges are more than twice as likely as current elderly hospice patients to have had a catheter and/or an ostomy (see Table 14.8), which may reflect the more critical condition of the former group. Discharges are also more likely to have had bowel and/or bladder incontinence. However, this group needs much less ADL and IADL assistance than current patients, which may reflect their less mobile and severe conditions.

Given their more critical condition, discharges are more likely than current hospice patients to have been using a hospital bed, special mattress, and/or and oxygen (see Table 14.9). Discharges also are less likely to have used wheelchairs and/or walkers, again reflecting their less mobile condition.

TABLE 14.8

Percent Distribution of Elderly Hospice Care Discharges and Current Hospice Patients according to Functional Status: 1998

	Elderly Hospice Discharges	Current Hospice Patients	Ratio of Hospice Discharges to Current Hospice Patients
Has catheter or ostomy*	41%	19%	2.16
Has difficulty controlling:			
Bladder and/or bowels**	58	45	1.29
Bladder**	54	40	1.35
Bowels**	41	27	1.52
Receives help with ADLs*			
Bathing	69	75	0.92
Dressing	59	62	0.95
Transferring	40	55	0.73
Eating	31	29	1.07
Toilet room	29	45	0.64
Walking	24	41	0.59
Receives Help with IADLs*			
Taking medications	35	34	1.03
Doing light housework	19	31	0.61
Preparing meals	9.2	12	0.77

*Among those with known catheter, ostomy, bladder and bowel status.

**Due to the large difference in percent of catheter/ostomy usage between discharges and residents, these percentages are based on those without a catheter and/or ostomy to allow for a more accurate comparison.

***Based on those of known status.

Source: Special analysis conducted by Kris Hodges on data from National Center for Health Statistics, *1998 National Home and Hospice Care Survey*, CD-ROM series 13, no. 27 (Hyattsville, MD, October 2000).

TABLE 14.9

Percent Distribution of Elderly Hospice Care Discharges and Patients Using a Particular Aid: 1998

Aid	Discharges (Just Prior to Discharge)	Current Patients	Ratio of Discharges to Current Patients
Hospital bed	76%	59%	1.29
Wheelchair	33	44	0.74
Oxygen	51	40	1.27
Commode	33	38	0.86
Special mattress	43	32	1.35
Walker	19	31	0.59
No aids used	3.4	4.8	0.71

Source: Special analysis conducted by Kris Hodges based on data from National Center for Health Statistics, *1998 National Home and Hospice Care Survey*, CD-ROM series 13, no. 27 (Hyattsville, MD, October 2000).

NOTES

All percents in data are based on totals that exclude missing values and those of unknown status.

1. National Hospice and Palliative Care Organization, "NHPCO Facts and Figures" (December 10, 2001). Available online at www.hospiceinfo.org.
2. Special analysis conducted by Kris Hodges based on data from National Center for Health Statistics, *1998 National Home and Hospice Care Survey*, CD-ROM series 13, no. 27 (Hyattsville, MD, October 2000).
3. RoperASW, 1999.
4. National Hospice and Palliative Care Organization, "NHPCO Facts and Figures."
5. National Center for Health Statistics, *1998 National Home and Hospice Care Survey*.
6. Ibid.
7. Ibid.
8. Special analysis conducted by Kris Hodges on data from National Center for Health Statistics, *1998 National Home and Hospice Care Survey*.

CHAPTER 15

Causes, Places, and Timing of Death

Life is pleasant. Death is peaceful. It's the transition that's troublesome.

—Isaac Asimov

I'm not afraid to die. I just don't want to be there when it happens. It is impossible to experience one's death objectively and still carry a tune.

—Woody Allen

We didn't lose the game; we just ran out of time.

—Vince Lombardi

As discussed in Chapter 1, today's elderly are healthier than their peers in any previous generation. Many conditions that were not curable decades ago can now be treated before they do permanent damage or take a life. In other words, seniors are dying less and living longer.

When life does end, the elderly are most likely to succumb to one of five conditions: heart disease, cancer, stroke, chronic lower respiratory disease, or pneumonia or influenza. They are most likely to die in a hospital. Interestingly, the elderly's death rate varies considerably by place of residence and the time of year.

This chapter presents the recent data supporting these and other trends on deaths among the elderly. Highlights of this chapter include:

- During the twentieth century, death rates for all Americans, including seniors, have declined, contributing to longer life expectancy.
- Three-quarters of all deaths in the United States are among seniors.
- Heart disease is the leading killer of seniors overall, but cancer is the leading cause of death for most of the youngest-old.
- Pulmonary-related death rates among senior women are catching up to those for senior men.
- Most accident-related deaths among seniors are from injuries due to falls.

- Senior men are the most likely group to commit suicide.
- The elderly in Hawaii have, by far, the lowest death rates of all seniors.
- Elderly deaths peak in winter months and are lowest in summer months.

OVERALL DEATHS

■ Three-quarters of all deaths in the United States are among seniors

As would be expected, seniors account for the vast majority of the deaths in the United States; 75 percent of the 2.4 million deaths in 2000 were among seniors. Quantifiably, this can be stated as:[1]

- 1,801,459 seniors dying during the year,
- 4,922 seniors dying every day,
- 205 seniors dying every hour, or
- 3.4 seniors dying every minute.

■ About 1 in 20 seniors dies each year

In the year 1999, 5.6 percent of elderly men and 4.9 percent of elderly women died.[2] By the time seniors enter their mid-nineties, 1 in 4 dies each year (see Table 15.1).[3] A significant gender difference exists in elderly death rates, which narrows at the older age groups. Specifically, up until age 95, senior men are substantially more likely to die than senior women are (see Chart 15.1).

TABLE 15.1
Elderly Death Rates (per 100,000 Persons) for All Causes, by Age and Sex: 1997

	Men	Women	Ratio of Men to Women	Ratio of Death Rate to Prior 5-Year Age Group	
				Men	Women
65+ years	5,621	4,692	1.20	NA	NA
65–69	2,557	1,530	1.67	NA	NA
70–74	3,949	2,426	1.63	1.54	1.59
75–79	5,831	3,764	1.55	1.48	1.55
80–84	9,320	6,325	1.47	1.60	1.68
85–89	15,262	11,203	1.36	1.64	1.77
90–94	21,366	17,572	1.22	1.40	1.57
95+	26,078	25,556	1.02	1.22	1.45

Note: NA = Not Applicable.
Sources: National Center for Health Statistics, Health, United States, 1999 with Health and Aging Chartbook (Hyattsville, MD, 1999); National Vital Statistics Reports 47, no. 19 (June 30, 1999): Figure 7.

CHART 15.1   Elderly Death Rates for All Causes, by Age and Sex: 1997

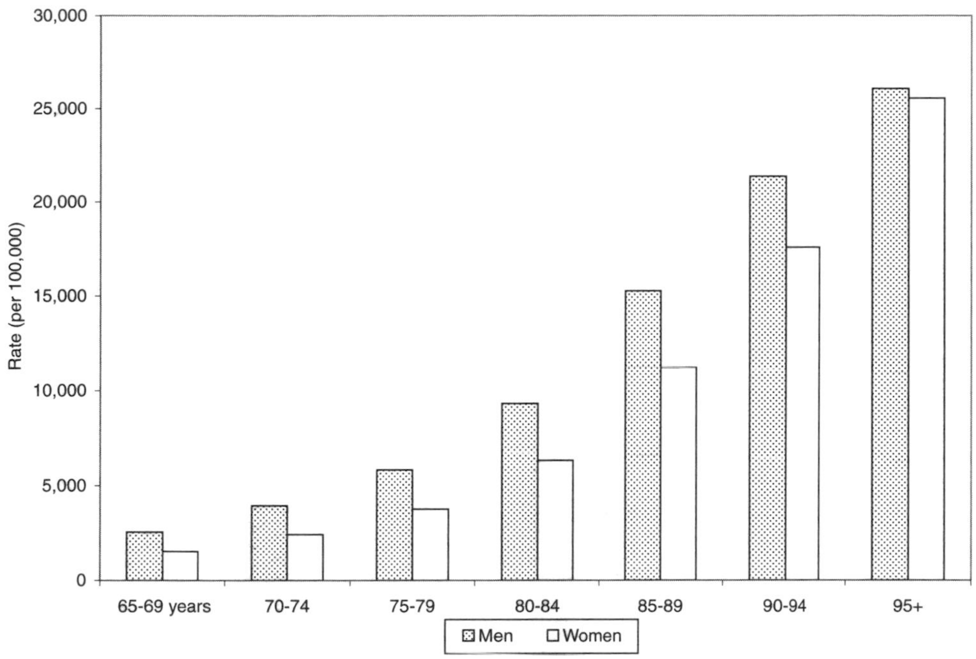

Source: National Center for Health Statistics, *Health, United States, 1999 with Health and Aging Chartbook* (Hyattsville, MD, 1999).

With each successive 5-year age increment from age 65 to 95, the likelihood of dying is approximately 1.5 times higher (see Table 15.1). The greatest increase in the risk of dying occurs between the age groups of 80–84 and 85–89.[4]

Death rates for seniors are declining

During the twentieth century, death rates for all Americans, including seniors, have declined contributing to increased life expectancy. At the end of the twentieth century, elderly men were about one-third less likely to die than their similarly aged,

Most older adults are not afraid of their own deaths

Two-thirds (66 percent) of adults aged 60+ are not at all afraid of their own deaths; one-quarter (24 percent) are slightly bothered, and only 7 percent are truly afraid of it.[5] In actuality, older adults are more afraid of public speaking (28 percent) or walking outside alone at night (29 percent) than they are of their own deaths. Proportionately fewer older adults are afraid of their own deaths than younger adults (7 percent compared to 17 percent).

TABLE 15.2
Death Rates (per 100,000 Persons) among Seniors for All Causes by Age and Sex: 2000 versus 1950 and 1985

	Men			Women		
		Percent Change			Percent Change	
	2000	1950 to 2000	1985 to 2000	2000	1950 to 2000	1985 to 2000
65–74 years	3,020	–39%	–22%	1,950	–41%	–7%
75–84	6,858	–34	–19	4,910	–42	–5
85+	16,614	–23	–11	14,769	–23	2

Sources: Arialdi M. Minino, "Deaths: Preliminary Data for 2000," *National Vital Statistics Reports* 49, no. 12 (National Center for Health Statistics, National Vital Statistics System, October 19, 2001): Table 1; National Center for Health Statistics, *Health, United States, 2001 with Urban and Rural Health Chartbook* (Hyattsville, MD, 2001), Table 36.

midcentury counterparts (see Table 15.2). Declines in death rates for elderly women are somewhat greater than for elderly men over the same period. However, during the more recent past (1985–2000), the reverse is true, with elderly men having double-digit declines versus single-digit declines (or even increases) for elderly women.

■ Black seniors aged 65–84 are more likely to die than their white counterparts

In a 1-year time period, black men and women aged 65–84 are more likely to die than their white counterparts (see Table 15.3).[6] However, among the oldest-old (aged 85+), the reverse is true, with white men and women more likely to die.

TABLE 15.3
Death Rates for All Causes, by Age, Sex, and Race: 2000

	White	Black	Ratio of Black to White
Men			
65–74 years	2,955	4,058	1.37
75–84	6,827	8,190	1.20
85+	16,919	15,428	0.91
Women			
65–74 years	1,900	2,648	1.39
75–84	4,871	5,948	1.22
85+	14,958	14,351	0.96

Source: Arialdi M. Minino, "Deaths: Preliminary Data for 2000," *National Vital Statistics Reports* 49, no. 12 (National Center for Health Statistics, National Vital Statistics System, October 19, 2001): Table 1.

TABLE 15.4
Death Rates (per 100,000 Persons) for All Causes, by Age, Sex, and Race: 1985 and 2000

	White			Black		
	1985	2000	Percent Change 1985–2000	1985	2000	Percent Change 1985–2000
Men						
65–74 years	3,771	2,955	–22%	5,172	4,058	–22%
75–84	8,486	6,827	–20	9,262	8,190	–12
85+	18,980	16,919	–11	15,774	15,428	–2
Women						
65–74 years	2,027	1,900	–6	2,968	2,648	–11
75–84	5,112	4,871	–5	6,078	5,948	–2
85+	14,745	14,958	1	12,703	14,351	13

Sources: Arialdi M. Minino, "Deaths: Preliminary Data for 2000," *National Vital Statistics Reports* 49, no. 12 (National Center for Health Statistics, National Vital Statistics System, October 19, 2001): Table 1; National Center for Health Statistics, *Health, United States, 2001 with Urban and Rural Health Chartbook* (Hyattsville, MD, 2001), Table 36.

Among the elderly, white men have experienced the most dramatic declines in death rates since 1985 (see Table 15.4). Elderly black men, except the oldest-old, have also experienced significant declines in death rates. Death rates for elderly white and black women have declined less dramatically. In fact, the oldest-old black women have actually experienced double-digit increases in death rates since 1985.

■ Never-married elderly have the highest death rates

The elderly who have never been married are substantially more likely to die than their counterparts who have ever been married (see Chart 15.2 and detailed data in Table 15.5). In fact, compared to their presently married counterparts, the never-marrieds are as much as three times more likely to die.

Among those who have ever been married, those who are presently married have the lowest death rates. Among the younger of these ever-married elderly (aged 65 to 74), those who are presently married have the lowest death rates followed by the widowed and then the divorced, who have the highest death rates. However, among the older of the ever-married elderly (aged 75+), those who are widowed have the highest death rates. This relationship holds for both men and women.

SPECIFIC CAUSES OF DEATH

In this section on specific causes of death, a departure is taken in presenting trend data for the following reason. In 1999, a major revision of the International Classification of Diseases (ICD) occurred, and as a result, breaks exist in comparability with previous vital statistics data. We have chosen to show trends based on National Vital

CHART 15.2   Death Rates for All Causes, by Age and Marital Status: 1999

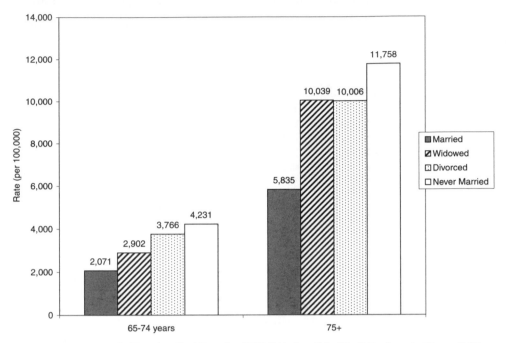

Source: Donna L. Hoyert et al., "Deaths: Final Data for 1999," *National Vital Statistics Reports* 49, no. 8 (National Center for Health Statistics, National Vital Statistics System, September 21, 2001): Table 22.

TABLE 15.5
Death Rates (per 100,000 Persons) for All Causes, by Age, Sex, and Marital Status: 1999

	Never Married	Ever Married				Ratio of Never Married to:	
		Total Ever Married	Presently Married	Widowed	Divorced	Ever Married	Presently Married
Total							
65–74 years	4,231	2,404	2,071	2,902	3,766	1.76	2.04
75+	11,758	8,076	5,835	10,039	10,006	1.46	2.02
Men							
65–74 years	6,055	2,975	2,605	4,556	4,937	2.04	2.32
75+	12,081	8,863	7,320	13,148	11,756	1.36	1.65
Women							
65–74 years	2,779	1,936	1,450	2,528	2,901	1.44	1.92
75+	11,570	7,604	3,764	9,361	9,091	1.52	3.07

Source: Donna L. Hoyert et al., "Deaths: Final Data for 1999," *National Vital Statistics Reports* 49, no. 8 (National Center for Health Statistics, National Vital Statistics System, September 21, 2001): Table 22.

Statistics data between 1985 and 1998 (years with comparable ICD data). However, 1999 data are provided but not included in any trend calculations. In addition, in several cases (all of which are indicated), title changes in causes of death occurred in 1999.

■ Four conditions account for 7 in 10 elderly deaths

In 1999, the elderly incurred 1,797,331 deaths.[7] Heart disease, cancer, stroke, and chronic lower respiratory diseases (e.g., bronchitis, emphysema, asthma) account for 70 percent of those deaths (see Chart 15.3).

Heart disease and cancer consistently are the top two causes of death among elderly blacks and whites as well as men and women.[8] The greatest difference between races is that hypertension is in the top 10 causes of death for black elderly people, but not for their white counterparts. For elderly black men, hypertension replaces Alzheimer's disease, and for elderly black women, it replaces accidents.

Heart Disease–related Deaths

■ Heart disease is the leading killer of seniors

The elderly account for 75 percent of all deaths but 84 percent of all heart-related deaths.[9] Heart disease is the leading cause of death among seniors; one-third of all deaths among seniors in 1999 were due to heart disease (see Chart 15.3). Deaths due

CHART 15.3   Leading Causes of Death among the Elderly: 1999

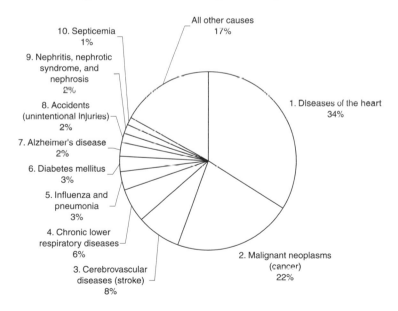

Source: Robert N. Anderson, "Deaths: Leading Causes for 1999," *National Vital Statistics Reports* 49, no. 11 (National Center for Health Statistics, National Vital Statistics System, October 12, 2001): Table 1.

TABLE 15.6
Death Rates (per 100,000 Persons) for Diseases of the
Heart, by Age and Sex: 1999

	Men	Women	Ratio of Men to Women
65+ years	1,884	1,669	1.13
65–74	962	503	1.91
75–84	2,309	1,563	1.48
85+	6,313	5,914	1.07

Source: Robert N. Anderson, "Deaths: Leading Causes for 1999,"
National Vital Statistics Reports 49, no. 11 (National Center for
Health Statistics, National Vital Statistics System, October 12,
2001): Table 1.

to heart disease become more prevalent with age. Twenty-nine percent of deaths among the youngest-old were heart disease–related, compared with 39 percent of deaths among the oldest-old in 1999.[10]

In 1999, 1.9 percent of elderly men and 1.7 percent of elderly women died of heart-related diseases (see Table 15.6). Significant gender differences exist, primarily at younger ages. Among the youngest-old, men are nearly twice as likely as women to die of heart disease. Among the oldest-old, though, the difference narrows such that men are only 7 percent more likely than women to die of such causes.

■ Heart disease–related deaths are more likely among younger blacks

Black men and women aged 65 to 84 are more likely to die from heart-related causes than their white counterparts (see Table 15.7).[11] However, among the oldest-old (aged 85+), the reverse is true: white men and women have higher death rates than blacks from heart disease.

TABLE 15.7
Death Rates (per 100,000 Persons) for Diseases of the Heart, by Age, Sex, and Race: 1999

	Men			Women		
	White	Black	Ratio of Black to White	White	Black	Ratio of Black to White
65+ years	1,898	2,003	1.06	1,683	1,820	1.08
65–74	942	1,294	1.37	474	833	1.76
75–84	2,314	2,560	1.11	1,535	2,070	1.35
85+	6,462	5,433	0.84	6,006	5,526	0.92

Source: Robert N. Anderson, "Deaths: Leading Causes for 1999," *National Vital Statistics Reports* 49, no. 11 (National Center for Health Statistics, National Vital Statistics System, October 12, 2001): Table 1.

TABLE 15.8

Death Rates (per 100,000 Persons) for Diseases of the Heart, by Age, Sex, and Race: 1985 and 1998

	Men			Women		
	1985	1998	Percent Change 1985–1998	1985	1998	Percent Change 1985–1998
Total						
65–74 years	1,536	997	–35%	746	523	–30%
75–84	3,497	2,377	–32	2,220	1,580	–29
85+	8,252	6,331	–23	7,038	5,877	–17
White						
65–74 years	1,523	981	–36	713	494	–31
75–84	3,527	2,382	–32	2,208	1,556	–30
85+	8,482	6,479	–24	7,170	5,971	–17
Black						
65–74 years	1,839	1,313	–29	1,150	859	–25
75–84	3,437	2,649	–23	2,533	2,045	–19
85+	6,394	5,447	–15	5,687	5,373	–6

Source: National Center for Health Statistics, *Health, United States, 2000 with Adolescent Chartbook* (Hyattsville, MD, 2000), Table 37.

■ The elderly are less likely to die of heart disease than their predecessors were

The likelihood of the elderly dying from heart disease declined dramatically between 1985 and 1998 (see Table 15.8).[12] However, the declines are somewhat greater for men than for women, and for whites than for blacks.

Cancer Deaths—An Overview

■ Cancer is the second leading cause of death among all seniors, but the leading cause among virtually all of the youngest-old

Compared with heart disease–related deaths, those due to cancer are less skewed toward the elderly. The elderly account for 71 percent of all cancer deaths.[13] Cancer is the second leading cause of death among the elderly, accounting for 22 percent of all senior deaths in 1999 (see Chart 15.3).[14] However, cancer is the leading cause of death among the youngest-old, except for black women, for whom heart disease still ranks as the number one killer (see Table 15.9). Cancer deaths are more likely among the youngest-old; 34 percent of this age group succumb to cancer. This declines to 23 percent of the middle-old and 12 percent of the oldest-old.

In 1999, 1.4 percent of elderly men and 0.9 percent of elderly women died of cancer (see Table 15.10). Gender differences are also evident with cancer and widen at

TABLE 15.9

Death Rates (per 100,000 Persons) for Heart Disease and Cancer, by Age, Sex, and Race: 1999

	White			Black		
	Heart Disease	Cancer	Ratio of Cancer to Heart Disease	Heart Disease	Cancer	Ratio of Cancer to Heart Disease
Men						
65–74 years	942	1,017	1.08	1,294	1,316	1.02
75–84	2,314	1,732	0.75	2,560	2,303	0.90
85+	6,462	2,613	0.40	5,433	3,098	0.57
Women						
65–74 years	474	677	1.43	833	767	0.92
75–84	1,535	1,068	0.70	2,070	1,194	0.58
85+	6,006	1,453	0.24	5,526	1,560	0.28

Source: Robert N. Anderson, "Deaths: Leading Causes for 1999," *National Vital Statistics Reports* 49, no. 11 (National Center for Health Statistics, National Vital Statistics System, October 12, 2001): Table 1.

older ages. Among the youngest-old, men are 52 percent more likely than women to die of cancer. At the other end of the age spectrum, the oldest-old men are 81 percent more likely than women to succumb to such causes. Racial differences also exist: elderly black women, and especially elderly black men, are more likely to die of cancer than their white counterparts (see Table 15.11).

Although cancer is more likely to claim elderly men than elderly women, cancer death rates have increased for elderly women since 1985 (see Table 15.12).[15] Increases for black women have been somewhat more than for white women during this period. Except for the oldest-old men, death rates for elderly men have generally declined. However, some racial differences exist, with all but the youngest-old black men losing ground to cancer relative to their white counterparts.

TABLE 15.10

Death Rates (per 100,000 Persons) for Cancer, by Age and Sex: 1999

	Men	Women	Ratio of Men to Women
65+ years	1,412	930	1.52
65–74	1,031	677	1.52
75–84	1,746	1,068	1.63
85+	2,619	1,449	1.81

Source: Robert N. Anderson, "Deaths: Leading Causes for 1999," *National Vital Statistics Reports* 49, no. 11 (National Center for Health Statistics, National Vital Statistics System, October 12, 2001): Table 1.

TABLE 15.11
Death Rates (per 100,000 Persons) for Cancer, by Age, Sex, and Race: 1999

	Men			Women		
	White	Black	Ratio of Black to White	White	Black	Ratio of Black to White
65+ years	1,400	1,751	1.25	935	1,003	1.07
65–74	1,017	1,316	1.29	677	767	1.13
75–84	1,723	2,303	1.34	1,068	1,194	1.12
85+	2,613	3,098	1.19	1,453	1,560	1.07

Source: Robert N. Anderson, "Deaths: Leading Causes for 1999," *National Vital Statistics Reports* 49, no. 11 (National Center for Health Statistics, National Vital Statistics System, October 12, 2001): Table 1.

TABLE 15.12
Death Rates (per 100,000 Persons) for Cancer, by Age, Sex, and Race: 1985 and 1998

	Men			Women		
	1985	1998	Percent Change 1985–1998	1985	1998	Percent Change 1985–1998
Total						
65–74 years	1,105	1,046	–5%	645	675	5%
75–84	1,840	1,746	–5	938	1,049	12
85+	2,452	2,563	5	1,281	1,413	10
White						
65–74 years	1,077	1,030	–4	645	676	5
75–84	1,817	1,722	–5	938	1,051	12
85+	2,449	2,554	4	1,285	1,415	10
Black						
65–74 years	1,533	1,345	–12	704	770	9
75–84	2,230	2,285	2	986	1,138	15
85+	2,629	3,051	16	1,284	1,514	18

Source: National Center for Health Statistics, *Health, United States, 2000 with Adolescent Chartbook* (Hyattsville, MD, 2000), Table 39.

Specific Cancers

Lung cancer is the leading cause of cancer-related deaths among seniors, followed by breast cancer (for women) and prostate cancer (for men). The third leading cause of cancer-related deaths for seniors is colorectal cancer. Unless otherwise noted, the following cancer death statistics for specific types of cancer are from the Surveillance, Epidemiology, and End Results (SEER) program of the National Cancer Institute. These statistics provide greater detail by age, sex and race for specific types of cancer deaths than do readily available National Vital Statistics figures.

■ Lung cancer death rates have increased substantially among senior women

Lung cancer, including bronchus, is the leading cause of cancer-related deaths among seniors, accounting for about 30 percent of all elderly cancer deaths in 1998.[16] Seniors account for 71 percent of all lung cancer deaths.[17]

Elderly men of all ages are substantially more likely than elderly women to die of lung cancer (see Table 15.13). Racial differences also exist, with elderly black men more likely to die of lung cancer than their white counterparts (see Table 15.14). The opposite is true of elderly women. White women are more likely to die of such causes than black women are.

From 1973 to 1996, the likelihood of dying from lung cancer increased dramatically, especially for elderly women, who, in 1996, were 3.7 times more likely than their 1973 counterparts to die from lung cancer.[18] Elderly men had a 30 percent greater chance of dying from lung cancer in 1996 compared to 1973. Despite the significant increase, elderly women are still one-third to one-half as likely to die from lung cancer as are elderly men of comparable ages (see Table 15.13).

■ Breast cancer is the second leading cause of cancer deaths among senior women

Breast cancer is the second leading cause of cancer deaths among senior women, except among women 85+. In that age group, it is the leading cause of cancer deaths, surpassing lung cancer (see Table 15.15).[19] Six in ten breast cancer deaths (59 percent) are among senior women.[20]

During the years 1994 to 1998, elderly black women were somewhat more likely than their white counterparts to die from breast cancer (see Table 15.16).[21] This situation is the opposite of that in 1973. From 1973 until 1996, breast cancer death rates

TABLE 15.13
Death Rates (per 100,000 Persons) for Lung Cancer, by Age and Sex: 1994–1998

	Men	Women	Ratio of Men to Women	Ratio of Women to Men
65+ years*	458	215	2.13	0.47
65–69	357	181	1.97	0.51
70–74	471	231	2.04	0.49
75–79	526	247	2.13	0.47
80–84	577	243	2.37	0.42
85+	521	186	2.80	0.36

*Age-adjusted.

Note: Figures include bronchus.

Source: National Cancer Institute, SEER Cancer Statistics Review 1973–1998 (Bethesda, MD, 2001), Table XV-6.

TABLE 15.14

Death Rates (per 100,000 Persons) for Lung Cancer, by Age, Sex, and Race: 1994–1998

	White	Black	Ratio of White to Black	Ratio of Black to White
Men				
65+ years*	454	568	0.80	1.25
65–69	354	449	0.79	1.27
70–74	465	621	0.75	1.34
75–79	522	645	0.81	1.24
80–84	576	685	0.84	1.19
85+	524	552	0.95	1.05
Women				
65+ years*	219	197	1.11	0.90
65–69	186	172	1.08	0.92
70–74	235	228	1.03	0.97
75–79	253	211	1.20	0.83
80–84	248	200	1.24	0.81
85+	188	168	1.12	0.89

*Age-adjusted.

Note: Figures include bronchus.

Source: National Cancer Institute, SEER Cancer Statistics Review 1973–1998 (Bethesda, MD, 2001), Table XV-6.

for elderly black women caught up and surpassed those of elderly white women.[22] Specifically, elderly black women in 1996 were 38 percent more likely to die from breast cancer than their counterparts were in 1973, whereas elderly white women were only 7 percent more likely.

TABLE 15.15

Death Rates (per 100,000 Persons) among Elderly Women for Lung and Breast Cancers, by Age: 1994–1998

	Lung Cancer**	Breast Cancer	Ratio of Breast Cancer to Lung Cancer
65+ years*	215	118	0.55
65–69	181	89	0.49
70–74	231	110	0.48
75–79	247	127	0.51
80–84	243	153	0.63
85+	186	199	1.07

*Age-adjusted

**Figures include bronchus.

Source: National Cancer Institute, SEER Cancer Statistics Review 1973–1998 (Bethesda, MD, 2001), Tables IV-3 and XV-6.

TABLE 15.16
Death Rates (per 100,000 Persons) among Elderly Women for
Breast Cancer, by Age and Race: 1994–1998

	All Women	White	Black	Ratio of Black to White
65+ years*	118	118	131	1.11
65–69	89	90	99	1.10
70–74	110	110	131	1.19
75–79	127	128	138	1.08
80–84	153	154	171	1.11
85+	199	200	206	1.03

*Age-adjusted.
Source: National Cancer Institute, SEER Cancer Statistics Review 1973–
1998 (Bethesda, MD, 2001), Table IV-3.

■ For senior men, prostate cancer is the second leading cause of cancer deaths

Prostate cancer is the second most common cause of cancer-related deaths among senior men. Senior men account for 92 percent of all prostate cancer deaths.[23] Elderly black men are more than twice as likely as their white counterparts to die of prostate cancer (see Table 15.17).[24] Additionally, elderly black men are substantially more likely than their 1970s counterparts to die from prostate cancer. This trend is not seen for white men. Specifically, between 1973 and 1996, prostate cancer death rates for elderly black men increased significantly more than for elderly whites (42 percent versus 13 percent).[25]

TABLE 15.17
Death Rates (per 100,000 Persons) among Elderly Men for
Prostate Cancer: 1994–1998

	All Men	White	Black	Ratio of Black to White
65+ years*	217	200	466	2.33
65–69	71	62	168	2.71
70–74	142	127	357	2.81
75–79	248	227	555	2.44
80–84	433	404	922	2.28
85+	760	723	1,324	1.83

*Age-adjusted.
Source: National Cancer Institute, SEER Cancer Statistics Review 1973–
1998 (Bethesda, MD, 2001), Table XXII-2.

TABLE 15.18
Death Rates (per 100,000 Persons) for Colorectal Cancer,
by Age and Sex: 1994–1998

	Men	Women	Ratio of Men to Women
65+ years*	147	100	1.47
65–69	88	54	1.63
70–74	125	80	1.56
75–79	164	112	1.46
80–84	234	166	1.41
85+	324	261	1.24

*Age-adjusted.
Source: National Cancer Institute, *SEER Cancer Statistics Review 1973–1998* (Bethesda, MD, 2001), Table VI-6.

■ Colorectal cancer is the third most common cause of cancer deaths among the elderly

Three-quarters (77 percent) of colorectal cancer deaths are among seniors.[26] Colorectal cancer deaths are more likely among men than women, and among blacks than whites (see Tables 15.18 and 15.19).[27]

Elderly white men and women were less likely in 1996 to die from colorectal cancer than their 1970s counterparts, with a 20 percent decline in death rates for white men and 26 percent decline for women from 1973 to 1996.[28] Elderly black men and women, however, were more likely to die from colorectal cancer, with a 24 percent increase among black men and an 8 percent increase among black women over the same time period.

Cerebrovascular Deaths

■ Nearly 3 in 4 people who suffer a stroke are seniors

Seniors account for about 72 percent of the people who suffer a stroke each year.[29] They also account for 89 percent of all cerebrovascular deaths each year.[30] Cerebrovascular disease is the third leading cause of death among seniors, accounting for 8.3 percent of all senior deaths (see Chart 15.3).[31]

Overall, elderly women are more likely than elderly men to die from cerebrovascular disease, but that is the situation only among the oldest-old (see Table 15.20). Up through age 84, elderly men are more likely than elderly women to die of such circumstances. All but the oldest-old blacks (both men and women) are more likely to die from cerebrovascular disease than their white counterparts are (see Table 15.21).

The likelihood of the elderly dying from cerebrovascular disease declined dramatically for both sexes between 1985 and 1998 (see Table 15.22). Elderly men and

TABLE 15.19

Death Rates (per 100,000 Persons) for Colorectal Cancer, by Age, Sex, and Race: 1994–1998

	White	Black	Ratio of Black to White
Men			
65+ years*	145	180	1.24
65–69	86	109	1.27
70–74	122	170	1.39
75–79	163	201	1.23
80–84	233	282	1.21
85+	327	342	1.05
Women			
65+ years*	98	132	1.35
65–69	52	76	1.46
70–74	78	115	1.47
75–79	111	146	1.32
80–84	163	214	1.31
85+	260	288	1.11

*Age-adjusted.
Source: National Cancer Institute, *SEER Cancer Statistics Review 1973–1998* (Bethesda, MD, 2001), Table VI-6.

women of both major racial groups have also experienced substantial declines in the likelihood of stroke-related deaths.[32]

Chronic Lower Respiratory Disease Deaths

Prior to 1999, chronic lower respiratory disease was called chronic obstructive pulmonary disease. Therefore, in this section, although not necessarily specified by the

TABLE 15.20

Death Rates (per 100,000 Persons) for Cerebrovascular Disease, by Age and Sex: 1999

	Men	Women	Ratio of Men to Women	Ratio of Women to Men
65+ years	380	466	1.23	0.82
65–74	149	119	0.80	1.25
75–84	495	458	0.93	1.08
85+	1,456	1,671	1.15	0.87

Source: Robert N. Anderson, "Deaths: Leading Causes for 1999," *National Vital Statistics Reports* 49, no. 11 (National Center for Health Statistics, National Vital Statistics System, October 12, 2001): Table 1.

TABLE 15.21
Death Rates (per 100,000 Persons) for Cerebrovascular Disease, by Age, Sex, and Race: 1999

	Men			Women		
	White	Black	Ratio of Black to White	White	Black	Ratio of Black to White
65+ years	375	461	1.23	469	494	1.05
65–74	138	264	1.91	110	200	1.82
75–84	485	635	1.31	450	582	1.29
85+	1,476	1,343	0.91	1,693	1,559	0.92

Source: Robert N. Anderson, "Deaths: Leading Causes for 1999," *National Vital Statistics Reports 49,* no. 11 (National Center for Health Statistics, National Vital Statistics System, October 12, 2001): Table 1.

authors, all 1999 data relate to the chronic lower respiratory terminology, and earlier data relate to the chronic obstructive pulmonary terminology.

■ Pulmonary-related death rates among senior women are catching up to those of senior men

The elderly account for 87 percent of all deaths due to chronic lower respiratory diseases (e.g., emphysema, asthma, and bronchitis), which are the fourth leading cause of death among seniors (see Chart 15.3).[33] As a group, elderly women of all

TABLE 15.22
Death Rates (per 100,000 Persons) for Cerebrovascular Disease, by Age, Sex, and Race: 1985 and 1998

	Men			Women		
	1985	1998	Percent Change 1985–1998	1985	1998	Percent Change 1985–1998
Total						
65–74 years	201	146	−28%	151	117	−22%
75–84	661	475	−28	566	443	−22
85+	1,730	1,347	−22	1,919	1,563	−19
White						
65–74 years	186	135	−27	138	109	−21
75–84	650	465	−28	553	434	−21
85+	1,766	1,366	−23	1,945	1,590	−18
Black						
65–74 years	380	256	−33	286	197	−31
75–84	814	621	−24	754	560	−26
85+	1,429	1,243	−13	1,657	1,398	−16

Source: National Center for Health Statistics, *Health, United States, 2000 with Adolescent Chartbook* (Hyattsville, MD, 2000), Table 38.

TABLE 15.23
Death Rates (per 100,000 Persons) for Chronic Lower
Respiratory Disease, by Age and Sex: 1999

	Men	Women	Ratio of Men to Women	Ratio of Women to Men
65+ years	378	267	1.42	.71
65–74	213	151	1.41	.71
75–84	507	329	1.54	.65
85+	959	509	1.88	.53

Source: Robert N. Anderson, "Deaths: Leading Causes for 1999,"
National Vital Statistics Reports 49, no. 11 (National Center for Health
Statistics, National Vital Statistics System, October 12, 2001): Table 1.

races, especially those aged 85+, have experienced the greatest increases in pulmonary-related death rates since 1985.[34]

The death rates for elderly women attributable to this disease increased 50 percent or more from 1985 to 1998 (see Table 15.25).[35] Nevertheless, death rates from this cause for senior women still are about one-half to three-quarters that of their male counterparts (see Table 15.23). Elderly white people, especially women, are substantially more likely than their black counterparts to die of pulmonary-related causes (see Table 15.24).

Influenza and Pneumonia Deaths

■ Elderly black women are the least likely elderly group to die from pneumonia or influenza

The elderly account for 90 percent of all pneumonia and flu deaths.[36] Of the two diseases, pneumonia is by far the most prevalent cause of death, accounting for 98

TABLE 15.24
Death Rates (per 100,000 Persons) for Chronic Lower Respiratory Disease, by Age, Sex, and Race: 1999

	Men			Women		
	White	Black	Ratio of Black to White	White	Black	Ratio of Black to White
65+ years	392	288	1.36	285	138	2.07
65–74	221	177	1.25	162	88	1.84
75–84	520	424	1.23	347	174	1.99
85+	998	651	1.53	535	263	2.03

Source: Robert N. Anderson, "Deaths: Leading Causes for 1999," *National Vital Statistics Reports* 49, no. 11 (National Center for Health Statistics, National Vital Statistics System, October 12, 2001): Table 1.

TABLE 15.25
Death Rates (per 100,000 Persons) for Chronic Obstructive Pulmonary Disease, by Age, Sex, and Race: 1985 and 1998

	Men			Women		
	1985	1998	Percent Change 1985–1998	1985	1998	Percent Change 1985–1998
Total						
65–74 years	219	201	–8%	96	143	49%
75–84	505	472	–7	163	296	81
85+	758	870	15	209	445	113
White						
65–74 years	225	209	–7	101	153	51
75–84	526	486	–8	171	313	83
85+	798	905	13	218	467	114
Black						
65–74 years	178	164	8	48	85	76
75–84	322	372	16	77	149	94
85+	374	571	53	94	231	146

Source: National Center for Health Statistics, *Health, United States, 2000 with Adolescent Chartbook* (Hyattsville, MD, 2000), Table 42.

percent of the combined deaths in 1999. Elderly men are more likely than elderly women to die from pneumonia or influenza (see Table 15.26). Black and white elderly men are overall equally as likely to die from pneumonia or flu, and except among the oldest-old men, black men are more likely than white males to die of these diseases (see Table 15.27). Except among the youngest-old elderly women, white women are more likely than black to die of influenza or pneumonia.

TABLE 15.26
Death Rates (per 100,000 Persons) for Influenza and Pneumonia, by Age and Sex: 1999

	Men	Women	Ratio of Men to Women
65+ years	168	164	1.02
65–74	48	30	1.60
75–84	194	134	1.45
85+	861	700	1.23

Source: Robert N. Anderson, "Deaths: Leading Causes for 1999," *National Vital Statistics Reports* 49, no. 11 (National Center for Health Statistics, National Vital Statistics System, October 12, 2001): Table 1.

TABLE 15.27
Death Rates (per 100,000 Persons) for Influenza and Pneumonia, by Age, Sex, and Race: 1999

	White	Black	Ratio of White to Black	Ratio of Black to White
Men				
65+ years	169	168	1.01	0.99
65–74	45	74	0.61	1.64
75–84	194	209	0.93	1.08
85+	878	745	1.18	0.85
Women				
65+ years	170	137	1.24	0.81
65–74	29	38	0.76	1.31
75–84	135	132	1.02	0.98
85+	715	591	1.21	0.83

Source: Robert N. Anderson, "Deaths: Leading Causes for 1999," *National Vital Statistics Reports* 49, no. 11 (National Center for Health Statistics, National Vital Statistics System, October 12, 2001): Table 1.

Diabetes Deaths

■ Black seniors, especially women, are most affected by diabetes

The elderly account for 76 percent of all diabetes deaths.[37] Elderly men are more likely than elderly women to die of diabetes, and elderly blacks (men and women alike) are substantially more likely than their white counterparts to die of the disease (see Tables 15.28 and 15.29).[38] Elderly black women are even more likely than their male counterparts to die of diabetes.

TABLE 15.28
Death Rates (per 100,000 Persons) for Diabetes, by Age and Sex: 1999

	Men	Women	Ratio of Men to Women
65+ years	153	148	1.03
65–74	101	86	1.17
75–84	196	168	1.17
85+	333	309	1.08

Source: Robert N. Anderson, "Deaths: Leading Causes for 1999," *National Vital Statistics Reports* 49, no. 11 (National Center for Health Statistics, National Vital Statistics System, October 12, 2001): Table 1.

TABLE 15.29

Death Rates (per 100,000 Persons) for Diabetes, by Age, Sex, and Race: 1999

	Men			Women		
	White	Black	Ratio of Black to White	White	Black	Ratio of Black to White
65+ years	146	241	1.65	134	292	2.18
65–74	94	179	1.90	74	193	2.61
75–84	188	307	1.63	152	360	2.37
85+	323	469	1.45	288	555	1.93

Source: Robert N. Anderson, "Deaths: Leading Causes for 1999," *National Vital Statistics Reports* 49, no. 11 (National Center for Health Statistics, National Vital Statistics System, October 12, 2001): Table 1.

Alzheimer's Disease

■ Virtually all Alzheimer's deaths are among the elderly

Ninety-nine percent of all Alzheimer's deaths are attributable to the elderly.[39] In 1999, Alzheimer's disease claimed 92 of every 100,000 elderly men. Elderly women were 66 percent more likely to succumb to such a death, with 153 of every 100,000 dying due to Alzheimer's disease. The gender gap narrows a bit among the oldest-old: women in this group are 40 percent more likely than men to die from Alzheimer's disease (654 versus 467 per 100,000).

Accidental Deaths

In 1999, the National Vital Statistics terminology was changed from "accidents and adverse effects" to "accidents (unintentional injuries)." In this section, the reference is to "accidental deaths," regardless of the year of the data.

■ Accidental deaths are less skewed toward the elderly

Although the elderly account for three-quarters of all deaths, they account for only one-third of all accident-related deaths (such as falls or motor vehicle-related accidents).[40] Elderly men of all ages are more likely than elderly women to have an accidental death (see Table 15.30).[41]

■ Falls are the major source of accidental deaths among the elderly

Unintentional falls are the single largest cause of accidental deaths among the elderly, accounting for 31 percent of such deaths in 1999.[42] Three-quarters of all fall-related deaths (77 percent) are attributable to seniors. Elderly men are more likely than women to die as a result of a fall (see Table 15.31).[43] However, that likelihood narrows somewhat among older age groups. White men and women are substantially more likely than their black counterparts to die of fall-related injuries.

TABLE 15.30
Death Rates (per 100,000 Persons) for Accidents and
Unintentional Injuries: 1999

	Men	Women	Ratio of Men to Women
65+ years	111	81	1.37
65–74	61	32	1.90
75–84	131	81	1.61
85+	361	247	1.46

Source: Robert N. Anderson, "Deaths: Leading Causes for 1999,"
National Vital Statistics Reports 49, no. 11 (National Center for
Health Statistics, National Vital Statistics System, October 12,
2001): Table 1.

■ Motor vehicle deaths are less skewed toward the elderly

Although seniors account for 75 percent of all deaths, they account for only 18 percent of all motor vehicle–related deaths.[44] Motor vehicle–related deaths account for 24 percent of elderly accidental deaths. The vast majority of seniors who died in motor vehicle–related crashes in 1997 were occupants of passenger vehicles rather than pedestrians (nearly 80 percent versus 16 percent).[45]

The elderly may be more susceptible to motor vehicle–related accidents due to age-related declines in vision or hearing and cognitive functions.[46] Medical conditions, physical impairments, and medications may also affect driving ability. In 1999, 22 seniors per 100,000 died from motor vehicle–related injuries, with the likelihood increasing among older age groups (from 18 per 100,000 for ages 65–74, to 27 per 100,000 for ages 75–84, to 30 per 100,000 for ages 85+).[47] Only young adults aged 15–24 and 25–34 have comparable death rates (27 and 17 per 100,000, respectively).

TABLE 15.31
Death Rate (per 100,000 Persons) of Fall-Related Deaths,
by Age, Sex, and Race: 1998

	Men	Women	Ratio of Men to Women
65+ years	31	26	1.19
65–74	12	6.5	1.91
75–84	39	25	1.54
85+	135	97	1.38
Race			
White, 65+	33	28	1.18
Black, 65+	18	11	1.54

Source: National Vital Statistics, unpublished data, Work Table 1, 1998.

TABLE 15.32

Death Rates (per 100,000 Persons) for Motor Vehicle–Related Injuries, by Age, Sex, and Race: 1985 and 1998

	Men			Women			Ratio of Men to Women, 1998
	1985	1998	Percent Change 1985–1998	1985	1998	Percent Change 1985–1998	
65+ years	30.4	32.1	5.6%	15.8	17.8	13%	1.80
65–74	23.0	23.5	2.2	14.0	14.5	3.6	1.62
75–84	41.3	39.7	–3.9	19.2	21.8	14	1.82
85+	55.3	61.2	11	15.0	19.2	28	3.19
Race							
White, 65+	29.9	31.9	6.7	16.2	18.1	12	1.76
Black, 65+	35.2	36.0	2.3	11.2	13.8	23	2.61

Source: National Center for Health Statistics, *Health, United States, 2000 with Adolescent Chartbook* (Hyattsville, MD, 2000), Table 45.

■ Men 85+ are the most likely seniors to die from a motor vehicle–related accident

Elderly men are substantially more likely than similarly aged women to incur a motor vehicle–related fatality (see Table 15.32).[48] The difference is greatest among the oldest-old group—men are more than three times as likely as women to have such a fatality. Elderly black men are somewhat more likely than elderly white men to die from a motor vehicle–related accident, but elderly black women are somewhat less likely than elderly white women to do so. For the most part, motor vehicle–related deaths among seniors have increased since 1985.

■ Seniors are more likely to be injured than killed in motor vehicle–related accidents

The likelihood of nonfatal motor vehicle–related injuries among the elderly increased 9 percent between 1990 and 1997 (from 684 to 748 injuries per 100,000 persons).[49] Seniors are 31 times more likely to incur a nonfatal motor vehicle–related injury than they are to die from one (748 injuries per 100,000 versus 24 deaths per 100,000 in 1997).[50]

Suicide

■ Suicides are highest among elderly men

Senior men of all ages have the highest suicide rates of any age group.[51] In fact, elderly men are as likely to commit suicide as they are to die in a motor vehicle–related accident. From ages 25 to 64, men incur about 23 suicides per 100,000 persons (see Chart 15.4). That rate increases slightly among men aged 65 to 74 and

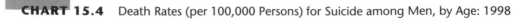

CHART 15.4   Death Rates (per 100,000 Persons) for Suicide among Men, by Age: 1998

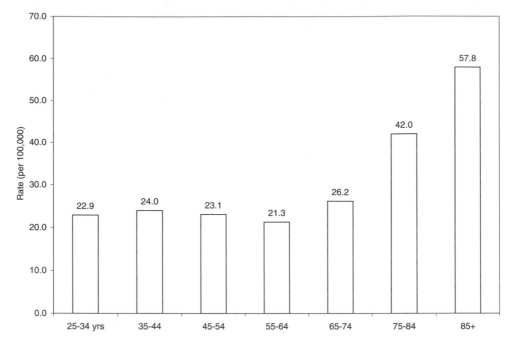

Source: National Center for Health Statistics, *Health, United States, 2000 with Adolescent Chartbook* (Hyattsville, MD, 2000), Table 47.

then dramatically increases 62 percent among the middle-old, and an additional 38 percent among the oldest-old. The result is that the oldest-old men are more than twice as likely as the youngest-old men to commit suicide.

Men account for the vast majority (82 percent) of suicides among seniors[52] and are about seven times more likely than women to commit suicide (see Table 15.33).[53] Elderly white men and women are substantially more likely than their black counterparts to commit suicide. Suicide rates for all but the oldest-old men and women have declined since 1985.

■ Firearms are the top suicide method among seniors; poisoning is second

Seven in ten suicides among seniors are committed with a firearm.[54] However, firearm usage for suicide is twice as prevalent among elderly men as among elderly women (77 percent of suicides among men are with a firearm versus 34 percent among women). Elderly women are more likely to use poisoning (29 percent of suicides among elderly women are by poisoning versus 12 percent among men).

TABLE 15.33
Death Rates (per 100,000 Persons) for Suicide, by Sex and Age: 1985 and 1998

	Men			Women		
	1985	1998	Percent Change 1985–1998	1985	1998	Percent Change 1985–1998
65+ years	41	34	−17%	6.6	4.7	−28%
65–74	34	26	−23	6.9	4.3	−38
75–84	53	42	−21	6.7	4.9	−27
85+	56	58	3	4.7	5.8	23
Race						
White, 65+	44	37	−16	6.9	5.0	−28
Black, 65+	16	12	−27	2.7	1.2	−56

Source: National Center for Health Statistics, *Health, United States, 2000 with Adolescent Chartbook* (Hyattsville, MD, 2000), Table 47.

WHERE AND WHEN PEOPLE DIE

■ **The elderly are more than twice as likely to die in a hospital as at home**

About one-half of the elderly die in a hospital, most often as inpatients (see Chart 15.5).[55] Nursing homes are the next most common place of death for seniors, followed by residences. Where the elderly die varies considerably by age group and gender. Hospitals and residents become less prominent and nursing homes become more prominent for older seniors (see Chart 15.6). Among the oldest-old women, nursing homes are the most common place of death; nearly one-half of all their deaths occur there (see Table 15.34). This is not surprising because the oldest-old women are the most likely age and gender group to be nursing home residents. Among all other age and gender groups, hospitals are the most common place of death.

TABLE 15.34
Percent of All Deaths Occurring According to Place of Death, by Age and Sex: 1998

	Men			Women		
Place of Death	65–74 Years	75–84 Years	85+ Years	65–74 Years	75–84 Years	85+ Years
Hospital or medical center	59%	54%	44%	56%	49%	36%
Hospital inpatient	46	45	38	47	42	31
Hospital outpatient, emergency room, or other	12	9	6	9	7	5
Nursing home	11	20	35	14	27	47
Residence	28	23	18	26	20	14
Other places or unknown	3	3	3	3	3	2

Source: National Vital Statistics, unpublished 1998 data, Table 309.

CHART 15.5 Where the Elderly Die: 1998

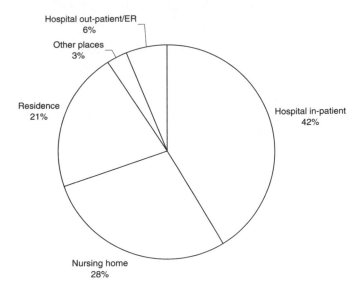

Source: National Vital Statistics, unpublished 1998 data, Table 309.

CHART 15.6 Where the Elderly Die, by Age: 1998

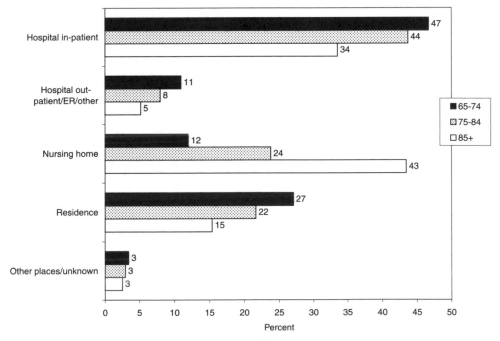

Source: National Vital Statistics, unpublished 1998 data, Table 309.

ELDERLY DEATHS BY STATE OF RESIDENCE AND DATE

■ Is Hawaii the Fountain of Youth?

Death rates among the elderly vary considerably by state of residence (see Table 15.35).[56] The elderly in Hawaii have, by far, the lowest death rates of all other elderly Americans. In fact, the next closest elderly death rates are 14 to 22 percent higher than the death rates for elderly Hawaiians.

■ The elderly are least likely to die in the summer and most likely to die in the winter

Across the three elderly age categories, elderly residents of warm-climate states such as Hawaii, California, and Florida, as well as the northeastern states of New York and Connecticut and the cold-weather state of North Dakota, are consistently among the states with the 10 lowest elderly death rates.

At the other end of the spectrum are states such as Oklahoma, Georgia, Louisiana, Mississippi, West Virginia, Tennessee, and Kentucky, which are consistently among the states with the 10 highest elderly death rates across the three elderly age categories.

CHART 15.7   Number of Elderly Deaths per Day: December 1999 to December 2000

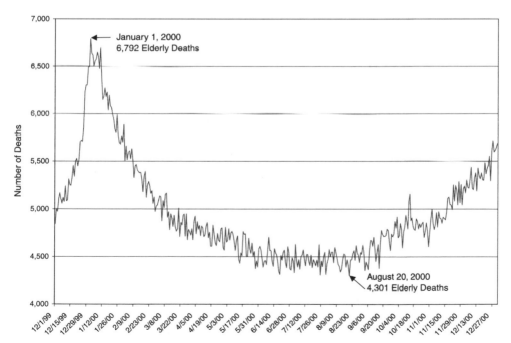

Source: National Vital Statistics, unpublished 1999 and 2000 data, Working Table 306.

TABLE 15.35

Death Rates (per 100,000 Persons) by State: 2000 (Listed by Death Rate Ranking of 65–74-Year-Olds)

	Death Rates			Rankings		
	65–74 Years	75–84 Years	85+ Years	65–74 Years	75–84 Years	85+ Years
Total U.S.	2,428.6	5,688.4	15,321.5	NA	NA	NA
Hawaii	1,738.8	4,097.6	12,080.6	1	1	1
Utah	1,980.9	5,445.5	15,216.3	2	15	18
California	2,074.4	5,001.7	13,822.0	3	3	2
Minnesota	2,083.7	5,154.3	15,147.7	4	4	17
Colorado	2,115.4	5,301.4	15,264.6	5	9	21
North Dakota	2,116.8	5,276.4	13,958.0	6	8	3
Florida	2,141.5	5,000.0	14,166.0	7	2	4
Connecticut	2,177.0	5,231.0	14,540.8	8	5	9
New York	2,225.8	5,270.8	14,257.2	9	7	7
New Mexico	2,240.8	5,353.4	14,252.4	10	13	6
Washington	2,240.8	5,453.1	15,093.5	11	16	14
South Dakota	2,251.3	5,243.6	14,984.1	12	6	11
Rhode Island	2,261.8	5,411.7	15,121.7	13	14	15
New Hampshire	2,267.5	5,781.8	16,031.7	14	25	34
Nebraska	2,268.6	5,331.0	14,864.5	15	12	10
Alaska	2,275.0	6,200.0	14,285.7	16	38	8
Iowa	2,275.8	5,315.8	15,225.6	17	10	19
Massachusetts	2,291.8	5,533.7	15,311.2	18	18	22
Idaho	2,299.2	5,515.6	15,136.7	19	17	16
Oregon	2,310.6	5,659.8	15,532.7	20	22	25
Wyoming	2,312.3	5,940.2	15,261.5	21	29	20
Arizona	2,333.1	5,329.0	14,178.7	22	11	5
Kansas	2,336.3	5,607.7	16,060.0	23	20	35
Montana	2,338.7	5,725.5	15,029.4	24	23	12

The differential in death rates between the "best" and "worst" states is substantial. Even if the extremely low death-rate state of Hawaii is dropped, Mississippi's youngest-old elderly are 54 percent more likely to die than their Utah counterparts. Among the middle-old, Georgia residents are 34 percent more likely to die than their Florida counterparts. And the oldest-old West Virginia residents are 26 percent more likely to die than their California counterparts.

Elderly deaths peak in the winter months and are lowest in the summer months (see Chart 15.7).[57] The elderly are most likely to die in January and least likely to die in August. In 2000, January 1 was the day the elderly were most likely to die. On this day, the elderly were 58 percent more likely to die than on August 20, the day they were least likely to die (6,792 elderly deaths versus 4,301 deaths).

A plot of elderly deaths by day from December 1999 through February 2000 reveals an interesting pattern around Christmas Day (see Chart 15.8). For this time pe-

TABLE 15.35
Continued

	Death Rates			Rankings		
	65–74 Years	75–84 Years	85+ Years	65–74 Years	75–84 Years	85+ Years
Wisconsin	2,341.5	5,544.1	15,488.9	25	19	24
New Jersey	2,358.3	5,633.8	15,557.9	26	21	26
Vermont	2,397.9	6,034.3	15,993.8	27	34	31
Delaware	2,447.9	5,855.9	16,460.6	28	27	43
Pennsylvania	2,472.7	6,022.1	16,008.8	29	33	32
Texas	2,491.4	5,963.3	15,962.7	30	31	29
Maine	2,495.4	6,100.0	16,621.4	31	36	45
Maryland	2,527.8	5,871.5	15,802.3	32	28	28
Illinois	2,530.8	5,739.5	15,067.3	33	24	13
Michigan	2,548.1	5,850.3	15,427.0	34	26	23
Virginia	2,578.5	5,951.2	16,120.0	35	30	36
Missouri	2,612.7	6,047.0	16,026.6	36	35	33
Ohio	2,644.9	6,153.7	16,211.2	37	37	38
North Carolina	2,660.7	6,231.6	16,404.4	38	39	42
Indiana	2,737.6	6,233.6	16,132.3	39	40	37
Arkansas	2,742.6	6,495.4	16,360.2	40	45	40
Oklahoma	2,761.9	6,294.0	16,962.2	41	41	48
Nevada	2,765.3	5,977.3	15,564.7	42	32	27
South Carolina	2,774.6	6,339.7	15,985.1	43	43	30
Georgia	2,853.0	6,685.9	16,538.3	44	50	44
Tennessee	2,853.7	6,624.7	16,925.4	45	48	47
Alabama	2,888.6	6,475.5	16,300.0	46	44	39
Louisiana	2,914.2	6,307.3	16,395.4	47	42	41
West Virginia	2,938.5	6,605.0	17,423.4	48	47	50
Kentucky	2,966.0	6,571.6	17,165.4	49	46	49
Mississippi	3,055.3	6,674.3	16,698.3	50	49	46

Source: National Vital Statistics, unpublished 2000 data, Table 23a.

riod, a trend of increasing numbers of daily elderly deaths in December leads up to Christmas Day, after which the rate of change dramatically increases up to January 1, the day in 2000 on which the most elderly died. From January 1–10, the number of elderly deaths plateaus and then begins the decline toward the more favorable summer months.

These "eyeball" assessments are revealed in the data themselves. From December 1 to December 25, 1999, the average daily increase in deaths was 0.7 percent versus 2.5 percent from December 25 to January 1, 2000. This same basic pattern is observed during Decembers in 1997, 1998, and 2000.

Throughout the year, elderly deaths by day of the week are evenly distributed with no particular day appearing more likely than another.

CHART 15.8   Number of Elderly Deaths per Day: December 1999 to February 2000

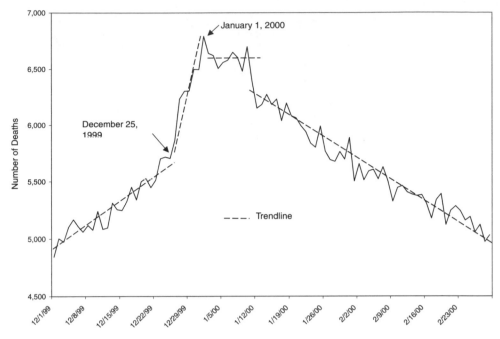

Source: National Vital Statistics, unpublished 1999 and 2000 data, Working Table 306.

NOTES

1. Arialdi M. Minino, "Deaths: Preliminary Data for 2000," *National Vital Statistics Reports*, 49, no. 12 (National Center for Health Statistics, National Vital Statistics System, October 19, 2001): Table 1.
2. Robert N. Anderson, "Deaths: Leading Causes for 1999," *National Vital Statistics Reports* 49, no. 11 (National Center for Health Statistics, National Vital Statistics System, October 12, 2001): Table 1.
3. National Center for Health Statistics, *Health, United States, 1999 with Health and Aging Chartbook* (Hyattsville, MD, 1999).
4. Ibid.
5. RoperASW, 1996.
6. Minino, "Deaths: Preliminary Data for 2000," Table 1.
7. Anderson, "Deaths: Leading Causes for 1999," Table 1.
8. Ibid.
9. Donna L. Hoyert et al., "Deaths: Final Data for 1999," *National Vital Statistics Reports* 49, no. 8 (National Center for Health Statistics, National Vital Statistics System, September 21, 2001): Table 9.
10. Anderson, "Deaths: Leading Causes for 1999," Table 1.
11. Ibid.
12. National Center for Health Statistics, *Health, United States, 2000 with Adolescent Chartbook* (Hyattsville, MD, 2000), Table 37.
13. Hoyert et al., "Deaths: Final Data for 1999," Table 9.
14. Anderson, "Deaths: Leading Causes for 1999," Table 1.
15. National Center for Health Statistics, *Health, United States, 2000,* Table 39.

16. Sherry L. Murphy, "Deaths: Final Data for 1998," *National Vital Statistics Reports* 48, no. 11 (National Center for Health Statistics, National Vital Statistics System, July 24, 2000): Table 10.
17. National Cancer Institute, *SEER Cancer Statistics Review 1973–1998* (2001), Table I-15.
18. National Cancer Institute, *SEER Cancer Statistics Review 1973–1996* (1999), Table XV-1.
19. National Cancer Institute, *SEER Cancer Statistics Review 1973–1998* (2001), Tables IV-3 and XV-6.
20. Ibid., Table I-15.
21. Ibid., Table IV-3.
22. National Cancer Institute, *SEER Cancer Statistics Review 1973–1996* (1999), Table IV-1.
23. National Cancer Institute, *SEER Cancer Statistics Review 1973–1998* (2001), Table I-15.
24. Ibid., Table XXII-2.
25. National Cancer Institute, *SEER Cancer Statistics Review 1973–1996* (1999), Table XXII-1.
26. National Cancer Institute, *SEER Cancer Statistics Review 1973–1998* (2001), Table I-15.
27. Ibid., Table VI-6.
28. National Cancer Institute, *SEER Cancer Statistics Review 1973–1996* (1999), Table VI-1.
29. American Heart Association, "Older Americans and Cardiovascular Diseases; Biostatistical Fact Sheets" (2000). Available online at www.americanheart.org/statistics/biostats.
30. Hoyert et al., "Deaths: Final Data for 1999," Table 9.
31. Anderson, "Deaths: Leading Causes for 1999," Table 1.
32. National Center for Health Statistics, *Health, United States, 2000*, Table 38.
33. Anderson, "Deaths: Leading Causes for 1999," Table 1.
34. Ibid.
35. National Center for Health Statistics, *Health, United States, 2000*, Table 42.
36. Hoyert et al., "Deaths: Final Data for 1999," Table 9.
37. Ibid.
38. Anderson, "Deaths: Leading Causes for 1999," Table 1.
39. Hoyert et al., "Deaths: Final Data for 1999," Table 9.
40. Ibid.
41. Anderson, "Deaths: Leading Causes for 1999," Table 1.
42. Hoyert et al., "Deaths: Final Data for 1999," Table 9.
43. National Vital Statistics, unpublished data, Work Table 1, 1998.
44. Hoyert et al., "Deaths: Final Data for 1999," Table 9.
45. Centers for Disease Control and Prevention, "Surveillance for Injuries and Violence among Older Adults," *MMWR, CDC Surveillance Summaries* 48, no. SS-8 (December 17, 1999).
46. Centers for Disease Control and Prevention, "Motor Vehicle–Related Deaths among Older Americans Fact Sheet," *National Center for Injury Prevention and Control Fact Sheet* (October 25, 1999).
47. Hoyert et al., "Deaths: Final Data for 1999."
48. National Center for Health Statistics, *Health, United States, 2000*, Table 45.
49. Centers for Disease Control and Prevention, "Surveillance for Injuries and Violence."
50. Ibid. and National Center for Health Statistics, *Health, United States, 2000*, Table 45.
51. National Center for Health Statistics, *Health, United States, 2000*, Table 47.
52. Centers for Disease Control and Prevention, "Surveillance for Injuries and Violence." 1990–1996 data.
53. National Center for Health Statistics, *Health, United States, 2000*, Table 47.
54. Centers for Disease Control and Prevention, "Surveillance for Injuries and Violence." 1990–1996 data.
55. National Vital Statistics, unpublished 1998 data, Table 309.
56. National Vital Statistics, unpublished 2000 data, Table 23a.
57. National Vital Statistics, unpublished 1999 and 2000 data, Working Table 306.

CHAPTER 16

Paying for Health Care: Health Care Spending, Medicare, Medicaid, and Supplemental Insurance

Medicare came into being in 1965 as a means of providing health insurance for older people. Most Americans breathed a sigh of relief, feeling confident that basic health care for their families and themselves in old age was now assured. Unfortunately, this was soon revealed to be far from the truth.

—Robert Butler, Why Survive?
Growing Old in America

Medicaid plays a critical role in the health care system by purchasing health care for certain low-income populations. However, its impact is often overlooked.

—Nancy-Ann DeParle, former
administrator, Health Care
Financing Administration

Health costs and financing play a dominant role in the lives of seniors. Central to any discussion of the health expenditures of the elderly is Medicare, which covers 95 percent of seniors. While Medicare is the cornerstone of health care for persons aged 65 and older, it covers only 57 percent of the elderly's health care costs. At the time of this writing, it does not pay for long-term care or prescription drugs.

Medicaid, which provides benefits to the elderly with low incomes, is also an important player in the elderly's health care coverage. It provides medical coverage to 12 percent of elderly Americans and covers the cost of long-term care for many of the low-income and middle-class elderly.

This chapter covers the elderly's health care spending and key elements of Medicare and Medicaid, including how the programs are different and how they can work together.

Highlights of this chapter include:

- Health care expenses account for 12 percent of the average senior's household spending.

- Older Americans have a high opinion of the Medicare program. However, many Medicare beneficiaries have difficulty understanding the program and getting the information they need.
- Medicare is projected to run out of funds in 2029.
- Medicare spent $5,657 per enrollee in 1999. Such spending is expected to increase to $10,257 in 2009.
- Medicare pays only 57 percent of the health costs of the elderly.
- Medicaid is the primary source of public funds for nursing home care.

HEALTH CARE SPENDING BY THE ELDERLY

■ Twelve percent of the average senior's household spending is for health care

According to data from the 2000 Consumer Expenditure Survey health care expenses account for 12 percent of the average senior's household spending (see Table 16.1).[1] Health spending is even more of a burden for people aged 75+, consuming 15 percent of their household expenditures. In contrast, people under age 65 spend 4 percent of their household expenditures on health care.[*] Given the elderly's smaller household size, the differential in spending on a per-person basis is even greater.

TABLE 16.1
Distribution of Average Household Spending, by Age: 2000

	Under 65 Years		65+ Years		65–74 Years		75+ Years	
Total average annual household spending	$40,942		$26,533		$30,782		$21,908	
	Percent Spending for Health	Average Annual Household Spending	Percent Spending for Health	Average Annual Household Spending	Percent Spending for Health	Average Annual Household Spending	Percent Spending for Health	Average Annual Household Spending
Total health care	100%	$1,766	100%	$3,247	100%	$3,163	100%	$3,338
Health insurance	46	821	50	1,619	51	1,608	49	1,631
Medical services	31	541	21	672	22	686	20	658
Drugs*	18	314	25	822	24	744	27	908
Medical supplies	5	90	4	133	4	126	4	141

*Includes prescription and nonprescription drugs.

Note: Percentages may not total to 100 due to rounding.

Source: U.S. Department of Labor, Consumer Expenditure Survey, 2000. Available at www.bls.gov.

---

[*] Based on age of reference person.

Half of the average senior household's health care spending is for insurance. Prescription and nonprescription drugs account for an additional 25 percent. Medical services, such as physician's services, lab tests, and nursing home care, make up another 21 percent.

FEDERAL SPENDING FOR THE ELDERLY'S HEALTH CARE

■ Medicare accounts for one-sixth of all health spending

National health spending is projected by actuaries at the Centers for Medicare and Medicaid Services (CMS), formerly the Health Care Financing Administration (HCFA), to reach $1.6 trillion in 2003.[2] This figure includes all spending by individuals, Medicare, Medicaid, private health insurance, and other sources. National health expenditures are projected to be $2.6 trillion in 2010 and reach 15.9 percent of the gross domestic product (GDP). Medicare's share of national health expenditures in 2003 is projected to be 17 percent, or $276.6 billion.

According to CMS, the projected growth in health spending over the next decade is fueled in part by rapid increases in spending for prescription drugs. Experts, such as noted economist Victor Fuchs, attribute the increase to technology.[3]

■ Medicare and Medicaid spending equals 20 percent of the federal budget

Spending for Medicare and Medicaid, much of which benefits the elderly, plays a significant role in government spending. Together Medicaid and Medicaid account for 20 percent of the federal budget. The Congressional Budget Office (CBO) projected federal spending for 2001 to be $1.85 trillion.[4] Medicare was expected to spend $237 billion, equaling 13 percent of the federal budget. Spending for Medicaid was estimated at $130 billion for 2001, or 7 percent of the budget.

■ Medicare spending is growing faster than the overall economy

The CMS projects that Medicare spending will grow faster than the U.S. economy. Between 2000 and 2030, Medicare's share of the GDP is expected to double from 2.2 percent to 4.5 percent.[5]

■ Medicare and Medicaid costs for people with Alzheimer's disease are contributing to the rise in health care spending

Medicare and Medicaid spending for people with Alzheimer's disease made up about 14 percent of total Medicare spending in 2000, even though this group comprised less than 10 percent of Medicare beneficiaries.[6] A 50-state study by the Lewin Group for the Alzheimer's Association projected a jump of 54 percent by the year 2010 in Medicare costs for people with Alzheimer's. The study suggested that the cost to Medicare of treating people with Alzheimer's disease will soar from $31.9 billion in 2000 to $49.3 billion in 2010. The study found a similar impact on Medicaid, with program expenditures for nursing home care for people with Alzheimer's increasing from $18.2 billion in 2000 to an estimated $33 billion in 2010.

Most people who get Alzheimer's and related dementias are Medicare beneficiaries. Medicaid expenditures for people with Alzheimer's disease are high due to the uninsured cost of long-term care. According to the Alzheimer's Association, nearly half of Medicare beneficiaries with Alzheimer's disease also qualify for Medicaid because they have exhausted their own resources paying for long-term care.

MEDICARE

■ Medicare started in 1965

Medicare was signed into law in 1965 by President Lyndon Johnson as Title XVIII of the Social Security Act.

DEFINITION: Medicare is a federal social insurance program with benefits available to all insured participants without regard to income and assets. The Medicaid, program, in contrast, is income specific.

Social Security and Railroad Retirement beneficiaries automatically receive a Medicare card 3 months before their sixty-fifth birthdays. The card is the ticket to obtaining services by Medicare-approved suppliers.

Medicare's beneficiaries are certain disabled persons under age 65 and the aged. Most persons who need a kidney transplant or renal dialysis are also covered, regardless of age. This chapter covers Medicare benefits primarily as they relate to the elderly only.

■ Medicare is highly valued

The Commonwealth Fund surveyed 2,000 adults aged 50 to 70 in order to understand how Medicare is perceived.[7] They found that Americans in this age group have a high opinion of the Medicare program. Sixty-eight percent of current Medicare beneficiaries considered becoming eligible for Medicare an important event in their lives. The survey also found that nearly two-thirds (63 percent) of individuals in the group aged 50 to 70 who are not eligible for Medicare would be interested in enrolling before age 65 if the option were offered.

Medicare was found to be important for individuals with low incomes and health problems as well as those who are better off and have higher incomes. Eight in ten low-income Medicare beneficiaries and those with health problems said that becoming a beneficiary was "very important" to them. One-half of better-off beneficiaries (living above 250 percent of the poverty level) and 47 percent of those who rate their health as excellent reported becoming eligible as "very important."

■ Medicare is confusing to most

Although most beneficiaries consider the Medicare program valuable, many have difficulty understanding it and getting the information they need about it. A recent survey found that 37 percent of Americans aged 65+ think Medicare covers outpatient prescription drugs, and 56 percent think that Medicare covers long-term care, when the program actually covers neither.[8]

Older Americans fear that Medicare will run out of money. Survey data from RoperASW found that 52 percent of Americans aged 60+ agreed with the statement "Medicare will run out of money and won't be available when I need it."[9]

■ What does Medicare cover?

One major criticism of Medicare is that it has not kept up with the times. Medicare covers only those services that are "medically reasonable and necessary for the diagnosis and treatment of illness or injury or to improve the functioning of a malformed body member."[10] Two major health care costs not covered by Medicare are long-term care and prescription drugs, which together account for almost 60 percent of senior's out-of-pocket spending for health care. Medicare also does not cover other important costs, such as routine eye exams and annual physicals (see sidebar).

Medicare does not cover:

- Acupuncture
- Deductibles, coinsurance, copayments
- Dental care and dentures
- Cosmetic surgery
- Custodial care
- Health care while traveling outside the United States
- Hearing aids
- Orthopedic shoes
- Outpatient prescription drugs
- Routine or yearly physical exams
- Routine care for the feet
- Routine care for the eyes
- Screening tests, with the exception of bone mass measurements, colorectal screening, diabetes services, mammograms, Pap smears and pelvic exams, and prostate cancer screening.
- Immunizations, with the exception of flu, pneumonia, and hepatitis B shots.

Medicare Parts A and B

The Medicare program consists of two parts: Part A, hospital insurance (HI); and Part B, supplementary medical insurance (SMI).

Part A Coverage

Part A pays only part of the costs of the services it covers. Beneficiaries must pay deductibles and coinsurance. With limitations and copays, Part A covers inpatient hospital care, skilled nursing facility care (up to 100 days following hospitalization), home health visits (for persons who need skilled nursing care on an intermittent basis, physical therapy, or speech therapy), and hospice care (for terminally ill beneficiaries with a life expectancy of 6 months or less for two 90-day periods, followed by an unlimited number of 60-day periods).

Part B Coverage

Part B of Medicare generally pays 80 percent of an approved amount set by CMS for covered services after the beneficiary pays an annual deductible ($100). Services covered include:

- Consultations, as well as home, office, and institutional visits. Limitations apply for services rendered by dentists, podiatrists, and chiropractors, as well as for the treatment of mental illness.

- Other medical and health services, including laboratory and other diagnostic tests, X-ray and other radiation therapy, outpatient hospital services, rural health clinic services, durable medical equipment, home dialysis supplies and equipment, artificial devices (other than dental), physical and speech therapy, and ambulance services.

- Specified preventive services, including an annual screening mammography for all women over age 40; a screening Pap smear and a screening pelvic exam once every 3 years, and more often for women who are at high risk of developing cervical cancer; specified colorectal screening procedures; diabetes self-management training services; bone mass measurement for high-risk persons; glaucoma screening; and prostate cancer screening.

- Drugs and vaccines, including immunosuppressive drugs for a minimum of 36 months following a covered organ transplant; erythropoietin (EPO) for treatment of anemia for persons with chronic kidney failure; and certain oral cancer drugs. The program also covers flu shots, pneumococcal pneumonia vaccines, and hepatitis B vaccines for those at risk.

Who is eligible for Medicare?

Part A

Most Americans aged 65+ are automatically entitled to Medicare Part A benefits because they or their spouses paid the HI payroll tax on their earnings covered by either the Social Security or Railroad Retirement systems. In addition, beginning on January 1, 1983, federal employment was included in determining eligibility for protection under Medicare Part A. Employees of state and local governments hired after March 31, 1986, are also liable for the HI tax. Persons aged 65+ who are not automatically entitled to Part A may obtain coverage, providing they pay a monthly premium. The 2002 monthly premium was $319 ($175 for persons who have at least 30 to 39 quarters of covered employment).[11]

Part B

Part B of Medicare is voluntary. All persons aged 65+ (even those not entitled to Part A) may elect to enroll in the SMI program by paying the monthly premium. The 2002 premium was $54.00 per month.[12] Persons who voluntarily enroll in Part A are required to enroll in Part B.

■ Medicare+Choice versus traditional Medicare

In 1997, Congress created the Medicare+Choice (M+C) program to let more private insurance companies offer coverage to Medicare beneficiaries. M+C offers alternatives to fee-for-service Medicare, which is often referred to as the "traditional" or "original" program.

Traditional Medicare is offered nationwide, and beneficiaries may go to any doctor, specialist, or hospital that accepts Medicare. Beneficiaries pay a fee for each health care service or supply they use. Beneficiaries stay in this plan unless they elect to join an M+C plan.

Medicare+Choice plans provide health care under contract to Medicare. Some plans may offer additional benefits, such as prescription drugs, and some may not charge a monthly fee. According to law, beneficiaries under M+C may receive services through Medicare health maintenance organizations (HMOs), preferred provider organizations (PPOs), provider-sponsored organizations (PSOs), private-fee-for-service plans (PFFS), and other alternative health delivery programs. Beneficiaries in M+C plans continue paying the Medicare Part B premium. Medicare pays M+C plans a fixed monthly amount to cover Medicare beneficiaries.

■ How is Medicare financed?

Medicare Part A is financed primarily through a payroll tax on current workers and their employers called the Hospital Insurance (HI) tax. Employers and employees each pay a tax of 1.45 percent on all earnings. The self-employed pay a single tax of 2.9 percent on earnings. Unlike the Social Security payroll tax, there is no limit on the amount that workers and their employers pay into the system. The HI tax is payable on all wages.

Medicare Part B is financed through a combination of monthly premiums paid by beneficiaries and federal general revenues. Beneficiary premiums have generally represented about 25 percent of Part B costs; general revenues (i.e., tax dollars) account for the remaining 75 percent. Part B premiums will increase significantly in future years. By 2007, the monthly premium is projected to be about $105. The premium for a beneficiary with a $10,000 annual income would therefore be about 9 percent of this income in 2007.[13]

In a RoperASW survey, 7 in 10 people aged 60+ agreed or strongly agreed that Medicare will run out of money and won't be available when they need it.[14]

MEDICARE BENEFICIARIES

■ Medicare covers 95 percent of elderly

Medicare covers 95 percent of the elderly as well as many people who are on Social Security due to disability.[15] The passage of Medicare in 1965 greatly increased the use of health care services by the elderly. In 1964, hospital discharges averaged 190 per 1,000 elderly. Over a period of 9 years, discharges for the elderly almost doubled to an average of 350 per 1,000 in 1973. Additionally, the proportion of elderly using physician services jumped from 68 percent to 76 percent between 1963 and 1970.

■ Thirty-four million elderly are enrolled in Medicare Part A, and 33 million are enrolled in Medicare Part B

When Medicare began on July 1, 1966, approximately 19 million people enrolled. In 2001, about 40 million people were enrolled in the Medicare program.[16] About 34 million elderly and 5 million disabled beneficiaries were enrolled in Medicare Part A in 2000, and approximately 22 percent of these individuals actually received medical services covered by HI during the year. The total number of Part A beneficiaries increased by 16.2 percent over the last 10 years.[17]

About 33 million aged and 5 million disabled persons were enrolled in Medicare Part B in 2000.[18] Approximately 87 percent of these individuals received medical services covered by Part B during the year. The total number of enrollees in Part B increased by 14.5 percent from 1990 to 2000.

■ Beneficiaries with poor health status are the biggest spenders

Not surprisingly, Medicare spending for beneficiaries who report poor health status is 6.5 times greater than for those reporting excellent health. In 1997, average Medicare spending for beneficiaries of all ages in excellent health was $1,620, compared with $11,812 for those in poor health (see Chart 16.1).[19]

CHART 16.1   Medicare Spending, by Health Status of Beneficiaries of All Ages: 1997

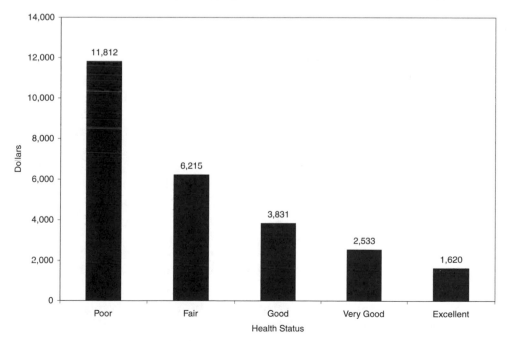

Source: Health Care Financing Administration, *Profile of Medicare Beneficiaries: 1998* (Washington, DC: Health Care Financing Administration, 1998).

CHART 16.2   Medicare Recipients, by Sex and Age: 1996

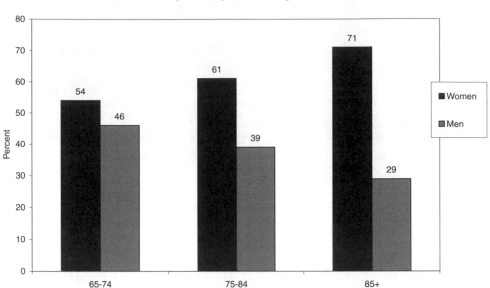

Source: Urban Institute Analysis of the Medicare Current Beneficiary Survey, 1996. Reported in "Medicare and Women," The Henry V. Kaiser Family Foundation. Available at www.kff.org.

■ Women rely on Medicare for many more years than men do

Because women live an average of 7 years longer than men do, the elderly Medicare population includes a disproportionate share of women (see Chart 16.2). Seventy-one percent of Medicare beneficiaries aged 85+ are female.

Older women are also more likely to have chronic diseases and physical limitations requiring long-term care. Two-thirds of Medicare beneficiaries with functional limitations are women, as are two-thirds of all Medicare beneficiaries who receive home health services.[20]

Female elderly Medicare beneficiaries are more likely than their male counterparts to be poor, making additional health care costs prohibitive. Seven in ten Medicare beneficiaries with incomes below the poverty level are women.[21] Individuals who are poor are more likely to be in worse health than their wealthier peers. Of all poor female beneficiaries, 43 percent report being in fair or poor health, compared with 20 percent of those with incomes more than 200 percent above the poverty level.[22]

■ Medicare beneficiaries are more satisfied with health care coverage than those without Medicare

Medicare recipients express greater satisfaction with many aspects of their health care than do non-Medicare patients (who also have health coverage).[23] In addition, Medicare patients are more satisfied with both the quality and availability of medi-

TABLE 16.2
Percent of Patients with Opinions about Various Aspects of Health Care

Opinion	Medicare Patients	Non-Medicare Patients (with Health Coverage)	Percentage Point Difference (Medicare–Non-Medicare)
Very satisfied with:			
Availability of medical care	51%	40%	11
Quality of medical care	47	36	11
Arrangements for paying for medical care	43	32	11
Cost of medical care is very reasonable	27	23	4

Source: RoperASW, 1998.

cal care they receive and the arrangements they have for paying for medical care (see Table 16.2). Medicare and non-Medicare patients have nearly equal feelings, however, about the reasonableness of medical care costs.

When asked to rate their overall experiences with their health care plans, Medicare patients rate their overall experiences higher than non-Medicare patients do. On a scale of 0 (the worst possible) to 10 (the best possible), 59 percent of Medicare patients give a rating of 8 or higher, compared to 48 percent of non-Medicare patients.[24] Medicare patients also give higher ratings to the health care they received from all health care providers in the past 12 months (67 percent versus 47 percent).

Most Medicare beneficiaries (94 percent) have a personal or family doctor.[25]

MEDICARE FINANCING AND EXPENDITURES

■ Medicare Part A could run out of funds in 2029

The future financing for Part A of Medicare through the HI trust fund has been threatened in recent years because hospital spending has increased faster than revenues. In March 2001, the board of trustees for Medicare projected that Medicare Part A will be solvent until 2029.[26] The projected depletion date extends by 14 years the previous forecast of 2015 the trustees made in 1999.

■ Hospital payments and physician services account for 6 out of every 10 Medicare dollars

The Congressional Budget Office (CBO) estimates that Medicare benefits totaled $237 billion in 2001.[27] Fifty-five percent of Medicare benefit payments in 2001 were for inpatient hospital and physicians' services (see Chart 16.3). Services provided by skilled nursing facilities (SNFs), home health agencies, and hospices accounted for

CHART 16.3   Where the Medicare Dollar Goes: 2001

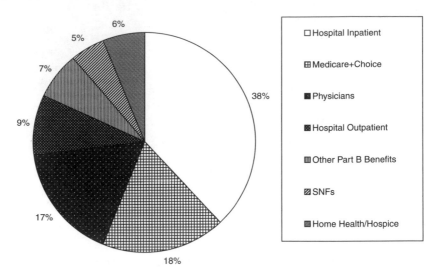

Source: Congressional Budget Office, April 2001 baseline.

11 percent, and 16 percent of Medicare benefit payments went to outpatient hospital services and other medical and health services. Eighteen percent of payments went to M+C.

■ Medicare spent $5,657 per elderly beneficiary in 1999

Total per capita Medicare spending per enrollee (including administrative costs) was estimated at $5,657 in 1999 and is expected to increase to $10,257 in 2009, for an average annual rate of increase of 6.1 percent over the 10-year period. Health care analyst Victor Fuchs projects that Medicare spending per beneficiary will reach $14,000 in 2020.[28]

■ Five percent of Medicare beneficiaries account for 45 percent of Medicare spending

Medicare spending is unevenly distributed among beneficiaries. Five percent of elderly beneficiaries account for 45 percent of Medicare spending for this population group, and only 14 percent of beneficiaries account for close to three-fourths (73 percent) of all spending for elderly beneficiaries.[29]

■ More than a quarter of Medicare outlays are for beneficiaries in their last year of life

An analysis of Medicare claims and related data from 1993 through 1998, published in the journal *Health Affairs*, found that more than one-fourth (27.4 percent) of Medicare outlays are spent for beneficiaries in their last year of life.[30] The share of Medicare spending for the last year of life has been stable for two decades. Thirty-eight percent of beneficiaries have some nursing home stay in the year of their death. Medicare outlays for beneficiaries who died were about six times higher than for survivors.

The analysis also found that Medicare paid 61 percent of the costs of health care prior to death. Medicaid paid 10 percent, out-of-pocket costs accounted for 18 percent, and other sources paid 12 percent.

Another study on the last year of life, published in the *Journal of the American Medical Association,* found that Medicare expenditures for the elderly in the last year of life decrease as age increases.[31] The study used data from two states, Massachusetts and California. The researchers found that each additional year of age was associated with a $413 decrease in cost in Massachusetts and a $408 decrease in California. Each of these effects was statistically significant.

■ Medicare beneficiaries get back more than they contribute

Medicare recipients typically get back considerably more in benefits than they contribute to the program in payroll taxes and premiums during their lifetimes.

The Congressional Budget Office has estimated the extent to which Medicare enrollees' contributions during their working years cover the expected value of their benefits under the program.[32] The CBO specifically looked at the contributions of the self-employed (which they refer to as "self-insured") because their personal contributions are higher than for people who are employees. For a self-insured man who worked continuously at an average wage from 1966, when Medicare began, until retirement in 1985, the present value of his contributions is about 29 percent of the expected value of his lifetime Medicare benefits. For self-insured women, it is 26 percent.

In comparison, younger generations will pay more into Medicare in relation to what they can expect to get back when they become beneficiaries. For self-insured men retiring in 1995, contributions represented about 37 percent of benefits; for those retiring in 2005, contributions will represent about 41 percent. For self-insured women retiring in 1995, contributions represented about 32 percent of benefits; for those retiring in 2005, contributions will represent about 36 percent.

■ Medicare has contributed to a reduction in poverty among the elderly

Along with Social Security, Medicare has helped to reduce poverty among the elderly. The elderly poverty rate has declined steadily from 17.9 percent in 1966 (the year following enactment of Medicare).[33] In 2000, the poverty rate for this group was 10.2 percent.

Out-of-Pocket Costs

One-half of older adults (49 percent) say the rising cost of health care is one of the top two or three concerns they have, significantly more than the 31 percent of younger adults who have the same concerns.[34]

■ Medicare covers only 57 percent of the elderly's health care costs

Medicare has significant gaps in coverage; it pays only 57 percent of the health costs of the elderly.[35]

Forty-five percent of older adults are concerned about the ability to pay for catastrophic health care expenses, but only 24 percent are concerned about paying ordinary medical bills.[36]

■ The elderly's out-of-pocket spending for health care equals about one-fifth of their income

The U.S. Congress Committee on Ways and Means estimated that out-of-pocket spending by the elderly totaled $2,430, or 19 percent of income, in 1999. Payments for Medicare cost-sharing charges and items not covered by Medicare (such as prescription drugs and dental care) represented 54 percent of average out-of-pocket spending in 1999 (see Chart 16.4). The remaining 44 percent was for premium payments for Medicare Part B, Medicare+Choice plans, and private insurance.

Out-of-pocket spending varies greatly by source of supplementary coverage (see Table 16.3). Based on 1999 statistics, beneficiaries who do not receive Medicaid, do not have Medigap insurance, and have no other supplemental coverage spend 22

CHART 16.4   Out-of-Pocket Spending for Noninstitutionalized Medicare Beneficiaries Aged 65+: 1999

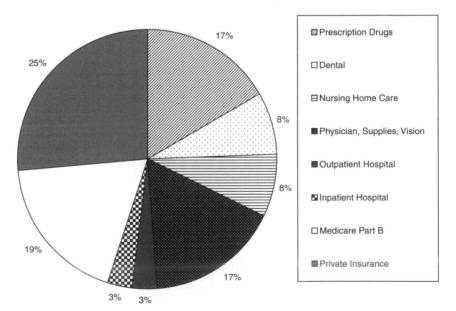

Source: American Association of Retired Persons, as reported in U.S. Congress, Committee on Ways and Means, *2000 Green Book* (Washington, DC, 2001).

TABLE 16.3
Average Out-of-Pocket Spending on Health Care by
Noninstitutionalized Medicare Beneficiaries Aged 65+, by
Supplemental Health Insurance Status: 1999 Projections

Source of Supplemental Coverage	Average Out-of-Pocket Costs	Percent of Income*
Medicare-only	$2,505	22%
Employer	2,545	16
Medigap	3,250	26
Medicare+Choice	1,630	12
Medicaid	280	5
QMB program**	840	13
SLMB program**	2,630	30
All beneficiaries	2,430	19

*Average out-of-pocket spending as a percent of income is calculated as the average of each beneficiary's share of income spent out of pocket for health care. Full year coverage.

**The QMB (Qualified Medicare Beneficiary) and SLMB (Specified Low Income Beneficiary) programs for low-income beneficiaries pay Medicare Part B costs.

Sources: U.S. Congress, Committee on Ways and Means, *2000 Green Book* (Washington, DC: U.S. Government Printing Office Online). For age 65+: 1999 Projections, IB#41, December 1999.

percent of their income on health care. Surprisingly, those with Medigap insurance spend an even greater share of their income on health care—26 percent of income.

■ Poor beneficiaries spend one-third of their income on health care

According to AARP's estimates, beneficiaries with incomes below the poverty level spent 33 percent of their incomes on health care in 1999. Those with incomes at the poverty level and up to twice that level spent about one-fourth of their incomes on health care that same year.[37] Poor persons without Medicaid coverage were expected to spend about 49 percent of their annual income out-of-pocket for health care.

SUPPLEMENTING MEDICARE

■ Options to supplement Medicare are becoming increasingly limited

The cost of supplementing Medicare is an increasing strain on the elderly's wallets. The following facts cited by the Kaiser Family Foundation describe the major contributing factors to the problem:[38]

- The Part B premium is prohibitively expensive for many elderly low-income beneficiaries.
- The costs of premiums for Medigap insurance are rising to the point that the coverage is out of reach for the low- to middle-income elderly. (See section on Medigap later in this chapter.)
- Many elderly Medicare beneficiaries do not live in areas where they have access to Medicare managed care.
- Only one-half of eligible older adults and people with disabilities get help through the federal "buy-in" program designed to help low-income beneficiaries with medical costs not paid for by Medicare (see section, "Buy-In Benefits" later in this chapter).
- Many elderly have low incomes but are not close enough to poverty to qualify for Medicaid. Medicaid reaches only one-half of all poor Medicare beneficiaries (see section on Medicaid later in this chapter).

■ Nine in ten Medicare beneficiaries have supplemental coverage

Although the cost of supplementing Medicare is high, estimates indicate that more than 9 in 10 elderly beneficiaries have some type of supplemental coverage, either through private sources or government-sponsored programs. Just 8 percent of beneficiaries have Medicare only.[39] Twenty-seven percent of Medicare beneficiaries purchase Medigap insurance privately, and 37 percent purchase Medigap insurance through their employers (see Table 16.4).

Medigap

Medigap policies fill in the gaps in traditional Medicare coverage. These supplemental plans offered by private insurance companies pay most or all of the costs of coinsurance and copayments. They may also pay deductibles. Some policies will also cover extra benefits that Medicare does not cover, such as prescription drugs. All states except three—Massachusetts, Minnesota, and Wisconsin—offer 10 standardized Medigap policies called Plans A through J.

By law, beneficiaries have the right to purchase Medicare supplemental policies during open enrollment, which starts on their sixty-fifth birthday and lasts for 6 months. They also have a right by law to buy a Medigap policy if they lose certain types of health coverage, such as due to the closure of a Medicare+Choice plan.

■ Beneficiaries with Medigap policies pay the highest out-of-pocket costs

Average out-of-pocket spending by Medicare beneficiaries varies, depending on the type of supplemental coverage. AARP estimated that in 1999 beneficiaries with Medigap policies had the highest out-of-pocket costs, at $3,250.[40] Estimates for beneficiaries with full-year Medicaid coverage were the lowest, at $280. Among

TABLE 16.4
Supplemental Coverage of Medicare
Beneficiaries: 1999

Type of Coverage	Percent of Beneficiaries Using Coverage
Employer	37%
Medigap insurance	27
Medicare+Choice plan	16
No supplemental coverage	8
Medicaid (full year)	4
QMB*	4
SLMB/Part year Medicaid*	3

*The QMB (Qualified Medicare Beneficiary) and
SLMB (Specified Low Income Beneficiary) programs pay Medicare Part B costs.

Source: CARP Public Policy Institute, *Out-of-Pocket
Spending on Health Care by Medicare Beneficiaries
Age 65 and Older: 1999 Predictions.* Available at
www.aarp.org.

TABLE 16.5
Out-of-Pocket Spending on Health Care by
Medicare Beneficiaries Aged 65+: 1999
Predictions

Type of Insurance	Average Out-of-Pocket Spending
Medigap	$3,250
SLMB*/Part Year Medicaid	2,630
Employer	2,545
Medicare Only	2,505
Medicare+Choice	1,630
Full Year QMB*	840
Full Year Medicaid	280
Average	2,430

*The QMB (Qualified Medicare Beneficiary) and
SLMB (Specified Low Income Beneficiary) pro-
grams for low-income beneficiaries pay Medicare
Part B costs.

Source: AARP Public Policy Institute, *Out-of-Pocket
Spending on Health Care by Medicare Beneficiaries
Age 65 and Older: 1999 Predictions.* Available at
www.aarp.org.

beneficiaries without Medicaid coverage, enrollees in M+C plans were projected to
have the lowest out-of-pocket costs, at $1,630 (see Table 16.5).

■ One-fourth of fee-for-service beneficiaries buy Medigap insurance

Most Medicare beneficiaries receive care through the traditional fee-for-service
program. In 1999, about 10.7 million Medicare beneficiaries, or 27 percent of all
beneficiaries, had a Medigap policy.[41]

■ Medigap costs are high

The cost of Medigap policies strains the budgets of many elderly Americans. In
1999, the average annual premium was about $1,300.[42] According to the General Ac-
counting Office (GAO), premiums for the three Medigap plans offering prescription
drug coverage have increased the most rapidly—by 17 percent to 34 percent from
1999 to 2000.[43] Premiums for Medigap plans without prescription drug coverage
rose from 4 percent to 10 percent from 1999 to 2000.

According to GAO, the dollar amount of Medigap premiums varies dramatically
by state and within states.[44] In 1999, average premiums for standardized Medigap
plans in California were $1,600—more than twice as high as Utah's average of $706.
This variation in premium is also evident for specific plan types: Average annual pre-

miums for Plan J of Medigap were $646 in New Hampshire and $2,802 in New York; for Plan C, they were $751 in New Jersey and $1,656 in California.

Also according to GAO, beneficiaries in the same state may pay widely varying rates for a given type of Medigap plan from different insurers. For example, in Texas the annual Plan A premium for a 65-year-old ranged from $300 to $1,683, depending on the insurer.

Employer-based Retiree Health Benefits

■ Employer-based retiree health benefits are declining

Employer-based health benefits have played an important role for retired workers and their spouses since Medicare was enacted: 34.1 percent of Americans aged 65+ had such coverage in 1999.[45] Fewer employers are providing retiree health benefits, however, or they are reducing their contribution to save costs. According to a Mercer/Foster Higgins National Survey of Employer-Sponsored Health Plans, the share of employers with more than 500 workers that provide health coverage to retirees aged 65+ fell from 40 percent in 1993 to 23 percent in 2001 (see Chart 16.5).[46] This represents a 1 to 2 percent drop each year from 1993 to 2000.

Employers also are asking retirees to pay an increasingly larger share of the cost of coverage. According to 1998 data from the Mercer/Foster Higgins National Survey of Employer-Sponsored Health Plans, 41 percent of employers paid the full cost of premiums for early retirees in 1993, but only 36 percent covered the total amount in 1998.[47]

CHART 16.5 Percent of Employers with More Than 500 Workers Providing Health Coverage to Retirees: 1993 to 2001

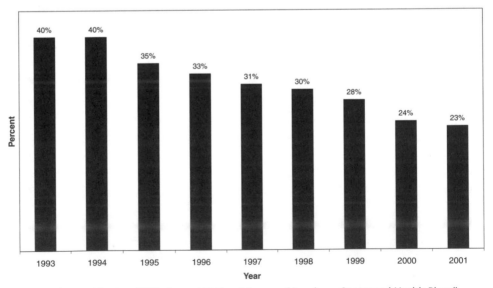

Source: Mercer/Foster Higgins, "15th Annual National Survey of Employer Sponsored Health Plans" (Chicago, IL, 2000).

Buy-In Benefits

■ Only one-half of people who qualify get buy-in benefits

In 1988, Congress created several Medicare "buy-in" programs to help low-income beneficiaries with growing medical costs. Through these programs, Medicaid helps pay costs such as Medicare premiums and deductibles. Beneficiaries with Medicare Part A with limited income and financial resources (under $4,000 for an individual or $6,000 for a couple) may qualify for assistance as a Qualified Medicare Beneficiary (QMB) or Specified Low Income Medicare Beneficiary (SLMB). The QMB program pays the Medicare monthly Part B premium, deductibles, and coinsurance. The SLMB program helps pay the Medicare monthly Part B premium for qualified Medicare beneficiaries.

In 1998, however, only one-half of eligible older adults and people with disabilities succeeded in getting QMB and SLMB benefits.[48] In a report on the buy-in problem, the Families USA Foundation said lack of knowledge about the program by beneficiaries and caseworkers is the major reason for low participation in the program.

A survey conducted in New York by the Medicare Rights Center (MRC) confirmed this finding. It found that low-income people with Medicare are not enrolling in the QMB and SLMB programs for two critical reasons: The majority (88 percent) are unaware that these programs exist, and even when they learn about these programs, they are not willing or able to undertake the effort to apply for them.[49]

Unlike Medicare, in which people are enrolled automatically at age 65, the Medicare assistance programs depend on states to do program outreach. They also usually require applicants to go to local Medicaid offices to complete applications and present income and resources documentation. Nationally, only 57 percent of eligible Medicare beneficiares have taken advantage of the assistance programs since the first one began in 1988.[50]

Medicare+Choice

■ Medicare+Choice is out of reach for many

The number of HMOs participating in Medicare has decreased substantially in recent years. There were 179 Medicare HMOs in 2001, down from 346 in 1998.[51]

In 2001, 5.6 million Medicare beneficiaries were enrolled in the M+C program (see Chart 16.6). According to CMS, 90 percent of beneficiaries were able to continue in their M+C plan in 2002. A total of 58 M+C contracts withdrew from the program or reduced their service areas in 2001, affecting approximately 536,000 Medicare beneficiaries, or 10 percent of M+C enrollees. Thirty-eight thousand beneficiaries had no option but to return to the Medicare fee-for-service program.[52] In 2002, Medicare introduced a pilot project that will provide care to about 11 million beneficiaries through PPO plans. PPOs will be offered in 241 counties in 23 states.

CHART 16.6   Enrollment in Medicare HMOs: 1985 to 2001

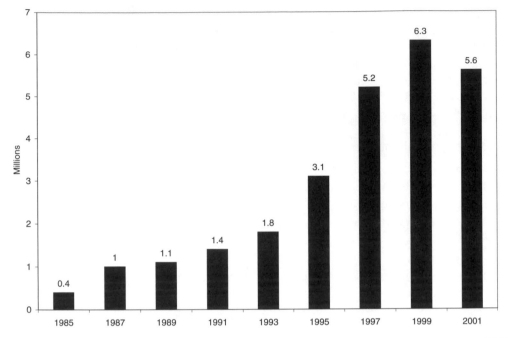

Source: Centers for Medicare and Medicaid Services, *Medicare Managed Care Contract Summary Report* (2001).

■ **Beneficiaries in metropolitan areas are most likely to have an M+C plan available to them**

Medicare beneficiaries in metropolitan statistical areas (MSAs) * with populations of more than 1 million are more than 10 times more likely as beneficiaries living in rural areas to have an M+C plan in their county.[53] In 2001, 94 percent of beneficiaries in MSAs of more than 1 million had a M+C plan available to them. In contrast, 57 percent of beneficiaries in cities with populations less than 1 million had an M+C plan available. Comparable figures for people in towns with populations greater than 10,000 and people in rural areas were 28 percent and 9 percent, respectively.

DEFINITION: Rural areas are defined as counties adjacent to MSAs when their population is less than 10,000 or counties not adjacent to an MSA.

■ **Medicare HMO enrollment decreases with age**

Enrollment in Medicare HMOs decreases with age, from 13 percent among persons aged 65 to 74, to 9 percent among persons aged 85+. Enrollment for the 65+ population is about equal for men and women. However, at the older ages, women

---
* Data are for metropolitan statistical areas (MSAs).

are slightly less likely than men to be HMO members. Enrollment is similar for blacks and whites, although blacks have slightly lower rates of participation at the oldest ages.[54]

■ Many HMOs offer additional benefits beyond the basic Medicare coverage

According to the Kaiser Family Foundation, in 1999, Medicare HMO plans provided physical exams (97 percent), eye exams (89 percent), outpatient prescription drug coverage (74 percent), and dental care (42 percent).[55]

■ More than half of Medicare HMOs charge premiums

In recent years, Medicare HMOs were able to offer their services with no premiums attached to them. However, due in part to changes in plan reimbursement, 54 percent of plans charged a monthly premium in 2001. The average monthly cost to beneficiaries was $42.52 in 2001.[56]

SATISFACTION WITH HEALTH CARE PLANS

Older adults find many elements to be essential in choosing their personal health care plan. Most important are access to immediate care, communication with health care providers, quality of care, and flexibility in choosing a doctor (see Table 16.6). However, satisfaction with their health care provider on these aspects falls considerably short of the importance placed on them.

TABLE 16.6

Rating of Elements in Choosing a Personal Health Care Plan among the 60+ Population, by Importance to the Consumer and Satisfaction with the Current Plan: 1998

Element of Care Plan	Percent Rating Element as Absolutely Essential	Percent Extremely Satisfied with This Element in Plan	Percentage Point Difference*
Access to immediate care when need it	71%	53%	−18
Communication between you and doctors about your condition/care	69	52	−17
Quality of doctors/hospitals available	68	55	−13
Ability to visit any doctor	66	56	−10
Clear explanation of payments can claim	62	40	−22
Ability to see specialist if think it necessary	62	50	−12
Total cost of plan to you	60	35	−25
Ease of getting convenient appointment with doctor	59	48	−11
Ability to go to any hospital	58	52	−6
Ability to provide prescription coverage	56	39	−17

*Difference between satisfaction and importance; a negative score means that the level of satisfaction is less than the level of importance.
Source: RoperASW, 1998.

MEDICAID

DEFINITION: Medicaid is a government-sponsored health care provider funded jointly by the states and federal government to make services available to the poorest persons.

■ Few adults understand Medicaid's role

Many adults lack understanding about the Medicaid program. A nationally representative survey conducted by *Family Circle* magazine and the Kaiser Family Foundation found that only 37 percent of respondents correctly stated that Medicaid is the program for low-income families.[57]

■ The Medicaid program varies from state to state

Medicaid provides medical and health-related services to America's poorest people. The program became law in 1965 under Title XIX of the Social Security Act as a jointly funded cooperative venture between the federal and state governments. Today it covers 12 percent of the total U.S. population.

Within broad national Medicaid guidelines, which the federal government provides, each of the states:

- establishes its own eligibility standards;
- determines the type, amount, duration, and scope of services;
- sets the rate of payment for services; and
- administers its own program.

Thus, services in the Medicaid program vary considerably from state to state, as well as within each state over time. The state-by-state variation in eligibility that Medicaid allows can mean persons with identical circumstances may be eligible to receive Medicaid benefits in one state but not in another.

■ Medicare and Medicaid are often confused

Medicare and Medicaid are often confused even though they differ greatly, as shown in the Table 16.7. For example, Medicare is an insurance program, but Medicaid is an entitlement program. Medicare has uniform standards, but, within certain guidelines, Medicaid leaves standards up to the states. Medicare covers almost all elderly Americans, whereas Medicaid covers only 12 percent of elderly Americans.

Medicaid is important to low-income Medicare beneficiaries because it can help pay for out-of-pocket costs. For example, in 1995, Medicare beneficiaries who were also Medicaid recipients paid 21 percent of their drug costs out-of-pocket, compared with 80 percent for Medicare beneficiaries with traditional Medigap insurance and 35 percent for those in Medicare HMOs.[58]

Medicaid also plays an important role for the frail elderly in need of long-term care. It is the largest insurer of long-term care for all Americans, including all Medicare beneficiaries and the middle class.

TABLE 16.7
Medicare versus Medicaid

Medicare	Medicaid
Social Insurance	Entitlement
Eligibility by Social Security and Railroad Retirement	Eligibility by very low income
Run by the federal government; CMS contracts with carriers and intermediaries	Run by state governments; CMS runs the federal participation
Services are the same throughout the country	Services vary by state
Funded by federal taxes and general revenues	Funded by federal and state governments
Designed to cover only acute and skilled care	Covers acute, skilled, and long-term care
Covers 39 million elderly	Covers 4 million elderly
Pays only one-half of the elderly's health care expenses	Covers most costs for very low income beneficiaries
Many beneficiaries buy Medigap insurance or join an HMO to supplement	Medicaid can act as a supplement to Medicare

■ What does Medicaid cover?

The federal government contributes between 50 percent and 88 percent of the payments for services provided under each state Medicaid program.[59] Among the services that Medicaid covers are inpatient and outpatient hospital services, laboratory and X-ray services, skilled nursing home services, physicians' services, physical therapy, hospice care, and rehabilitative services.

Medicaid patients are restricted to selecting from preapproved physicians and other providers of medical care. Because physicians are not fully reimbursed for services provided to Medicaid patients, many limit the number of Medicaid patients they see.

The most significant trend in Medicaid's service delivery is the rapid growth in managed care enrollment. In 1999, 56 percent of all Medicaid recipients were enrolled in managed care plans, up from 23 percent in 1994.[60]

■ One in eight elderly receives Medicaid

In 1998, Medicaid enrolled 3.9 million elderly persons, or 12 percent of those aged 65+.[61] The elderly Medicaid population has been growing at a smaller rate than the total elderly population. In 1998, 11 percent of Medicaid beneficiaries were elderly, down from 19 percent in 1978.[62]

■ Elderly Medicaid beneficiaries receive 31 percent of expenditures

Elderly Medicaid beneficiaries use a disproportionate share of the program's expenditures due to the high cost of services they receive. In 1998, 11 percent of all Medicaid beneficiaries were elderly, but 31 percent of total expenditures were spent on them.[63] In 1998, an average of $10,243 was spent on the average elderly Medicaid beneficiary.[64]

■ States have discretion in coverage eligibility

Individual states have some discretion in determining which groups their Medicaid programs cover and the financial criteria for Medicaid eligibility. To be eligible for federal funds, states are required to provide Medicaid coverage for most individuals who receive federally assisted income maintenance payments, as well as for related groups not receiving cash payments.

Two examples of the mandatory Medicaid eligibility groups that include the elderly are:

- Supplemental Security Income (SSI) recipients and other aged, blind, and disabled residents with low incomes; and
- low-income Medicare beneficiaries; all Medicare beneficiaries with incomes below the poverty level are supposed to receive Medicaid assistance for payment of Medicare premiums, deductibles, and cost sharing, but, as mentioned previously, one-half of those eligible do not receive this assistance.

Individual states also have the option to provide Medicaid coverage for other "categorically needy" groups. Examples of the optional groups that states may cover as categorically needy and elderly under the Medicaid program are:

- certain aged, blind, or disabled adults who have incomes above those requiring mandatory coverage, but below the federal poverty level;
- institutionalized individuals with income and resources below specified limits;
- persons who would be eligible if institutionalized but who are receiving care under home and community-based services waivers;
- recipients of state supplementary payments; and
- individuals who are medically needy but may have too much income to qualify under the mandatory or optional categorically needy groups, who are allowed to "spend down" and receive benefits.

■ Medicaid can act as a supplement to Medicare

Medicare and Medicaid can work together to provide low-income beneficiaries with the health care coverage they need. In 1997, Medicaid acted as a supplement to Medicare for more than 6.4 million beneficiaries of all ages.[65]

■ Medicaid is a primary source for long-term care

Although Medicaid was intended originally to provide basic medical services to the poor and disabled, it has become the primary source of public funds for nursing home care. In fact, Medicaid covers 46 percent of nursing home costs.[66] In 1998, federal and state Medicaid expenditures for long-term care totaled $40.6 billion. The reasons behind these expenditures are the high cost of long-term care and limited coverage under Medicare or private insurance.*

Although Medicaid's long-term care payments are primarily for nursing home care, some coverage of home and community-based care is provided. In 1998, Medicaid accounted for 17 percent of total spending on home health care, up from 12 percent in 1978.[67]

About one-third of discharged nursing home residents originally admitted as private-pay patients eventually spend down to Medicaid. Just over one-quarter of Medicaid discharged residents began their nursing home stays as private-pay patients. One-fifth of all current residents run out of personal funds at some point during their stays.[68]

▌ All state Medicaid programs cover drugs

All 50 states and the District of Columbia cover drugs under the Medicaid program. Outpatient prescription drugs were provided to 19.3 million Medicaid recipients in 1998 as part of their comprehensive health and medical package under the program.[69]

Total Medicaid expenditures for prescription drugs were $11.7 billion in 1998.[70] In 1997, the average Medicaid prescription cost ranged from $28.82 in Alabama to $47.17 in Alaska. The average annual Medicaid drug payment per recipient for prescription drugs was $571 in 1997.

▌ Medicaid managed care enrollment varies by region

According to CMS, as of June 30, 1998, only two states (Alaska and Wyoming) had failed to enroll some portion of their Medicaid population in managed care, and more than one-half of the total Medicaid population was enrolled in managed care. Enrollment in Medicaid managed care varies by region. For example, in the Seattle area, 84 percent of Medicaid beneficiaries are enrolled in managed care, compared with only 24 percent the Dallas area.

▌ The PACE Program is a new Medicaid option

The Balanced Budget Act of 1997 included an important option for states to provide home and community-based services to persons who would otherwise require institutional care. This option, known as PACE (Programs of All-inclusive Care for the Elderly), allows eligible persons (generally very elderly frail individuals) to re-

---

* Medicaid's spending for long-term care is driven by its coverage for individuals who need long-term care but are not poor. They qualify for the program through "spending down" and other eligibility standards that states may take advantage of. One of these is the medically needy option: individuals with incomes that are too high to receive cash welfare, but incur medical expenses that deplete their assets and incomes to levels that make them needy by state standards can receive long-term care coverage.

States may also use a special income rule, referred to as the 300 percent rule, for extending Medicaid eligibility to persons needing nursing home care. Under this rule, states are allowed to cover persons needing nursing home care so long as their income does not exceed 300 percent of the basic Supplemental Security Income cash welfare payment.

ceive all health, medical, and social services they need in return for a monthly capitated payment. This care is provided largely through in-home and day health centers but also includes care provided by hospitals, nursing homes, and other practitioners as determined to be necessary by the PACE provider. Fourteen states now have approved PACE demonstration sites. PACE is a covered Medicare benefit as well.

■ Medicaid spending is increasing

Federal and state Medicaid spending (excluding spending for the State Children's Health Insurance Program) totaled nearly $202 billion in 2000, an increase of 8.3 percent from 1999. The Medicaid share of total health spending was 15.5 percent in 2000.[71]

NOTES

1. U.S. Bureau of Labor Statistics, "Consumer Expenditure Survey, 2000," Table 3. Available online at www.bls.gov.
2. Office of the Actuary, Centers for Medicare and Medicaid Services, "National Health Care Expenditures Projections: 2000–2010" (March 2001).
3. Victor R. Fuchs, "Health Care for the Elderly, How Much? Who Will Pay for It?" *Health Affairs* 18, no. 1 (January/February 1999).
4. Congressional Budget Office, "The Budget and Economic Outlook: Fiscal Years 2002–2011" (Washington, DC, 2001).
5. Centers for Medicare and Medicaid Services, "Annual Report of the Trustees of the Medicare Insurance Trust Fund" (April 2001).
6. Alzheimer's Association, "Medicare and Medicaid Costs for People with Alzheimer's Disease" (April 3, 2001). Available online at www.alz.org.
7. Cathy Shoen et al., "Counting on Medicare: Perspectives and Concerns of Americans Ages 50 to 70 (The Commonwealth Fund, July 2000). Available online at www.cmwf .org.
8. Henry J. Kaiser Foundation/Harvard School of Public Health, National Survey on Medicare (October 20, 1998), reported in Patricia Neuman and Kathryn M. Langwell, "Medicare's Choice Explosion," *Health Affairs* 18, no. 1 (January/February, 1999).
9. RoperASW, 1998.
10. Social Security Act.
11. Centers for Medicare and Medicaid Services, "Medicare Basics" (2002). Available online at www.cms.gov.
12. Ibid.
13. Marilyn Moon et al., "An Examination of Key Provisions in the Balanced Budget Act of 1997." Available online at www.cmwf.org.
14. RoperASW, 1998.
15. Centers for Medicare and Medicaid Services, *Annual Report of the Medicare Board of Trustees to Congress* (2001).
16. Ibid.
17. Ibid.
18. Ibid.
19. Health Care Financing Administration, *Profile of Medicare Beneficiaries: 1998* (Washington, DC: Health Care Financing Administration, 1998).
20. "Medicare and Women" (Washington, DC: Henry J. Kaiser Foundation, not dated).
21. Ibid.

22. Ibid.
23. RoperASW, 1998.
24. Ibid.
25. RoperASW, 1999.
26. Centers for Medicare and Medicaid Services, *2001 Annual Report of the Board of Trustees of the Federal Hospital Insurance and Supplementary Medical Insurance Trust Funds*. Available online at www.hcfa.gov.
27. Congressional Budget Office (2001). Reported in Kaiser Family Foundation, *Medicare Chartbook* (2001).
28. Mark McClellan and Johnathon Skinner, "Medicare Reform, Who Pays and Who Benefits," *Health Affairs* 18, no. 1 (January/February, 1999): 49.
29. U.S. Congress, Committee on Ways and Means, *Medicare and Health Care Chartbook* (Washington, DC: Government Printing Office, 1997).
30. Christopher Hogan et al., "Medicare Beneficiaries Cost of Care in the Last Year of Life," *Health Affairs* (July/August, 2001).
31. Norman G. Lewinsky et al., "Influence of Age on Medicare Expenditures and Medical Care in the Last Year of Life," *Journal of the American Medical Association* 286, no. 11 (September 19, 2001).
32. U.S. Congress, Ways and Means Committee, *1998 Green Book* (Washington, DC: U.S. Government Printing Office Online).
33. U.S. Census Bureau, Historical Poverty Tables, Table 16. Available at www.census.gov.
34. RoperASW, 2000.
35. U.S. Congress, Committee on Ways and Means, *2000 Green Book* (Washington, DC: U.S. Government Printing Office Online).
36. RoperASW, 1997.
37. AARP Public Policy Institute, 1999 Predictions.
38. Kaiser Family Foundation, "Medicare and Medicaid for the Elderly and Disabled Poor" (May 1999).
39. AARP Public Policy Institute, "Out-of-Pocket Spending."
40. AARP Public Policy Institute, 1999 Predictions. Available online at www.aarp.org.
41. General Accounting Office, "Medigap Insurance: Plans Are Widely Available but Have Limited Benefits and May Have High Costs" (Washington, DC, July 2001).
42. Ibid.
43. Ibid.
44. Ibid.
45. National Center for Health Statistics, *Health US Updated* (Hyattsville, MD, August 2001).
46. Mercer/Foster Higgins, "15th Annual National Survey of Employer Sponsored Health Plans" (Chicago, IL, 2000).
47. Special Committee on Aging, United States Senate, *Developments in Aging: 1997 and 1998, Volume 1*.
48. Families USA, "Shortchanged: Billions Withheld from Medicare Beneficiaries" (Washington, DC: Families USA, July 1998).
49. Medicare Rights Center, "Barriers to Enrolling in Medicare Assistance Programs Identified in Medicare Rights Center Study" (November 6, 2000). Available online at www.medicarerights.com.
50. Ibid.
51. Kaiser Family Foundation, *Medicare Chartbook*.
52. Statement of Tom Scully, Former Administrator, Centers for Medicare and Medicaid Services, "Preliminary Status of the Medicare+Choice Program for 2002." Availabe online at www.seniors.gov.
53. Kaiser Family Foundation, *Medicare Chartbook*.
54. Ibid.

55. Ibid.
56. Ibid.
57. Family Circle Magazine and the Kaiser Family Foundation, "National Survey on Health Care and Other Elder Care Issues," *Family Circle* (November 1, 2000).
58. Margaret Davis et al., "Prescription Drug Coverage, Utilization, and Spending among Medicare Beneficiaries," *Health Affairs* 13, no. 1 (1999): 231–243.
59. Health Care Financing Administration, "Profile of Medicaid, Chartbook 2000." Available online at www.hcfa.gov.
60. Health Care Financing Administration, "National Summary of Medicaid Managed Care Programs and Enrollment" (June 30, 1999). Available at www.hcfa.gov.
61. Health Care Financing Administration, "Profile of Medicaid."
62. Ibid.
63. Ibid.
64. Ibid.
65. Ibid.
66. Ibid.
67. Ibid.
68. U.S. Congress, *2000 Green Book*.
69. Health Care Financing Administration, "Profile of Medicaid."
70. Ibid.
71. Katharine Levit et al., "Inflation Spurs Health Spending in 2000," *Health Affairs* 18, no. 1 (January/February, 2002).

Selected Bibliography and Useful Web Sites

Adams, Patricia F., Gerry E. Hendershot, and Marie A. Marano, "Current Estimates from the National Health Interview Survey, 1996," series 10, no. 200 (National Center for Health Statistics, Vital and Health Statistics, October 1999).

Alexopoulos, George S., Ira R. Katz, Charles F. Reynolds III, Daniel Carpenter, and John P. Docherty, *Expert Consensus Pocket Guide to the Pharmacotherapy of Depressive Disorders in Older Patients* (White Plains, NY: Expert Knowledge Systems, 2001).

Alliance for Aging Research, "Will You Still Treat Me When I'm 65?" (May 1996).

Anderson, Robert N., "Deaths: Leading Causes for 1999," *National Vital Statistics Reports* 49, no. 11 (National Center for Health Statistics, National Vital Statistics System, October 12, 2001).

Bryson, Ken, and Lynne M. Casper, *Coresident Grandparents and Grandchildren* (Washington, DC: Bureau of the Census, 1998).

Bureau of the Census, *65+ in the United States* (Washington, DC: Bureau of the Census, 1996).

Bureau of the Census, *Age: 2000* (Washington, DC: Bureau of the Census, September, 2001).

Bureau of the Census, "Educational Attainment in the United States: March 1998," *Current Population Reports*, P-20-513 (Washington, DC: Bureau of the Census, October 1998).

Bureau of the Census, "Housing Vacancies and Home Ownership Annual Statistics" (Washington, DC: Bureau of the Census, 2001).

Bureau of the Census, "Projections of the Resident Population by Age, Sex, Race, and Hispanic Origin, 1999 to 2100" (Washington, DC: Bureau of the Census, 2000).

Bureau of the Census, "Resident Population Estimates of the United States by Age and Sex: April 1, 1990 to June 1, 1999" (Washington, DC: Bureau of the Census, 1999).

Bureau of the Census, *The 65 Years and Over Population* (Washington, DC: Bureau of the Census, 2001).

Bureau of the Census, *Statistical Abstract of the United States: 2001* (Washington, DC: Bureau of the Census, 2001).

Burger, Sarah Greene, et al., "Malnutrition and Dehydration in Nursing Homes: Key Issues in Prevention and Treatment," National Citizen's Coalition for Nursing Home Reform (June 2000).

Centers for Disease Control and Prevention, "Surveillance for Five Health Risks among Older Adults—United States, 1993–1997," *MMWR, CDC Surveillance Summaries* 48, no. SS-8 (December 17, 1999).

Centers for Disease Control and Prevention, "Surveillance for Injuries and Violence among Older Adults," *MMWR, CDC Surveillance Summaries* 48, no. SS-8 (December 17, 1999).

Centers for Disease Control and Prevention, "Surveillance for Morbidity and Mortality among Older Adults—United States, 1995–1996," *MMWR, CDC Surveillance Summaries* 48, no. SS-8 (December 17, 1999).

Centers for Disease Control and Prevention, "Surveillance for Sensory Impairment, Activity Limitation, and Health-Related Quality of Life among Older Adults—United States, 1993–1997," *MMWR, CDC Surveillance Summaries* 48, no. SS-8 (December 17, 1999).

Centers for Disease Control and Prevention, "Surveillance for Use of Preventative Health-Care Services by Older Adults, 1995–1997," *MMWR, CDC Surveillance Summaries* 48, no. SS-8 (December 17, 1999).

Centers for Medicare and Medicaid Services, "Annual Report of the Trustees of the Medicare Insurance Trust Fund" (Baltimore, MD, April 2001).

Centers for Medicare and Medicaid Services, "Medicare Basics" (Baltimore, MD, 2002).

Centers for Medicare and Medicaid Services, "National Health Care Expenditures Projections: 2000–2010" (March 2001).

Cole, Thomas R., *The Journey of Life* (New York: Cambridge University Press, 1992).

Congressional Budget Office, "The Budget and Economic Outlook: Fiscal Years 2002–2011" (Washington, DC, 2001).

Dychtwald, Ken, *Age Power* (New York: Tarcher, 1999).

Ernsberger, Paul, and Richard J. Koletsy, "Biomedical Rationale for a Wellness Approach to Obesity: An Alternative to a Focus on Weight Loss," *Journal of Social Issues* 55, no. 2 (1999): 221–260.

Federal Interagency Forum on Aging Related Statistics, *Older Americans 2000: Key Indicators of Well-Being* (Hyattsville, MD: Federal Interagency Forum on Aging Related Statistics, 2000).

Fischer, David Hackett, *Growing Old in America* (New York: Oxford University Press, 1978).

Foley, Lisa, and David Gross, "Are Consumers Well Informed about Prescription Drugs?" (Washington, DC: AARP Public Policy Institute, April 2000).

Fuchs, Victor R. "Health Care for the Elderly, How Much? Who Will Pay For It?" *Health Affairs* 18, no. 1 (January/February 1999).

Fullerton, Howard N., Jr. "Labor Force Projections to 2008: Steady Growth and Changing Composition," *Monthly Labor Review* (November 1999).

General Accounting Office, "Medigap Insurance: Plans Are Widely Available but Have Limited Benefits and May Have High Costs" (Washington, DC, July 2001).

Gerrior, Shirley, "Dietary Changes in Older Americans from 1977 to 1996: Implications for Dietary Quality," *Family Economics and Nutrition Review* 12, no. 2 (1999): 3–14.

Health Care Financing Administration, "The Characteristics and Perceptions of the Medicare Population (1998)," *Medicare Current Beneficiary Survey* (Baltimore, MD, 2001).

Health Care Financing Administration, *Profile of Medicaid, Chartbook 2000* (Baltimore, MD, September 2000).

Health Care Financing Administration, *Profile of Medicare Beneficiaries: 1998* (Baltimore, MD, 1998).

Health Insurance Association of America, "Who Buys Long-Term Care Insurance in 2000?" (Washington, DC, 2000)

Heiat, Asefeh, Viola Vaccarino, and Harlan M. Krumholz, "An Evidence-Based Assessment of Federal Guidelines for Overweight and Obesity as They Apply to Elderly Persons," *Archives of Internal Medicine* 161, no. 9 (May 14, 2001): 1194–1203.

Hoyert, Donna L., et al., "Deaths: Final Data for 1999," *National Vital Statistics Reports* 49, no. 8 (National Center for Health Statistics, National Vital Statistics System, September 21, 2001).

Kaiser Family Foundation, *Medicare Chartbook* (Washington, DC, 2001).

Kertzer, David I., and Peter Laslett (eds.), *Aging in the Past* (Berkeley: University of California Press, 1995).

Manton, Kenneth G., and XiLiang Gu, "Changes in the Prevalence of Chronic Disability in the United States Black and Nonblack Population above Age 65 from 1982 to 1999," *Proceedings of the National Academy of Sciences* 98, no. 11 (May 22, 2001): 6354–6359.

Mercer/Foster Higgins, "15th Annual National Survey of Employer Sponsored Health Plans" (Chicago, IL, 2000).

National Center for Health Statistics, *1998 National Home and Hospice Care Survey*, CD-ROM series 13, no. 27 (Hyattsville, MD, October 2000).

National Center for Health Statistics, *1999 National Nursing Home Survey*, CD-ROM series 13, no. 28 (Hyattsville, MD, November 2001).

National Center for Health Statistics, *Health, United States, 1999 with Health and Aging Chartbook* (Hyattsville, MD, 1999).

National Center for Health Statistics, *Health, United States, 2000 with Adolescent Chartbook* (Hyattsville, MD, 2000).

National Center for Health Statistics, *Health, United States, 2001 with Urban and Rural Health Chartbook* (Hyattsville, MD, 2001).

National Council on the Aging, "The Consequences of Untreated Hearing Loss in Older Persons" (Washington, DC, May 1999).

"National Survey on Prescription Drugs," *The NewsHour with Jim Lehrer*/Kaiser Family Foundation/Harvard School of Public Health (September 2000).

Paraprofessional Healthcare Institute, *Direct Care Health Workers: The Unnecessary Crisis in Long-Term Care* (Aspen, CO: Aspen Institute, January 2001).

Poisal, John, and Lauren Murray, "Growing Differences between Medicare Beneficiaries with and without Drug Coverage," *Health Affairs* 20, no. 2 (March/April 2001): 74–86.

Riche, Martha Farnsworth, "America's Diversity and Growth: Signposts for the 21st Century," *Population Bulletin* (Washington, DC: Population Reference Bureau, June 2000).

Rogers, Richard G., Robert A. Hummer, and Charles B. Nam, *Living and Dying in the USA* (San Diego, CA: Academic Press, 1995).

Rothschild, Jeffrey, and Lucian Leape, "The Nature and Extent of Medical Injury in Older Patients" (Washington, DC: Public Policy Institute, American Association of Retired Persons, September 2000).

Rowe, John W., and Robert L. Kahn, *Successful Aging* (New York: Random House, 1998).

SEER Cancer Statistics Review 1973–1996, National Cancer Institute (1999).

SEER Cancer Statistics Review 1973–1998, National Cancer Institute (2001).

Stone, Robyn I., *Long-Term Care for the Elderly with Disabilities: Current Policy, Emerging Trends, and Implications for the Twenty-First Century* (New York: Milbank Memorial Fund, 2000).

Stone, Robyn, and Joshua Wiener, "Who Will Care for Us?" (Washington, DC: Urban Institute; U.S. Department of Health and Human Services; America Association of Homes and Services for the Aged; and Robert Wood Johnson Foundation, October 2001).

Treas, Judith, "Older Americans in the 1990s and Beyond," *Population Bulletin* 50 (1995).

UN Population Division, "World Population Prospects: The 2000 Revision" (New York, 2000).

U.S. Administration on Aging, *Profile of Older Americans, 2001* (Washington, DC, December 2001).

U.S. Bureau of Labor Statistics, "Consumer Expenditure Survey, 2000" (Washington, DC, 2000).

U.S. Congress, Committee on Ways and Means, *Medicare and Health Care Chartbook* (Washington, DC: Government Printing Office, 1997).

U.S. Congress, Committee on Ways and Means, *1998 Green Book* (Washington, DC, 1998).

U.S. Congress, Special Committee on Aging, *Developments in Aging: 1997 and 1998, Volume 1* (Washington, DC, February 7, 2000).

U.S. Department of Agriculture, Food Surveys Research Group, Table Set 10, "Results from USDA's 1994–96 Continuing Survey of Food Intakes by Individuals and 1994–96 Diet and Health Knowledge Survey" (Beltsville, MD, 1997).

U.S. Department of Agriculture, Food Surveys Research Group, Table Set 19, "Results from USDA's 1994–96 Diet and Health Knowledge Survey" (Beltsville, MD, 2000).

U.S. Department of Health and Human Services, *Informal Caregiving: Compassion in Action* (Washington, DC, June 1998).

U.S. Department of Health and Human Services, "Older Adults and Mental Health," in *Mental Health: A Report of the Surgeon General* (Rockville, MD, 1999).

WEB SITES

The following Web sites provide online statistics, reports, and/or analyses on aging, demographics, health, nutrition, and related topics.

Alliance for Aging Research, www.agingresearch.org

Alzheimer's Association, www.alz.org

American Association of Homes and Services for the Aged, www.aahsa.org

American Association of Retired Persons (AARP), www.aarp.org

American Association of Retired Persons Research Center, www.research.aarp.org

American Geriatrics Society (AGS), www.americangeriatrics.org

American Medical Association (AMA), www.ama-assn.org

American Society on Aging (ASA), www.asaging.org

Center for Medicare and Medicaid Services (CMS), www.cms.gov

Center on an Aging Society, Georgetown University, www.aging-society.org

Committee on Ways and Means, U.S. House of Representatives, www.waysandmeans.house.gov

Congressional Budget Office, www.cbo.gov

The Commonwealth Fund, www.cmwf.org
(The Commonwealth Fund is a private foundation. Among other things, the foundation funds studies on the elderly. Many of the reports they support are available online.)

Families USA, www.familiesusa.org
(Families USA funds studies on Medicare and Medicaid and other key health care issues. Many of the reports they support are available online.)

Federal Inter Agency Forum on Aging Related Statistics, www.agingstats.gov

General Accounting Office (GAO), www.gao.gov

Gerontological Society of America (GSA), www.geron.org

Health Affairs, http://healthaffairs.org
(Health Affairs is a peer-reviewed quarterly journal, which is published bi-monthly. The journal's primary focus is domestic health care, including issues that affect the elderly. Health Affairs offers Web exclusives—papers published only on their Web site.)

Health Care Financing Administration (HCFA, now CMS), www.hcfa.gov

Health Insurance Association of America (HIAA), www.hiaa.org

Journal of the American Medical Association (JAMA), www.jama.ama-assn.org

Kaiser Family Foundation (KFF), www.kff.org
(The Henry J. Kaiser Family Foundation is an independent philanthropy focusing on the major health care issues facing the nation. The foundation is a valuable source of facts and analysis on such key issues as Medicare and Medicaid.)

Mediamark, www.mediamark.com
(Mediamark Research offers comprehensive demographic, lifestyle, product and media usage data from a single sample.)

Milbank Memorial Fund, www.milbank.org
(The Milbank Memorial Fund is a national foundation that funds publications on public health and health care policy. Many of their materials are relevant to the health care of the elderly. The foundation makes electronic articles available on its Web site.)

National Association for Home Care, www.nahc.org

National Cancer Institute SEER cancer statistics, http://seer.cancer.gov

National Center for Health Statistics (NCHS), www.cdc.gov/nchs

National Council of the Aging (NCOA), www.ncoa.org

National Hospice and Palliative Care Organization, www.hospiceinfo.org

National Institute on Aging (NIA), www.nia.nih.gov

New England Journal of Medicine (NEJM), www.nejm.org

Office of the Surgeon General, US Department of Health and Human Services, www.surgeongeneral.gov

RoperASW, www.roperasw.com
(RoperASW, formerly known as Roper Starch Worldwide, conducts an ongoing survey of American's attitudes and behavior called Roper Reports.)

Social Security Administration (SSA), www.ssa.gov

UN Population Division, www.un.org/esa/population/unpop.htm

Urban Institute, www.urban.org

U.S. Administration on Aging (AoA), www.aoa.dhhs.gov

U.S. Bureau of the Census, www.census.gov. and www.factfinder.gov

U.S. Bureau of Labor Statistics, www.bls.gov

U.S. Department of Agriculture, www.barc.usda.gov/bhnrc/foodsurvey

U.S. Department of Veterans Affairs (VA), www.va.gov

U.S. Food and Drug Administration, Center for Food Safety and Applied Nutrition, http://vm.cfsan.fda.gov

U.S. Senate Special Committee on Aging, www.aging.senate.gov

Index

About the Authors

Elizabeth Vierck is a well-known information specialist on health and aging. She spent over a decade as an analyst of the U.S. Senate Special Committee on Aging, as well as the U.S. Senate Committee on Labor and Human Resources. She is currently a freelance writer and information specialist. Vierck is widely published, with 10 mass-market books and numerous other publications to her credit. She is the originator of *Aging America* (U.S. Senate and AARP), a highly respected databook on aging. Other publications include *Paying for Healthcare After Age 65* (ABC-Clio), *Keys to Volunteering* (Barron's), *Health Smart* (Simon & Schuster), and *Factbook on Aging* (ABC-Clio). Vierck is a member of the American Society of Journalists and Authors.

Kris Hodges is a market research professional with 20 years of experience in survey and secondary data research. Currently, she provides freelance qualitative and quantitative research support for various clients and is a member of the Qualitative Research Consultants Association. Her analytical insights and industry perspective have added to the usability of the information presented in the book. Specifically, Hodges drew upon her food science and nutrition background to provide a thorough review and analysis of the nutritional status of the elderly. Her skills were also applied in integrating proprietary data from RoperASW and Mediamark Research and analyzing new data from the National Nursing Home Survey and the National Home and Hospice Care Survey.